COMMON PROBLEMS

in Gastrointestinal Radiology

COMMON PROBLEMS

in Gastrointestinal Radiology

William M. Thompson, M.D.
Professor and Chairman
Department of Radiology
University of Minnesota
Minneapolis, Minnesota

YEAR BOOK MEDICAL PUBLISHERS, INC.
CHICAGO • LONDON • BOCA RATON

1 2 3 4 5 6 7 8 9 0 YC 93 92 91 90 89

Library of Congress Cataloging-in-Publication Data
Common problems in gastrointestinal radiology / [edited by]
    William M. Thompson.
        p. cm.
    Includes bibliographies and index.
    ISBN 0-8151-8799-8
    1. Gastrointestinal system—Diseases—Diagnosis.
    2. Gastrointestinal system—Imaging. I. Thompson,
    William M. (William Moreau)
        [DNLM: 1. Gastrointestinal System—
    radiography.   WI 141 C734]
RC804.D52C65 1990   89-9021
616.3'30757—dc20   CIP
DNLM/DLC
for Library of Congress

Sponsoring Editor: James D. Ryan
Assistant Director, Manuscript Services: Frances M.
    Perveiler
Production Project Coordinator: Carol E. Reynolds
Proofroom Supervisor: Barbara M. Kelly

This work is dedicated to my parents, Dr. and Mrs. Charles M. Thompson, my wife Judy, and my two boys, Christopher and Thayer. All of you have contributed more than you know.

"In Medicine we have Diagnosis, which is a matter of faith, Prognosis, which is a question of hope, and Treatment, which is only too often an affair of charity, but the greatest of these is Diagnosis. For without accurate diagnosis it is impossible to forecast the course and outcome of a disease or to treat it satisfactorily."

Sir Robert Hutchison

CONTRIBUTORS

Nigel Anderson, M.B., Ch.B., F.R.A.C.R.
Fellow, Department of Radiology
Departments of Radiology and Medicine
University of California
San Diego Medical Center
San Diego, California

Howard J. Ansel, M.D.
Assistant Professor
Department of Radiology
University of Minnesota
Assistant Chief of Radiology
Veterans Administration Medical Center
Minneapolis, Minnesota

Mark E. Baker, M.D.
Assistant Professor of Radiology
Department of Radiology
Duke University Medical Center
Durham, North Carolina

Dennis M. Balfe, M.D.
Associate Professor of Radiology
Chief, Gastrointestinal Radiology
Mallinckrodt Institute of Radiology
Washington University School of Medicine
St. Louis, Missouri

Thomas C. Beneventano, M.D.*
Professor, Department of Radiology
Montefiore Medical Center
Albert Einstein College of Medicine
Bronx, New York

Michael E. Bernardino, M.D.
Professor of Radiology
Emory University School of Medicine
Atlanta, Georgia

Marcia K. Bilbao, M.D.
Professor of Radiology
University of Utah School of Medicine
Chief, Department of Radiology
Veterans Administration Medical Center
Salt Lake City, Utah

*Deceased

Russell A. Blinder, M.D.
Assistant Professor
Department of Radiology
Duke University Medical Center
Durham, North Carolina

Robert J. Boudreau, M.D., Ph.D.
Associate Professor
Department of Radiology
University of Minnesota
Minneapolis, Minnesota

Jeffrey C. Brandon, M.D.
Assistant Professor
Department of Radiology
Irvine Medical Center
Orange, California

Wilfrido Castaneda, M.D.
Professor, Department of Radiology
University of Minnesota
Minneapolis, Minnesota

Giovanna Casola, M.D.
Assistant Professor of Medicine
Departments of Radiology and Medicine
University of California
San Diego Medical Center
San Diego, California

Yu Men Chen, M.D.
Department of Radiology
Bowman Gray School of Medicine
Wake Forest University
Winstom-Salem, North Carolina

Michael Crain, M.D.
Clinical Instructor
Department of Radiology
The George Washington University Medical Center
Washington, D.C.

Wylie J. Dodds, M.D.
Professor of Radiology
Department of Radiology
Medical College of Wisconsin
Milwaukee, Wisconsin

Martin W. Donner, M.D.
Russell H. Morgan Department of Radiology and
  Radiologic Science
The Johns Hopkins Medical Institution
Baltimore, Maryland

N. Reed Dunnick, M.D.
Professor and Director
Division of Imaging
Department of Radiology
Duke University Medical Center
Durham, North Carolina

Jack Farman, M.D.
Professor, Department of Radiology
Columbia Presbyterian Hospital
New York, New York

Peter J. Feczko, M.D.
Staff Radiologist
Henry Ford Hospital
Detroit, Michigan

Michael P. Federle, M.D.
Professor and Chairman
Department of Radiology
University of Pittsburgh
Pittsburgh, Pennsylvania

David Frager, M.D.
Associate Professor of Radiology
Department of Radiology
Montefiore Medical Center
Albert Einstein College of Medicine
Bronx, New York

Patrick C. Freeny, M.D.
Clinical Associate Professor
University of Washington
Virginia Mason Clinic
Seattle, Washington

Gerald W. Friedland, M.D.
Professor, Radiology Department
Stanford University and Radiology Service
Palo Alto Veterans Administration Medical Center
Palo Alto, California

Richard Gadiner, M.D.
Professor, Senior Attending Physician
Rush Medical College
Rush-Presbyterian-St Luke's Medical Center
Chicago, Illinois

David W. Gelfand, M.D.
Professor of Radiology
Department of Radiology
Bowman Gray School of Medicine
Wake Forest University
Winston-Salem, North Carolina

Steven M. Genkins, M.D.
Associate, Department of Radiology
Duke University Medical Center
Durham, North Carolina

Stephen G. Gerzof, M.D., F.A.C.R.
Professor of Radiology
Boston Veterans Administration Medical Center
Boston, Massachusetts

Gary G. Ghahremani, M.D.
Professor of Radiology and Chairman
Department of Diagnostic Radiology
Evanston Hospital-McGaw Medical Center
Evanston, Illinois

Seth N. Glick, M.D.
Associate Professor of Radiology
Hahnemann University Hospital
Broad and Vine Streets
Philadelphia, Pennsylvania

Henry I. Goldberg, M.D.
Professor of Radiology
University of California at San Francisco
San Francisco, California

Marvin E. Goldberg, M.D.
Associate Professor
Department of Radiology
University of Minnesota
Minneapolis, Minnesota

Herbert F. Gramm, M.D.
Department of Radiology
New England Deaconess Hospital
Boston, Massachusetts

Cheryl H. Grandone, M.D.
Department of Radiology
Health Sciences Center
State University of New York at Stony Brook
Stony Brook, New York

Robert A. Halvorsen, Jr., M.D.
Associate Professor
Department of Radiology
University of Minnesota
Minneapolis, Minnesota

Roger K. Harned, M.D.
Professor, Department of Radiology
University of Nebraska Medical Center
Omaha, Nebraska

David F. Hunter, M.D.
Associate Professor
Department of Radiology
University of Minnesota
Minneapolis, Minnesota

C. Daniel Johnson, M.D.
Assistant Professor
Department of Radiology
Mayo Clinic
Rochester, Minnesota

Bronwyn Jones, M.B., B.S., F.R.A.C.P.,
F.R.C.P.
Associate Professor
Russell H. Morgan Department of Radiology and
  Radiologic Science
The Johns Hopkins Medical Institution
Baltimore, Maryland

Frederick M. Kelvin, M.D.
Department of Radiology, GI Section
Methodist Hospital of Indiana
Clinical Associate Professor of Radiology
Indiana University School of Medicine
Indianapolis, Indiana

Robert A. Kubicka, M.D.
Associate Professor
Rush Medical College
Associate Attending Physician
Department of Diagnostic Radiology and Nuclear
  Medicine
Rush-Presbyterian-St. Luke's Medical Center
Chicago, Illinois

Christopher C. Kuni, M.D.
Associate Professor
Department of Radiology
University of Minnesota
Minneapolis, Minnesota

John C. Lappas, M.D.
Associate Professor of Radiology
Indiana University School of Medicine
Indianapolis, Indiana

Igor Laufer, M.D.
Professor of Radiology
University of Pennsylvania Hospital
Philadelphia, Pennsylvania

Janis Gissel Letourneau, M.D.
Associate Professor
Department of Radiology
University of Minnesota Hospital
Minneapolis, Minnesota

Marc S. Levine, M.D.
Associate Professor of Radiology
University of Pennsylvania Hospital
Philadelphia, Pennsylvania

Joel E. Lichtenstein, M.D.
Professor of Radiology
University of Cincinnati
Cincinnati, Ohio

Robert L. MacCarty, M.D.
Associate Professor
Department of Radiology
Mayo Clinic
Rochester, Minnesota

Dean D. T. Maglinte, M.D.
Department of Radiology, GI Section
Methodist Hospital of Indiana
Clinical Professor of Radiology
Indiana University School of Medicine
Indianapolis, Indiana

William M. Marks, M.D.
Clinical Assistant Professor
University of Washington
Swedish Hospital
Seattle, Washington

R. Kristina Gedgaudas-McClees, M.D.
Associate Professor
Department of Radiology
Emory University School of Medicine
Atlanta, Georgia

Alec J. Megibow, M.D.
Associate Professor of Radiology
New York University Medical Center
New York City, New York

Morton A. Meyers, M.D.
Professor and Chairman
Department of Radiology
Health Sciences Center
State University of New York at Stony Brook
Stony Brook, New York

Matilde Nino-Murcia, M.D.
Assistant Professor
Radiology Department
Stanford University and Radiology Service
Palo Alto Veterans Administration Medical Center
Palo Alto, California

William W. Olmsted, M.D.
Professor and Director
Division of Diagnostic Radiology
The George Washington University Medical Center
Washington, D.C.
Visiting Scientist
Department of Radiologic Pathology
Armed Forces Institute of Pathology
Washington, D.C.

David J. Ott, M.D.
Department of Radiology
Bowman Gray School of Medicine
Wake Forest University
Winstom-Salem, North Carolina

Reed P. Rice, M.D.
Professor of Radiology
Department of Radiology
Duke University Medical Center
Durham, North Carolina

Charles A. Rohrmann, Jr., M.D.
Professor, Department of Radiology
University of Washington Hospital
Seattle, Washington

Stephen E. Rubesin, M.D.
Assistant Professor of Radiology
University of Pennsylvania Hospital
Philadelphia, Pennsylvania

Hal D. Safrit, M.D.
Instructor, Department of Radiology
Duke University Medical Center
Durham, North Carolina

Joel Sigeti, M.D.
Clinical Instructor of Radiology
University of California at San Francisco
San Francisco, California

Claire Smith, M.D.
Associate Professor
Rush Medical College
Associate Attending Physician
Director, Section of Gastrointestinal Radiology
Department of Diagnostic Radiology and Nuclear
    Medicine
Rush-Presbyterian-St. Luke's Medical Center
Chicago, Illinois

Stephen M. Smith, M.D.
Assistant Faculty
Rush Medical College
Department of Diagnostic Radiology and Nuclear
    Medicine
Rush-Presbyterian-St. Luke's Medical Center
Chicago, Illinois

David H. Stephens, M.D.
Professor, Department of Radiology
Mayo Medical School
Rochester, Minnesota

E. T. Stewart, M.D.
Professor of Radiology
Department of Radiology
Medical College of Wisconsin
Milwaukee, Wisconsin

Giles Stevenson, M.D.
Professor and Chairman
Department of Radiology
McMaster University Medical Center
Ontario, Canada

Steven K. Teplick, M.D.
Professor, Department of Diagnostic Radiology
University of Arkansas
Little Rock, Arkansas

William M. Thompson, M.D.
Professor and Chairman
Department of Radiology
University of Minnesota
Minneapolis, Minnesota

Mary Ann Turner, M.D.
Department of Radiology
Medical College of Virginia
Richmond, Virginia

Eric vanSonnenberg, M.D.
Associate Professor of Radiology and Medicine
Departments of Radiology and Medicine
University of California
San Diego Medical Center
San Diego, California

Robert R. Varney, M.D.
Assistant Professor of Radiology
Departments of Radiology and Medicine
University of California
San Diego Medical Center
San Diego, California

Hugh J. Williams, Jr., M.D.
Assistant Professor
Department of Radiology
Mayo Medical School
Consultant, Diagnostic Radiology
Mayo Clinic
Rochester, Minnesota

Susan M. Williams, M.D.
Associate Professor
Department of Radiology
University of Nebraska Medical Center
Omaha, Nebraska

Myron Wojtowycz, M.D.
Assistant Professor of Radiology
University of Wisconsin Hospital and Clinic
Madison, Wisconsin

FOREWORD

When Dr. Thompson first discussed the idea of a problem-oriented format for his book on gastrointestinal radiology I was frankly skeptical. It seemed unlikely that he would be able to define a sufficient number of reasonably common and concise specific imaging problems to really provide a worthwhile and comprehensive textbook. Having now seen the completed galley proofs I am very pleasantly surprised. I am, in fact, truly enthusiastic. I am proud to have contributed to several chapters. It should not have surprised me that he would choose a problem-oriented format for this book because Bill's forte as a clinical radiologist is his ability to recognize and cut through clinical problems expeditiously.

In picking contributors for the various chapters Dr. Thompson has chosen experts who approach specific problems as they would in everyday practice. The various imaging modalities are integrated logically. I believe this is a textbook that should be useful to the practicing radiologist when confronted with one of the specific problems addressed in the book. I also believe that the coverage is sufficiently comprehensive to serve as a basic textbook for a resident in training. Most of the chapters provide detailed differential diagnostic lists but also tell the reader how to take the "differential" out of the diagnostic problem. It is a readable text with logical sections, short pertinent chapters, excellent illustrations, and a comprehensive bibliography for each chapter. I am genuinely flattered to have been asked to write the foreword for this book which is a significant addition to the radiologic literature.

REED P. RICE, M.D.
Professor of Radiology
Department of Radiology
Duke University Medical Center
Durham, North Carolina

PREFACE

When I was first approached by Year Book to edit a problem-oriented textbook on gastrointestinal radiology, my first response was "no." However, through the persistence of Year Book Editor Jim Ryan, I was eventually convinced. Now that it is done I am delighted, but during the writing, while harassing my contributors and proofreading, I had my doubts that I had started something worthwhile.

The text contains 73 chapters arranged into 7 sections beginning with plain films of the abdomen (one of my favorites) and concluding with interventional radiology. Each chapter begins with a case presentation and a few questions. Some of the diagnoses are quite simple, with the main value of the chapter being the discussion. In other chapters the diagnosis is more elusive and the answer not revealed until the last paragraph. I anticipate these chapters will not only hold the readers' interest but will also be fun to read. While each chapter was edited, I purposely tried not to detract from the author's individual teaching style. The book is aimed principally at the resident, especially those studying for boards, and the private practitioner who has encountered a specific problem in his or her daily practice. While not every problem encountered in gastrointestinal radiology is included and not all the problems covered are common in every radiology practice, an attempt was made to focus on the more common diagnoses, differentials, and problems. The 72 co-authors made wonderful contributions to this text. They helped me accomplish my goal to provide a fun-to-read but educational treatise on gastrointestinal radiology.

With every project there are always a number of invaluable individuals who serve as an inspiration and others who keep the process moving. The readers should know that Reed Rice was my teacher, mentor, and eventual colleague. Hopefully, Reed's wonderful teaching style is clearly expressed throughout the book. I would like to acknowledge Joan Wallace, my good friend who edited each chapter, Audrey Chan for retyping each edited chapter, and my two wonderful secretaries, Linda Meyer and Judy Thompson (no relation) for their help in organizing and putting the final touches on each portion of the project. The Medical Media Service at the University provided excellent illustrations for all of the University of Minnesota authors. Finally, I want to thank my 72 co-authors whose expertise made the book much better than I ever could have done alone.

I hope you enjoy reading the book as much as I enjoyed writing and editing it.

WILLIAM M. THOMPSON, M.D.

CONTENTS

PART II   ESOPHAGUS   *85*

PART III   STOMACH-DUODENUM   *177*

PART I

Plain Films

CHAPTER 1

Right Upper Quadrant Calcification

William M. Thompson, M.D.

Case Presentation

A 42-year-old man was admitted with abdominal pain. On physical examination, the only abnormality was a fullness in his neck. Laboratory analysis revealed an elevated serum calcium level. As part of the evaluation an abdominal radiograph was obtained (Fig 1–1). What are the findings? What is the differential diagnosis?

DISCUSSION

Figure 1–1 shows a large number of irregular calcific densities ranging in size from a few millimeters to 1 cm. These calcifications are confined to the liver; other radiographs demonstrated calcifications located throughout the right and left lobes. Are there any other findings to help limit the diagnosis?

Radiographic demonstration of calcifications in the right upper quadrant of the abdomen is not infrequent (Table 1–1). Hepatic parenchymal disease causing these calcifications is relatively uncommon, and the differential diagnosis is not widely appreciated. Therefore appropriate procedures and thought processes should be undertaken to exclude calcifications in the lung base, skin and subcutaneous tissues, costal cartilage, retroperitoneal tumors, and lymph nodes as well as in adjacent structures such as the pancreas, kidney, and adrenal glands. The differential diagnosis also includes biliary calcifications, both within the gallbladder and in the extra- and intrahepatic biliary tree, and the arterial and venous circulation. The major focus of the discussion based on Figure 1 involves calcifications primarily in the region of the liver. Because the left lobe of the liver extends across the midline, calcifi-

cations within it must be differentiated from those within structures immediately adjacent. Hepatic calcifications (and general increases in density) are uncommon. When present, they always indicate an abnormality, even though the specific cause or nature of the abnormality is not apparent. Worldwide, the most common causes of hepatic calcifications are calcified granuloma (specifically, tuberculosis and histoplasmosis) and hydatid disease.

The gallbladder and bile ducts are a primary source of right upper quadrant calcification in 10% to 15% of cases.[1-3] The concentration of calcium in gallstones is sufficient to make the calculi radiopaque on plain abdominal radiographs. Gallstones vary from solitary ovoid calcifications, multiple tiny calcifications, or multiple faceted calcifications to vague linear areas of calcification. Occasionally gallstones can be recognized on plain abdominal radiographs by the appearance of distinctive stellate radiolucencies in the right upper quadrant. These radiolucencies are due to gas-containing fissures or faults within the gallstones. This phenomenon is referred to as the Mercedes-Benz sign, because the radiolucent cracks have a triradiate pattern similar to the symbol of the German automobile.[4] Recognition of this sign suggests cholelithiasis in the absence of

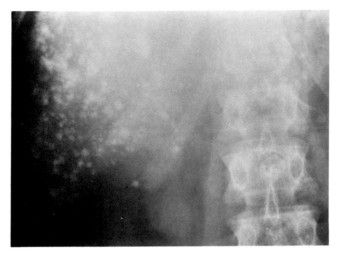

FIG 1–1.
Radiograph showing multiple calcifications within the liver. What is
the differential diagnosis? What are the most likely diagnoses?

calcification. Most authors agree that nitrogen fills the faults created by shrinkage of cholesterol crystals composing the gallstones.

Not all multiple faceted radiopaque densities in the right upper quadrant are in the gallbladder (Fig 1–2). Careful consideration must be given to calcification in the kidney due to a wide variety of renal diseases, including kidney stones, renal cysts, tuberculosis, and tumors. Rarely, calcified stones may pass from the gallbladder into the common duct. Calcified stones can develop in the common duct after cholecystectomy.[1]

Another interesting variant of calcium disease of the biliary tree is milk calcium bile,[1,2] usually associated with complete or incomplete obstruction of the cystic duct. Milk calcium bile consists primarily of calcium carbonate but also may contain magnesium carbonate in cholesterol. When the patient is erect, it may layer out or fill the gallbladder, mimicking a contrast-filled gallbladder (Fig 1–3). Differentiation requires knowledge of whether the patient was given a cholecystographic contrast material.

Extensive calcification of the gallbladder wall is called porcelain gallbladder, a term that emphasizes the characteristic blue discoloration and brittle consistency of the wall.[1] This rare finding is five times more common in women than in men; the mean age of patients is more than 50 years. Most authors consider the calcification to be a sequela of low-grade chronic inflammation; others suggest that it may be due to intramural hemorrhage or an imbalance of calcium metabolism. The plain abdominal radiograph shows a characteristic ring of calcification that conforms to the shape and location of the gallbladder. The thickness of the calcification varies and often is uneven and discontinuous (Fig 1–4). Differentiation of porcelain gallbladder from a single large calcified stone is important because there is a high association between carcinoma of the gallbladder and porcelain gallbladder.[5] Although porcelain gallbladder is uncommon in carcinoma of the gallbladder, the correlation of the two entities is striking; Polk[6] estimated the frequency of carcinoma in porcelain gallbladder to be 22%. Thus most clinicians agree that carcinoma occurs in the same portion of the gallbladder with sufficient frequency to warrant prophylactic cholecystectomy in patients with porcelain gallbladder, even if no symptoms are present. There are a number of case reports of primary carcinomas of the gallbladder calcifying, but this is a relatively rare occurrence.

Primary hepatic tumors, both benign and malignant, may show calcific change.[2,3,7-14] Primary hepatic tumors may calcify in a variety of patterns, ranging from spherical discrete calculi resembling cholelithiasis to irregular distinct stippled calcifications or spiculated calcifications. Calcification is more common in malignant hepatic tumors in children. Bile duct carcinoma may calcify, and has been described as an amorphous collection of calcium with sharply defined borders resembling calculi (Fig 1–5).[1,3] Tiny punctate stippled calcifications have been reported in patients with hemangio-

TABLE 1–1.
Right Upper Quadrant Calcification

Gallbladder and biliary tree
  Gallstones
  Common duct stones
  Milk of calcium bile
  Porcelain gallbladder
  Primary gallbladder carcinoma
Liver
  Neoplastic: Primary
    Hepatoma
    Cholangiocarcinoma
    Hepatoblastoma
    Hemangioendothelioma
    Hemangioma
  Neoplastic: Metastases
    Mucin-producing primary neoplasms: colon,
      stomach, pancreas, ovary
    Lung, osteogenic sarcoma, melanoma, breast
      lymphoma, neuroblastoma, and adrenal,
      thyroid, renal, testicular tumors
Infections
  Tuberculosis
  Histoplasmosis
  Brucellosis
  Coccidioidomycosis
  Hydatid disease
    Echinococcus granulosis (cystic hydatid
      disease)
    Echinococcus multilocularis (alveolar hydatid
      disease)
    Healed liver abscess
    Amebic abscess
    Pyogenic abscess
    Granulomatous disease of childhood
    Gumma
  Other parasitic infections
    Armillifer armillatus
    Ascaris lumbricoides
    Clonorchis sinensis
    Cysticercosis
    Filariasis
    Paragonimus westermani
    Toxoplasmosis
Vascular
  Hepatic artery aneurysm
  Portal vein thrombosis
  Miscellaneous
    Hematoma
    Congenital cyst
    Thorium contrast medium (Thorotrast) (mimics
      calcification)
Renal
  Stones
  Carcinoma
  Granulomatous infection
Adrenal
  Prior infection
  Prior hemorrhage

endotheliomas, and it is well known that hemangio-endotheliosarcoma can develop in patients who receive Thoratrast (thorium contrast medium).[10] The radiodensities in these patients can be due to the Thoratrast as well as to areas of calcification. Plachta[14] described a pattern of spicules in the form of numerous trabeculi irradiating from the central area toward the periphery (sunburst pattern) as characteristic of the calcification that occurs in cavernous hemangiomas.

Carcinoma of the colon is the most frequent primary tumor causing calcified metastases in the liver.[2, 3, 15–17] The calcifications are diffuse, finely granular, closely spaced, and occupy an irregular area of the liver. They are discrete, average 2 to 4 mm in diameter, have been likened to poppy seeds, and appear to be typical of colonic metastases. Not all colonic metastases, however, have this appearance. Calcifications may vary from tiny areas to large areas of irregular density. Calcified metastases to the liver have been reported in patients with thyroid, bronchogenic, pancreatic, adrenal, stomach, kidney, ovary, and breast carcinoma (Fig 1–6), osteogenic sarcoma, melanoma, mesothelioma, neuroblastoma, lymphoma, and embryonal tumors of the testes.[2, 3, 7–9, 18] Often the features of calcifications do not indicate whether they are caused by primary or metastatic neoplasms, and even differentiation from benign disease may be difficult. Calcification also may occur within focal areas of necrotic metastatic tumor in the liver after chemotherapy.

Inflammatory calcified granuloma secondary to tuberculosis and, more frequently, histoplasmosis is the most common cause of hepatic calcifications.[2, 3, 7–9, 19, 20] Calcifications have been associated with a large number of other infections (see Table 1–1). These calcifications may range in configuration and nature from miliary calcifications to solid, calcified granulomas that are moderately large (see Fig 1–6). The punctate, round calcifications that measure 1 to 3 mm and that may be seen in histoplasmosis are characteristic.[19, 20] When observed in the spleen and lungs, they are virtually diagnostic in an endemic area. Granuloma calcifications also may be nodular, popcorn-like, or solid, and even laminated hepatic calcifications may appear, as in the lungs. Brucellosis reportedly causes fluffy calcific densities that resemble snowflakes.[21] Similar lesions also may occur in the spleen.

When a calcified cystic lesion is shown to be intrahepatic, the first diagnosis must be hydatid disease.[22] The most common type, cystic hydatid disease, is caused by the larva of *Echinococcus granu-*

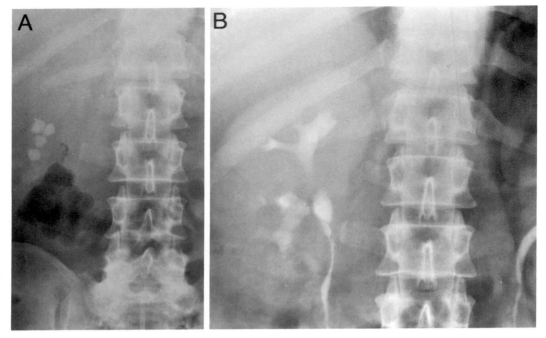

FIG 1–2.
A, radiograph of the abdomen demonstrating four faceted calcifications in the right upper quadrant, most consistent with gallstones. **B,** intravenous uro- gram demonstrating that the four calcifications are within the right kidney.

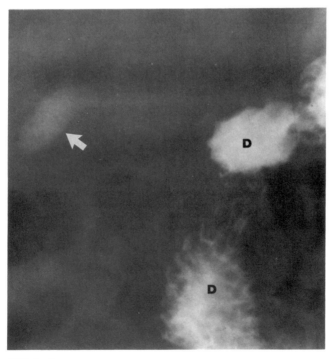

FIG 1–3.
Radiograph of right upper quadrant from an upper gastrointestinal examination. Calcific density in ovoid structure *(arrow)* is due to milk of calcium bile. *D,* duodenum.

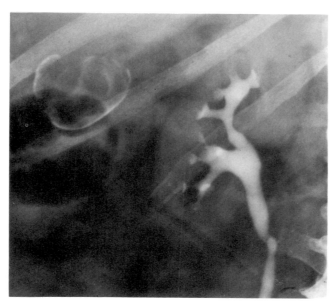

FIG 1–4.
Porcelain gallbladder. Coned view of right upper quadrant demonstrating calcification in gallbladder wall. Contrast agent in right pelvicaliceal system.

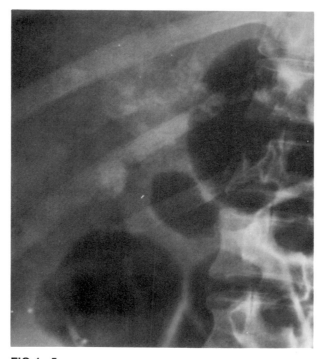

FIG 1–5.
Cholangiocarcinoma. Radiograph of right upper quadrant in a patient with jaundice. Calcification is due to an obstructing cholangiocarcinoma.

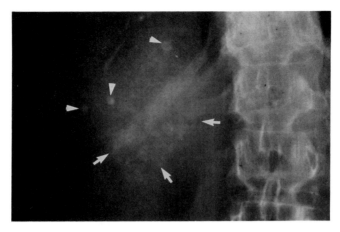

FIG 1–6.
Metastatic breast carcinoma. Radiograph of right upper quadrant demonstrating diffuse hazy calcification *(arrows)* due to tiny conglomerate calcifications (psammoma bodies). Large dense calcifications *(arrowheads)* are not due to metastases but probably to granulomas, such as histoplasmosis or tuberculosis.

losis, a parasite with worldwide distribution but found most often in the Mediterranean basin and in the Middle East. Humans are accidental intermediate hosts and acquire infestation by ingestion of the echinococcal ova. The calcification in an unruptured cyst usually is seen first as an arch, then gradually extends to form an oval or circle of calcium (Fig 1–7). Amorphous calcification occurs within the cyst. Polycystic calcification in an unruptured cyst is pathognomic of cystic hydatid disease. Not only is the mother cyst calcified but so are most of the daughter cysts. Ruptured cysts may have irregularly shaped calcification, but some of the calcium usually is arched. Calcification generally develops 5 to 10 years after the liver is infected and may appear in an active or inactive cyst. Extensive calcification, however, favors inactive cysts.

Alveolar hydatid disease, caused by *Echinococcus multilocularis,* is a rare and more malignant form of the disease. *E. multilocularis* does not appear as large cystic lesions. When the liver is involved, the patient usually has hepatomegaly. The pattern of calcification may resemble that seen in metastatic disease, with multiple solid densities that are amorphous.[23] Approximately two thirds of these patients have hepatic calcifications. In one series, more than half of the patients had calcifications characteristic of alveolar hydatid disease. These appear as small (2 to 4 mm in diameter) rings of calcification, usually in the region of large conglomerate calcifications (Fig 1–8). They may be isolated rings of calcification in some patients. Alveolar hy-

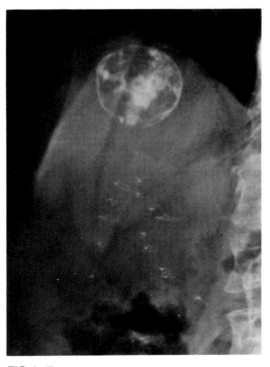

FIG 1–7.
Echinococcus granulosis (cystic hydatid disease). Right upper quadrant radiograph showing multiple circular calcifications within the liver, characteristic of calcified hydatid cysts.

CHAPTER 2

Left Upper Quadrant Calcification

Howard J. Ansel, M.D.

Case Presentation

A middle-aged woman came to the emergency room for the evaluation of abdominal pain. An abdominal radiograph (Fig 2–1) demonstrated a 9-cm spherical calcification in the left upper quadrant. What is the differential diagnosis? How might the diagnosis be confirmed?

DISCUSSION

Calcification within the abdomen generally is dystrophic; that is, it occurs in damaged or devitalized tissue. Except in nephrocalcinosis, it is unusual to see abdominal calcifications secondary to hypercalcemia.[1] In the case of a large spherical calcification, careful evaluation of the plain film, and possibly oblique or lateral films also, often helps in determining the organ of origin. Oral, rectal, or intravenous administration of contrast medium may be helpful in demonstrating the effect a mass has on adjacent viscera. Computed tomography and ultrasonography are often helpful in localizing mass lesions. Determining a site of origin reduces the number of potential causes for the abnormality.

The spleen is a frequent site of calcification. Splenic calcifications generally are small and punctate. Usually they are secondary to granulomas from tuberculosis or, in endemic areas, histoplasmosis. Large spherical calcifications are seen in splenic cysts (Fig 2–2). These may be epithelial-lined true cysts, echinococcal parasitic cysts, or in the majority of cases pseudocysts. Pseudocysts are not lined with epithelium and probably result from organiza-

tion of a splenic hematoma. All of these cysts may calcify and appear identical. If they become large, they tend to depress the splenic flexure of the colon and displace the stomach medially. In the case presented, the splenic flexure lies lateral to the calcified mass and does not appear to be affected by it.[2–5]

After trauma, infection, and infarction, the splenic capsule may calcify (Fig 2–3). Calcific perisplenitis outlines the spleen and conforms to the splenic contour; it is less spherical than the mass in the case presented.

In the case of smaller, ring-shaped calcifications in the left upper quadrant, aneurysms of the splenic artery must be considered. These calcifications generally are less than 3 cm in diameter and usually are due to atherosclerosis, although they may be secondary to trauma and infection. Splenic artery aneurysms are twice as common in women as in men, yet one the size of that in the case presented is extremely unlikely.[6]

The left lobe of the liver lies in the left upper quadrant. If this mass were hepatic in origin, it probably would represent an echinococcal cyst. Such a lesion might be expected to displace the

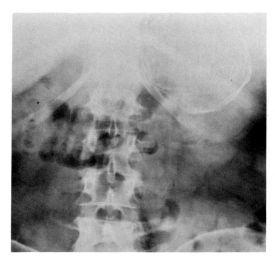

FIG 2–1.
A 9-cm diameter spherical calcification is present in the left upper quadrant.

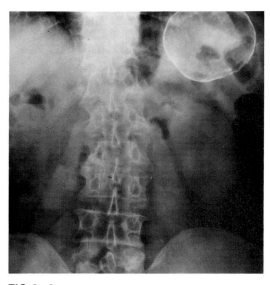

FIG 2–2.
Calcified splenic cyst. Separation of this mass from the renal margin would help exclude renal and supra-renal origin of this mass. In this case we might consider spleen, pancreas, and left lobe of liver as possible sites of origin of the mass.

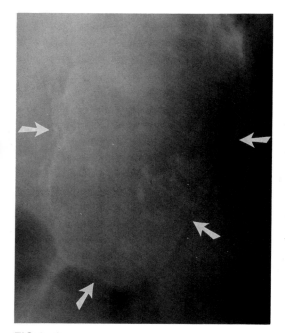

FIG 2–3.
Calcified perisplenitis. Calcification in the fibrous capsule *(arrows)* of the spleen secondary to an old flammatory process results in the development of a calcific rim around the spleen.

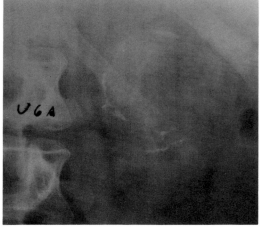

FIG 2–4.
Calcification within a hypernephroma. Although renal cysts calcify, the presence of calcification within the wall of an apparent cyst significantly increases the likelihood of malignancy. Biopsy is often necessary.

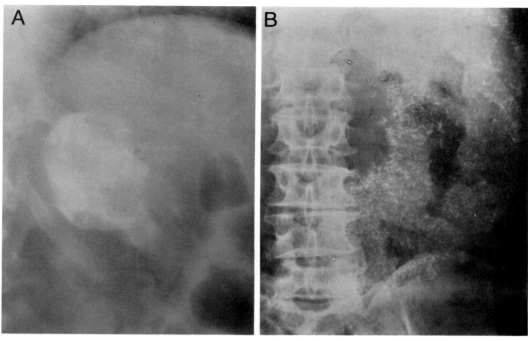

FIG 2–5.
A, gastric leiomyomas are largely exophytic. They are solid masses with dense, rather than curvilinear, rim calcification. **B,** mucinous adenocarcinoma of the stomach with thick infiltration of the gastric wall is outlined by punctate calcifications.

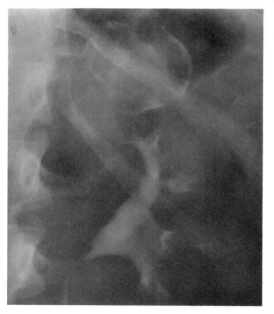

FIG 2–6.
Calcification within this adrenal cyst necessitated surgical exploration. Because benign and malignant adrenal neoplasms may calcify, exclusion of adrenal malignancy is important in the presence of an adrenal cystlike calcification. This patient also has ankylosing spondylitis.

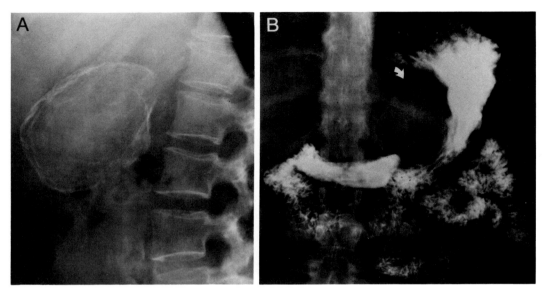

FIG 2-7.
The use of gastric contrast medium **(A)** and a lateral view **(B)** demonstrate the mass anterior to the spine, immediately adjacent and inferior to the splenic artery *(arrow)*. The mass bows the gastric body and antrum anteriorly, inferiorly, and laterally. The pancreas is the most likely site of origin.

stomach posteriorly, the transverse colon inferiorly, and the splenic flexure laterally.[7, 8]

Calcifications related to the kidney are another consideration. With intravenous administration of contrast material, this mass would be expected to distort the renal collecting system. Although benign renal cysts (whether simple, polycystic, multicystic, or parasitic) do calcify, more than 20% of such calcified lesions are malignant, and therefore malignancy must be excluded (Fig 2-4). Renal adenomas also may demonstrate peripheral calcification.[9-12]

Perinephric hematomas and abscesses rarely calcify. As with the splenic artery, renal artery aneurysms should be considered in the presence of small, ringlike calcifications.

It is unusual for gastric lesions to calcify, although calcification does occur within leiomyomas (Fig 2-5,A) and mucinous secreting adenocarcinomas (Fig 2-5,B). In both instances the calcification usually is distributed throughout the lesion rather than on the periphery, as in the case presented.[13] Leiomyomas tend to have dense calcifications, whereas mucinous adenocarcinomas often contain fine, sandlike calcifications.

Peripheral calcification within adrenal masses usually indicates a benign process. Simple adrenal cysts (Fig 2-6) and echinococcal cysts of the adrenal gland may calcify. Pheochromocytomas rarely calcify; however, when they do they frequently are malignant. Adrenal pseudocysts secondary to adrenal hemorrhage may have a similar configuration. Adrenal masses usually depress the kidney.[14-17]

Pancreatic masses arising from the body and tail of the pancreas displace the stomach forward or inferolaterally. The most likely cause of a spherical calcification arising from the pancreas is a pancreatic pseudocyst. Although pancreatic pseudocysts rarely calcify, the presence of calcification implies chronicity. The presence of punctate calcifications within the pancreatic parenchyma suggests chronic pancreatitis and is helpful in establishing the diagnosis of pseudocysts.

Pancreatic neoplasms occasionally contain calcium. Microcystic adenomas contain central, stellate calcifications; mucinous tumors contain random peripheral calcifications. Calcified phleboliths may be present in cavernous lymphangiomas.[18-20]

Cysts arising from the bowel mesentery and within the retroperitoneum also may calcify and should be considered in the differential diagnosis of this case.

The lateral abdominal film and the upper gastrointestinal examination (Fig 2-7,A and B) show that the mass arises posterior to the stomach yet anterior to the spine. This origin suggests the pancreas as the most likely site of origin. A diagnosis of pancreatic pseudocyst was confirmed at laparotomy.

In most instances, recognition of a calcified mass on plain film is followed by computed tomography or ultrasonography to determine its site of origin. Percutaneous cytologic or histologic biopsy study frequently provides the diagnosis.

REFERENCES

1. Baker SR, Elkin M: *Plain Film Approach to Abdominal Calcifications*. Philadelphia, WB Saunders Co, 1983, pp 65–80.
2. Whalen JP: Masses in the left upper quadrant, in *Radiology of the Abdomen: Anatomic Basis*. Philadelphia, Lea & Febiger, 1976.
3. Soler-Bechara J, Soscia JL: Calcified *Echinococcus* (hydatid) cyst of the spleen. *JAMA* 1964; 187:62–63.
4. Greene WW, Forough E: Calcified epidermoid cyst of the spleen. *Am Surg* 1963; 29:613–616.
5. Asbury GF: Calcified pseudocyst of the spleen. *Arch Surg* 1958; 76:148–150.
6. Culver GJ, Pirson HS: Splenic artery aneurysm. Report of 17 cases showing calcification on plain roentgenograms. *Radiology* 1957; 68:217–223.
7. Gonzalez LR, Marcos J, Illanos M: Radiologic aspects of hepatic *Echinococcus*. *Radiology* 1979; 130:21–27.
8. Bonakdarpour A: *Echinococcus* disease: Report of 112 cases from Iran and a review of 611 cases from the United States. *AJR* 1967; 99:660–667.
9. Daniel WW Jr, Hartman GW, Witten DM, et al: Calcified renal masses: A review of ten years' experience at the Mayo Clinic. *Radiology* 1972; 103:503–508.
10. Phillips TL, Chin FG, Palubinskas AJ: Calcification in the renal masses: An eleven-year survey. *Radiology* 1963; 80:786–794.
11. Kikkawa K, Lasser EC: "Ringlike" or "rimlike" calcification and renal cell carcinoma. *AJR* 1969; 107:737–742.
12. Cannon AH, Zanon B Jr, Karras BG: Cystic calcification in the kidney. Its occurrence in malignant renal tumors. *AJR* 1960; 84:837–848.
13. Crummy AB, Juhl JH: Calcified gastric leiomyoma. *AJR* 1964; 87:727–728.
14. Palubinskas AJ, Christensen WR, Harrison JH, et al: Calcified adrenal cysts. *AJR* 1959; 82:853–861.
15. Martin JF: Suprarenal calcifications. *Radiol Clin North Am* 1965; 3:129–138.
16. Wood JC: A calcified adrenal tumor. *Br J Radiol* 1952; 25:222–224.
17. Mitty HA, Yeh H: *Radiology of the Adrenals with Sonography and CT*. Philadelphia, WB Saunders Co, 1982.
18. Komaki S, Clark JM: Pancreatic pseudocyst. A review of seventeen cases with emphasis on radiologic findings. *AJR* 1974; 122:385–397.
19. Freeny PC, Lawson TL: *Radiology of the Pancreas*. New York, Springer-Verlag, 1982.
20. May G, Gardiner R: *Clinical Imaging of the Pancreas*. New York, Raven Press, 1987.

CHAPTER 3

Lower Abdominal Calcifications

Marvin E. Goldberg, M.D.
William M. Thompson, M.D.

Case Presentation

At noon a 49-year-old man came to the emergency room with lower abdominal pain. He had awakened with dull pain limited to the midepigastrium but without nausea, vomiting, or diarrhea. During the morning hours the pain gradually localized to the right lower quadrant. There was mild guarding on palpation of the abdomen and rebound tenderness on palpation of the right lower quadrant. Bowel sounds were normal. His white blood cell count was 15,600/uL with a left shift. The remainder of the laboratory values were normal. A supine film of the abdomen was obtained (Fig 3–1). What is the differential diagnosis? What diagnosis is most likely? What other radiographic studies might you consider? Are any needed?

DISCUSSION

Lower abdominal calcifications for differential diagnosis are listed in Table 3–1, and calcifications associated with acute conditions in Table 3–2. In the case presented the most likely diagnosis is acute appendicitis with possible perforation. The possible diagnoses are limited, and even though the calcification is unusual the symptoms fit the clinical diagnosis.

Differential diagnosis would include a ureteral or bladder stone, an enterolith in a loop of bowel or in Meckel's diverticulum, a gallstone, and a calcified mesenteric lymph node.[1-13] The calcification is large for a ureteral stone, but could be a stone in the bladder. Bladder calculi usually have a more homogeneous appearance (Fig 3–2), but can have a variety of atypical appearances (Fig 3–3). Ureteral calculi (Fig 3–4) can mimic appendicoliths (Fig 3–5), but the clinical and laboratory findings are considerably different; a barium contrast study or an intravenous urogram can easily differentiate between the two. An enterolith could appear similar to the calcification shown in Fig 3–1. A lateral film (Fig 3–6, B) or barium contrast study can specify the location of the enterolith. Gallstones can have a similar laminated appearance to the calcification seen in Fig 3–1; however, it would be unusual on a supine film for a gallstone to be so low in the pelvis unless it had traveled from the gallbladder into the gastrointestinal tract, especially into the hepatic flexure. Finally, calcified mesenteric lymph nodes do not have a laminated appearance. They are amorphous concretions, usually multiple, with no evidence of laminations (Fig 3–7).

Other radiographic studies to consider in the case presented are ultrasound, computed tomography, and barium enema contrast; however, in this

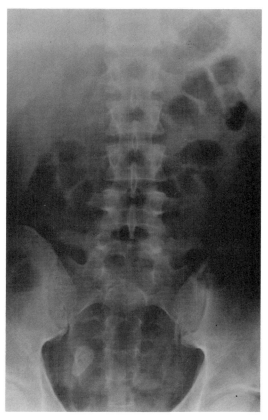

FIG 3–1.
Supine film of abdomen. What are the radiographic findings? What is the differential diagnosis?

patient the clinical findings were so characteristic that he was taken to surgery without additional radiographic studies.

Asymptomatic appendicoliths (see Fig 3–5,A and B) may be detected incidentally; however, it is important to search for these calcifications in certain clinical settings, such as acute appendicitis, because the appendix is frequently gangrenous and may be perforated (see Fig 3–5,C through E).[3–6] Calcification dense enough to be detected on abdominal radiographs has been reported to occur in 1% to 30% of patients whose appendices were examined for disease.[3] However, opaque calculi are of clinical importance because they are frequently associated with perforation, especially in children.[6] It is generally agreed that in a symptomatic patient with an appendiceal calculus on plain films, appendectomy should not be delayed.

The formation of appendicoliths requires inspissation of fecal material, which serves as a nidus

for calcium deposition.[3] With the stone fixed in the appendiceal lumen, concentric layers of calcium salts can form, giving the appendicolith a laminated appearance. Any nonabsorbable material can serve as a nidus, even including barium and BB shot (see Fig 3–5,F).[3]

Appendicoliths can occur wherever the appendix is located, usually the right lower quadrant. With a low-lying appendix the calcification can be quite low in the pelvis and can mimic a ureteral stone (see Fig 3–4), phlebolith, or dermoid calculus (Fig 3–8). When the appendix is retrocecal and posterior, the calcification can be demonstrated in the right upper quadrant. With malrotation the appendix could be located in the left upper quadrant.

Like other concretions, appendicoliths are sharply marginated, with curvilinear or faceted borders (see Fig 3–5).[3–6] Rarely, small irregularities may be noted on one surface, but usually appendicoliths assume a regular geometric shape. Appendicoliths are usually densely calcified, and approximately three fourths are clearly laminated. They can be large, up to 4 cm in diameter (see Fig 3–1), but are usually less than 1 or 2 cm in diameter (see Fig 3–5).

Most appendicoliths can be distinguished from calcified mesenteric lymph nodes, which have irregular margins and a mottled center (see Fig 3–7). Ureteral calculi are usually smaller and less laminated (see Fig 3–4,A). Occasionally an intravenous urogram or barium contrast study is needed to make this differentiation. Phleboliths are usually much smaller and have a central lucency, which is uncommon in appendicoliths. In addition, most phleboliths are located low in the pelvis, whereas most appendicoliths are located more superiorly (see Fig 3–2,C).

Calcification can occur in mucoceles and myxoglobulosis, both due to chronic obstruction of the appendix.[3, 14] However, the mucocele calcification resembles a cyst, and small calcifications in the globoside bodies appear as multiple concretions within the mucocele when myxoglobulosis is present.

In the course of viewing abdominal films the radiologist will see many types of calcifications in the abdomen (see Table 3–1). The ability to determine whether a given calcification is of clinical significance depends on previous experience and judgment within the framework of the location of organ containing the calcification.

Differential diagnosis of abdominal calcifications and other radiopacities on plain films is often a challenge. Occasionally, historical information is of

TABLE 3–1.

Lower Abdominal Calcifications*

I. Right lower quadrant
  A. Mesenteric nodes
  B. Appendix
    1. Calculi
    2. Pericecal abscess
    3. Mucocele
  C. Meckel's diverticulum
    1. Calculi
II. Median and paramedian
  A. Vascular system
    1. Aortic and iliac aneurysm
    2. Atherosclerosis aorta, celiac, iliac
    3. Phlebolith
  B. Pancreas
  C. Pelvic tumor
III. Pelvis
  A. Urinary tract
    1. Ureter
      a. Calculi
      b. Schistosomiasis (bilharziasis)
      c. Tuberculosis
    2. Bladder
      a. Calculi
      b. Schistosomiasis (bilharziasis)
      c. Tuberculosis
        (1) Encrusted cystitis
        (2) Carcinoma
      d. Precipitated silver (silver nitrate)
      e. Urachal calculus
      f. Urethral calculus
  B. Female genital tract
    1. Uterus
      a. Fibromyoma
      b. Lithopedion
      c. Calculi
        (1) Uterovesical
        (2) Vaginovesical
      d. Placenta
    2. Ovary
      a. Dermoid cyst
      b. Papillary cystadenoma
      c. Papillary cystadenocarcinoma
    3. Fallopian tubes
      a. Tuberculosis
      b. Calculi
  C. Male genital tract
    1. Prostate gland
      a. Calculi
      b. Metastatic calcification
      c. Tuberculosis
      d. Ochronosis

    2. Vas deferens
      a. Degenerative diabetes
      b. Tuberculosis
    3. Seminal vesicle
      a. Calculi
      b. Tuberculosis
  D. Rectum
    1. Fecaloma
    2. Mucinous adenocarcinoma
  E. Retrorectal tumor
  F. Other
    1. Phlebolith
    2. Mesenteric nodes
    3. Gallstones
    4. Omental fat deposits and free bodies
    5. Subperitoneal hematoma
IV. Radiopaque densities simulating calcification
  A. Skin lesion
    1. Papilloma
    2. Nevus
    3. Melanoma
    4. Colostomy stoma
    5. Tattoo
  B. Parasitic
    1. Cysticercosis
    2. Trichinosis
    3. Guinea worm
  C. Intramuscular injection
    1. Quinine
    2. Calcium gluconate
    3. Calcium penicillin
    4. Bismuth gold
  D. Operative scars
  E. Surgical wounds
    1. Iodoform gauze
    2. Drains and catheters
    3. Opaque sponge
    4. Metallic sutures or mesh
  F. Gastrointestinal tract
    1. Pills
    2. Paint fragments
    3. Retained barium, extraluminal barium
    4. Metallic foreign bodies
    5. Cholecystographic contrast medium
    6. Ingested bones or stones
    7. Fragments of dental fillings
  G. Spine
    1. Myelographic contrast medium
  H. Vagina
    1. Suppository, pessary
  I. Radiographic artifacts

*Modified from McAfee JG, Donner MW: *Am J Med Sci* 1962; 243:609–650.

TABLE 3–2.

Calcifications Associated With Acute Conditions*

Calcification	Acute Clinical Condition
Lower abdomen	
Appendiceal calculus	Appendicitis
Enterolith in Meckel's diverticulum or jejunal diverticulum	Acute inflammation or perforation
Ureteric calculus	Renal colic
Teeth or bone in ovarian dermoid	Torsion
Other abdominal areas	
Gallstones	Cholecystitis
	Pancreatitis
	Biliary colic
	Empyema of gallbladder
	Gallstone ileus
Milk of calcium bile	Cholecystis
Pancreatic calculi	Pancreatitis, chronic and acute
Calcified aneurysms	Rupture
Aorta	
Splenic artery	
Hepatic artery	
Renal artery	

*Modified from Grainger RG, Allison DJ: *Diagnostic Radiology, An Anglo-American Textbook of Imaging.* New York, Churchill Livingstone Inc, 1986, p 741.

value, and physical examination may contribute important information. Laboratory data such as the presence of microscopic hematuria can also be helpful. Frequently, however, the appearance of the opacity is unexplained. The plain film is in most cases the first radiographic examination, and often no further information is available to the radiologist. Hence the decision to order intensive diagnostic studies depends on evaluation of the nature of the calcification. Careful attention to morphologic features, location, and mobility can narrow the diagnostic possibilities considerably. The position and pattern of the calcification can be well established even before contrast studies or cross-sectional imaging tests are performed. To date there have not been many comprehensive classifications of abdominal calcification. In their excellent monograph on the plain film approach to abdominal calcifications, Baker and Elkin[3] proposed four categories based on morphologic findings: concretion, conduit wall calcification, cyst wall calcification, and solid mass calcification. Although there are potential pitfalls and notable exceptions to this classification, it does provide a nice overview.

The remainder of this chapter describes calcifications in the right and left lower quadrants of the abdomen, the midline, and the pelvis.

Right Lower Quadrant Calcifications

Ureteral calculi are common in the medial aspect of the right lower quadrant of the abdomen, as are calcified mesenteric lymph nodes. Appendicoliths are most often observed near the cecal gas pattern in the right lower quadrant (see Figs 3–1 and 3–5); however, their location varies depending on the position of the cecum and the length and direction of the appendix. Patients with enlarged livers can have calcified gallstones in the right lower quadrant.

Left Lower Quadrant Calcifications

The left lower quadrant of the abdomen is the least likely area to contain calcifications. Ureteral calculi can be located in the medial aspect (see Fig 3–4,B and C). Vascular calcifications, in particular, calcified aortic and iliac artery aneurysms, can occur (Fig 3–9). Calcified mesenteric nodes can be seen in the left lower quadrant, but for some reason,

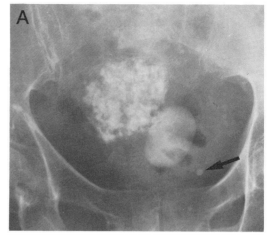

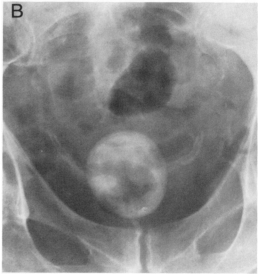

FIG 3–2.
Bladder calculi. **A,** radiograph of pelvis demonstrating a large smooth calculus within the bladder, a larger irregular calcification in a uterine leiomyoma, and a tiny calcification, which is a phlebolith, in the left true pelvis *(arrow).* **B,** large single bladder calculus and bilateral tubular calcification in the vas deferens. **C,** large circular calcification *(arrow),* which was proved on cystography to be in a bladder diverticulum. Note the multiple phleboliths.

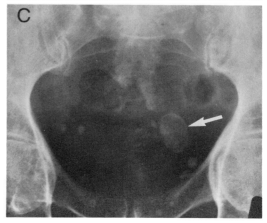

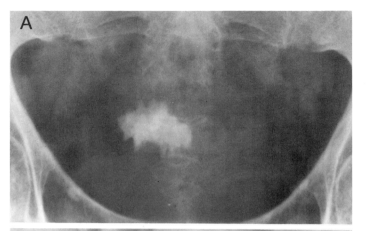

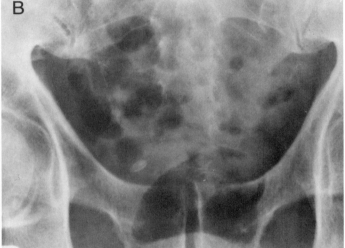

FIG 3–3.
Bladder calculi (atypical). **A,** large atypical "Jackstone"-type bladder calculus. **B,** small bladder calculus mimicking a phlebolith. **C,** irregular bladder calculi that formed around retained Foley catheter fragments.

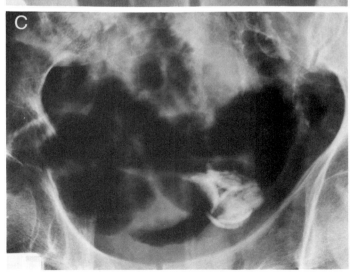

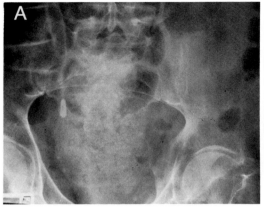

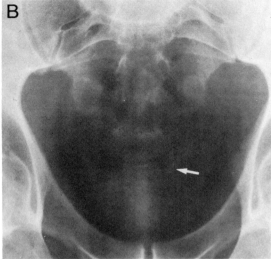

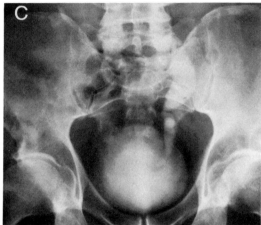

FIG 3–4.
Ureteral calcification. **A,** large right ureteral calculus.
B, faint calcification adjacent to coccyx *(arrow).* **C**
(same patient as in **A**), intravenous urogram
demonstrating that the calcification is in the distal left
ureter.

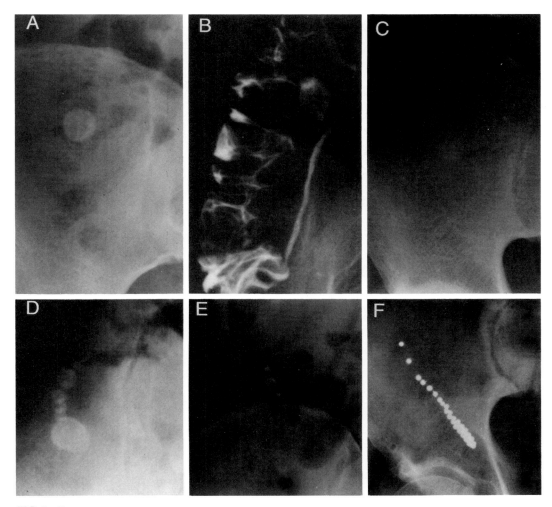

FIG 3–5.
Appendicoliths. Single appendicolith **(A)** and post-evacuation film **(B)** from a barium contrast study of the lower abdomen. The patient had no symptoms. **C,** two laminated appendoliths in a patient with acute appendicitis. **D,** multiple appendoliths in a patient with acute appendicitis. **E,** unusual shaped appendicolith in the presence of an appendiceal abscess. **F,** BB shot in the appendix. The patient had no symptoms.

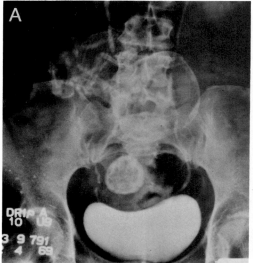 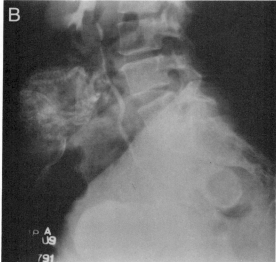

FIG 3–6.
Enterolith. **A,** radiograph during an intravenous urogram demonstrating a large calculus above the contrast-filled bladder. Note calcified fetus (a lithope-dion). **B,** lateral abdominal radiograph demonstrating that the large circular calculus is in the rectum. This elderly woman had severe rectal stenosis.

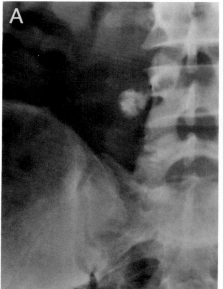 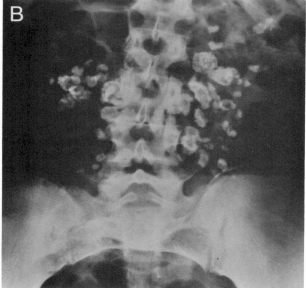

FIG 3–7.
Calcified lymph nodes. **A,** radiograph of right lower quadrant demonstrating a solitary calcified lymph node. Note irregular margin and mottled central portion of calcification. **B,** multiple calcified abdominal lymph nodes in a patient with known tuberculosis.

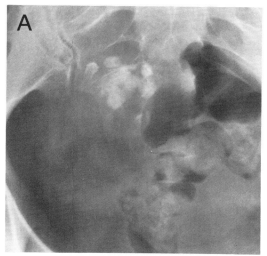

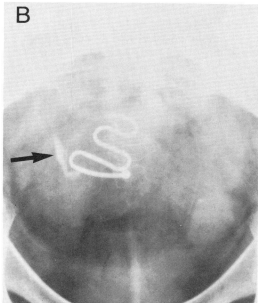

FIG 3–8.
Dermoid cyst (cystic teratoma). **A,** classic appearance with multiple toothlike calcifications. **B,** single calcification with an incisor-like appearance. Note the radiolucency and subtle thin wall *(arrow)* of the soft tissue component of the mass. The patient has an intrauterine device in place. **C,** small calcification within a radiolucent pelvic mass. Calcification does not have a toothlike appearance, but the diagnosis is suggested because the calcification is in the center of the radiolucent mass.

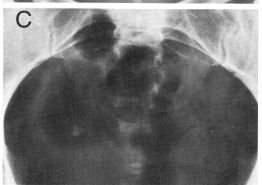

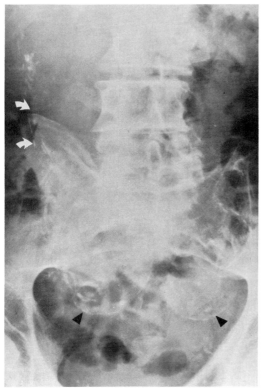

FIG 3–9.
Aortic and iliac artery aneurysms. Calcification in huge aortic aneurysm *(arrows)* and large bilateral iliac artery aneurysms *(arrowheads).* Note the linear nature of calcification in vessel walls.

appear more frequently in the right lower quadrant.[3, 11–13] Calcifications in the female genitourinary system, such as leiomyomas, may also extend into this area.

Midline

Calcifications in the midline of the lower abdomen can include pancreatic calculi in an enlarged pancreatic mass, aortic calcification (see Fig 3–9) on both sides of the vertebral bodies, and calcified tumors that grow out of the pelvis, particularly uterine leiomyoma.

Pelvis

By far the most common calcifications in the pelvis are phleboliths (see Fig 3–2,A and C).[3]

These can be seen at any site in the pelvis but characteristically are located just lateral to the lower part of the cecum at or below the level of the ischial spines (see Fig 3–6). Phleboliths can usually be differentiated by their central lucency and curvilinear margins. Also, phleboliths are relatively fixed, whereas ureteral calculi may be seen to have moved on successive films. Calcifications in the external iliac, arteries, and proximal portion of the hypergastric arteries and their branches are often noted in the elderly patient (see Fig 3–9). Occasionally appendicoliths can appear deep within the pelvis, particularly on the right side (see Fig 3–1). Bladder calculi, which are often solitary, large, and laminated, are seen in the lower midportion of the pelvis (see Fig 3–2). Prostatic calcifications most often appear as clusters of small fixed calculi in the midline at the level of the symphysis pubis. Occasionally these calcifications can be quite large and multiple. Calcifications in dermoid cysts are primarily noted in young women but can be seen at any age. Characteristically there is a radiopacity in the form of a tooth, within a relatively smoothly defined mass of decreased radiodensity (see Fig 3–8). Calcifications in uterine leiomyomas are seen particularly after the fourth decade and most commonly are a mottled type of calcification (see Fig 3–2,A). Infrequently, roughly curved linear rim calcification is seen. Psammomatous calcification in a female pelvis strongly suggests ovarian serous cystadenocarcinoma. Occasionally, noncystic or varied neoplasms show a regular calcification of the solid mass. Also, this type of calcification can be seen in adenocarcinoma of the rectosigmoid.

It is not uncommon in diabetic patients to see calcification in the vas deferens (see Fig 3–2,B). Calcification can also occur in other portions of the male genitourinary system, including the seminal vasicles and even the scrotum.

In the rectum, mucinous adenocarcinomas and fecalomas can calcify (see Fig 3–6).[15–17] Chronic inflammatory conditions may calcify any place in the body, as well as the rectum (Fig 3–10).

A variety of radiopaque densities can mimic calcifications (see Table 3–1). By close inspection, the radiologist can usually determine that these are too dense to be calcifications (Figs 3–11 and 3–12). Ingested or rectally placed medications can be radiodense and thus confused with calcifications (see Fig 3–11). Barium retained in the appendix or in colonic diverticuli or extravasated

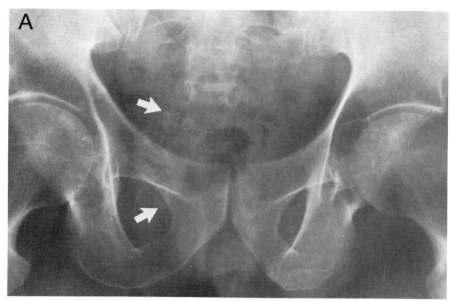

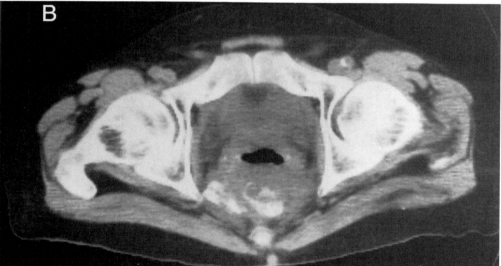

FIG 3–10.
Calcified chronic perirectal abscess (carbuncle). **A,** faint calcification superimposed over right pubic and ischial bones *(arrows)*. **B,** CT scan through rectum demonstrating that the calcification is perirectal and is a chronic perirectal abscess. The patient had a long history of perianal and perirectal fistulas.

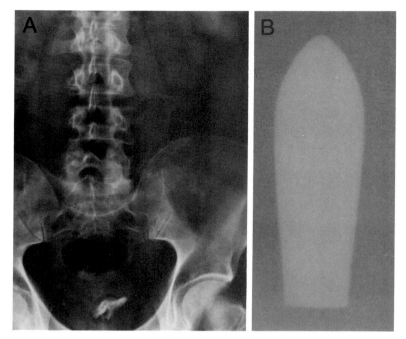

FIG 3–11.
Radiopaque suppositories. **A,** Radiograph demonstrating an irregular density, which is a partially dissolved bismuth suppository, in the lower pelvis. The patient had placed it in the rectum a few moments before the film was taken. **B,** Radiograph of a bismuth suppository.

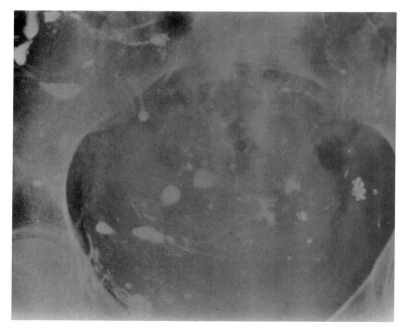

FIG 3–12.
Pelvic radiograph demonstrating multiple radiodensities due to extravasated barium contrast medium. The patient had undergone a barium enema study to detect a silent colon perforation.

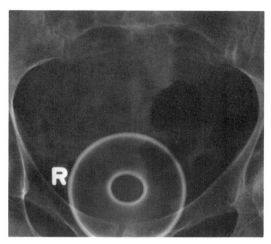

FIG 3–13.
Abdominal radiograph demonstrating a circular metallic density, which is the classic appearance of a pessary.

from the intestine can usually easily be distinguished from calcification. A number of iatrogenic conditions and surgical changes that produce radiodensity are listed in Table 3–1. Some of these, such as the pessary, have a characteristic appearance (Fig 3–13).

A pragmatic approach to abdominal calcification is taken by Grainger and Allison.[2] Table 3–2 lists acute conditions associated with various calcifications. Awareness of these clinical conditions will assist the radiologist in the differential diagnosis. This is a practical approach to the evaluation of an acute situation but does not lessen the need to maintain an overall awareness of the presence of calcifications and their significance.

REFERENCES

1. McAfee JG, Donner MW: Differential diagnosis of calcifications encountered in abdominal radiographs. *Am J Med Sci* 1962; 243: 609–650.
2. Grainger RG, Allison DJ: *Diagnostic Radiology, an Anglo-American Textbook of Imaging.* New York, Churchill Livingstone, 1986, p 741.
3. Baker SR, Eikin M: *Plain Film Approach to Abdominal Calcifications.* Philadelphia, WB Saunders Co, 1983.
4. Felson B, Bernhard CM: The roentgenologic diagnosis of appendiceal calculi. *Radiology* 1947; 49:178–191.
5. Berg RM, Berg HM: Coproliths. *Radiology* 1957; 68:839–844.
6. Brady BM, Carroll DS: The significance of the calcified appendiceal enterolith. *Radiology* 1957; 68:839–844.
7. Brenttner A, Euphrat E: Radiological significance of primary enterolithiasis. *Radiology* 1970; 94:283–288.
8. Dovey P: Calculus in a Meckel's diverticulum—A preoperative radiological diagnosis. *Br J Radiol* 1971; 44:888–890.
9. Burkitt DP: Pelvic phleboliths: Epidemiology and postulated etiology. *N Engl J Med* 1977; 296:1387–1391.
10. Schut JM, Mallens WM: Calcified enteroliths in regional enteritis. *Diagn Imaging Clin Med* 1986; 3:146–150.
11. Schechter S: Calcified mesenteric lymph nodes: Their incidence and significance in routine roentgen examination of the gastrointestinal tract. *Radiology* 1936; 27:485–493.
12. Fred HL, Eiband M, Collins LC: Calcifications in intraabdominal and retroperitoneal metastases. *AJR* 1964; 91:138–148.
13. Ghahremani GG, Staus FH II: Calcification of distant lymph node metastases from carcinoma of colon. *Radiology* 1971; 99:65–66.
14. Norman A, Leider LS, del Carman J: Mucocele of the appendix. *AJR* 1957; 77:647–651.
15. Fletcher BD, Morreals CL, Christian WH III, et al: Calcified adenocarcinoma of the colon. *AJR* 1967; 101:301–305.
16. Thompson R, Barry WF Jr: Rectal calculus. *Radiology* 1970; 96:411–412.
17. Zbornik RC: Large fecal stones—The sigmoid. *AJR* 1971; 113:355–359.

CHAPTER 4

Extraluminal Intraperitoneal Gas Collections

William M. Thompson, M.D.
Reed P. Rice, M.D.

Case Presentation

A 52-year-old man underwent a cholecystectomy and common duct exploration for gallstones. Five days after surgery, abdominal pain, fever, and an elevated white blood cell count developed. A supine radiograph of the abdomen was ordered (Fig 4–1).

DISCUSSION

The major radiographic abnormality in Figure 1 is the large radiolucency in the right upper quadrant. There is a thin curvilinear radiodense line, which probably represents the falciform ligament, and the T tube has lost its normal configuration and orientation. These findings indicate a large collection of extraluminal gas and raise the question of dislodgement of the T tube from the common bile duct.

What are the radiographic findings of pneumoperitoneum on a supine radiograph? What plain film radiographic findings suggest intra-abdominal abscess?

Even with the development of cross-sectional abdominal imaging methods, plain radiographs of the abdomen are the first radiographic study in the evaluation of most acute abdominal symptoms and many chronic abdominal complaints.[1-9] In many cases the plain films, in conjunction with the clini-cal findings, provide information useful in selecting appropriate subsequent imaging tests.

The recognition of extraluminal gas on plain abdominal films is almost always of clinical significance, except in the recent postoperative patient. When the diagnosis of spontaneous pneumoperitoneum is established, 90% of patients require emergency surgery.[1-3]

A properly performed plain film examination of the abdomen can detect as little as 1 ml intraperitoneal air.[5-7] The most sensitive studies are an upright view with the x-ray beam nearly tangential to the hemidiaphragm and a left lateral decubitus view centered over the lateral margin of the liver. Miller and Nelson[5] recommend that the patient be positioned in the left lateral decubitus position for 10 to 20 minutes before filming. The patient is then moved into the upright position for a chest film and upright abdominal film. A supine abdominal film is the last film in the series. This sequence optimizes the possibility of detection of a small quantity of

32

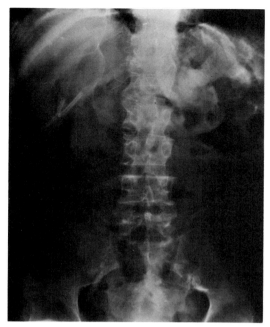

FIG 4−1.
Supine radiograph. What are the findings? What is the diagnosis? What further procedures are recommended to confirm the diagnosis?

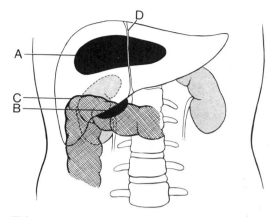

FIG 4−2.
Diagram of the location and signs of pneumoperitoneum on supine films. **A,** gas anterior to the liver. **B,** gas in the subhepatic space. **C,** outline of serosal and mucosal surfaces of the hepatic flexure. **D,** demonstration of the falciform ligament. (From Rice RP: The plain film of the abdomen, in Traveras JM, Ferrucci JT (eds): *Radiology: Diagnosis-Imaging-Intervention,* Vol 4. Philadelphia, JB Lippincott Co, 1986, pp 1−21. Used by permission.)

free air lateral to the liver on the decubitus view and above the liver in the upright views. Small quantities of free air are best seen under the right hemidiaphragm, because normal gas in the stomach and splenic flexure may obscure extraluminal collections under the left hemidiaphragm.

Some patients with a perforated viscus or penetrating abdominal injury are too ill for upright or prolonged decubitus positioning. In some cases the referring physician will request only a supine radiograph because the possibility of free peritoneal air has not been considered clinically. Pneumoperitoneum may be recognized on the supine film in more than 50% of patients (Fig 4−2). Menuck and Siemers[10] emphasize the importance of careful evaluation of the right upper quadrant to detect collections of air anterior to the liver and in the right subhepatic space on supine views (Figs 4−3 and 4−4). If there is a question about the possibility of pneumoperitoneum on the supine film, appropriate upright or left lateral decubitus views are warranted for confirmation.

In addition to the detection of a gas lucency superimposed over the liver and a linear collection of gas in the subhepatic space, a number of other radio-

graphic signs are indicative of free intraperitoneal air on the supine abdominal radiograph.[1−8, 10−13] The demonstration of both the inner and outer wall of the bowel (Rigler's sign) is a well-known radiographic sign of free air that may be identified on supine films (Fig 4−5,A and B), and usually indicates a large quantity of free intraperitoneal air. Another sign indicative of a large amount of free air is visualization of the falciform ligament, which appears as a linear density overlying the liver just to the right of and parallel to the spine (Fig 4−6). A large quantity of free air may outline the margins of major abdominal structures, such as the liver, gallbladder, stomach, and intestine. The inverted V sign (Fig 4−7) is the demonstration of air outlining the lateral umbilical ligaments, which contain the umbilical artery remnants.[12] The "football" sign is sometimes seen in infants with a large quantity of free peritoneal air collects under the protuberant anterior abdominal wall. In some patients small lucent triangles of gas can be identified outside the bowel wall, where three loops of distended bowel are in close proximity (see Fig 4−5,A).

When a perforated viscus is suspected in a patient with spontaneous pneumoperitoneum, the immediate use of water-soluble contrast material generally is easy and safe and frequently is rewarding.[1, 2] In 35% of patients with a perforated ulcer it

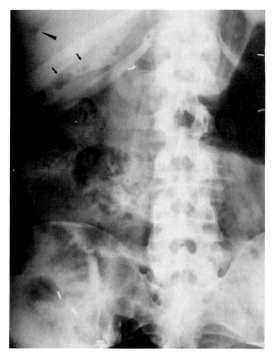

FIG 4−3.
Pneumoperitoneum: subtle free air in right upper quadrant. Supine radiograph in a 50-year-old man who had undergone renal transplantation 5 years earlier. The patient had abdominal pain without fever or significant elevation of the white blood cell count. Subtle extraluminal air is demonstrated under the free edge of the liver *(small arrows)* and anterior to the liver *(arrowhead).* At surgery, sigmoid diverticulitis was diagnosed.

is impossible to demonstrate pneumoperitoneum on routine films of the abdomen; a limited upper gastrointestinal study using water-soluble contrast medium can document the presence and location of a perforation.[1] When there is suspicion of an anastomotic leak or perforation of the colon, a water-soluble contrast enema may be useful.

The radiologist also has a large responsibility in suggesting or confirming the diagnosis of intra-abdominal abscess. The majority of intra-abdominal abscesses occur in postoperative patients, and morbidity and mortality are extremely high without expeditious diagnosis and appropriate drainage. In the postoperative patient the abscess may be totally unsuspected clinically and may first be suggested on a plain film of the abdomen obtained to evaluate prolonged postoperative ileus. Fever in these patients may be ascribed to pneumonia or other infection.

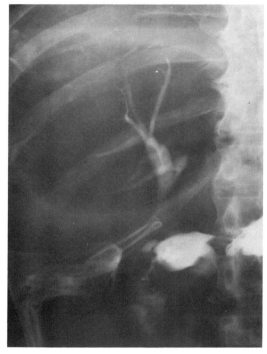

FIG 4−4.
Pneumoperitoneum: air anterior to liver. Radiograph of right upper quadrant during an upper gastrointestinal series. Barium in the common bile duct refluxes through a choledochoduodenostomy. Note the large circular gas collection.

Physical examination generally is limited by the recent abdominal incision. Many postoperative patients also are taking antibiotics or various immunosuppressive agents that may mask the clinical signs and symptoms of a potentially fatal abdominal abscess.[14,15] If there is plain film radiographic or other clinical evidence of intra-abdominal abscess, computed tomography, ultrasound, and radionuclide gallium- or indium-labeled leukocyte scans generally are needed for confirmation and localization of the abscess prior to surgical or percutaneous drainage.

The radiologist should be aware of the common sites at which intra-abdominal abscesses form and of the various pathways by which pus may extend from one area of the abdomen to another. A detailed description of these pathways is beyond the scope of this chapter but is available elsewhere.[16, 17] In brief, an upper abdominal abscess in either the right or left subphrenic space or the right subhepatic space may extend into the pelvis via the right or left

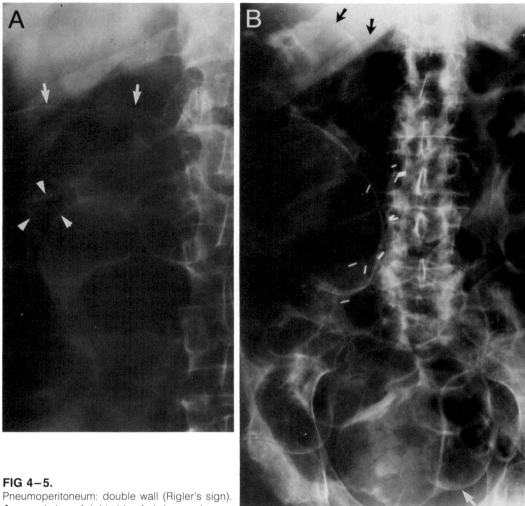

FIG 4–5.
Pneumoperitoneum: double wall (Rigler's sign).
A, coned view of right side of abdomen demonstrating free air in the right upper quadrant and
air on both sides of bowel *(arrows)*. Note triangle sign *(arrow-heads)*. **B,** supine abdominal radiograph demonstrating air on both sides of the bowel wall in the pelvis and right upper quadrant *(arrows)*.

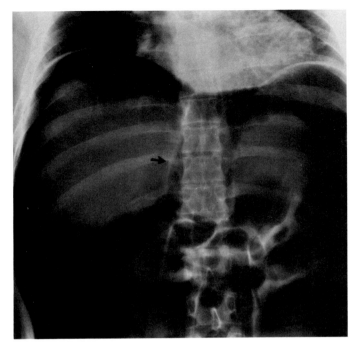

FIG 4–6.
Massive pneumoperitoneum: falciform ligament sign. Supine radiograph of the upper abdomen demonstrating free air surrounding the liver, gallbadder, and stomach and the falciform ligament *(arrow)*.

FIG 4–7.
(Same patient as in Fig 4–6). View of pelvis demonstrating the umbilical ligaments *(arrows)* and a large amount of free intraperitoneal air in the pericolic gutters.

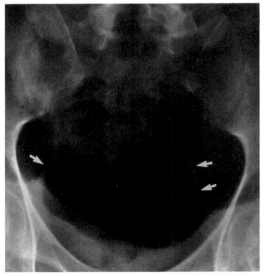

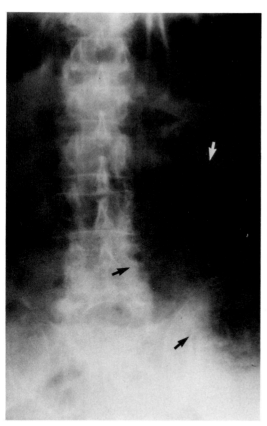

FIG 4–8.
Intra-abdominal abscess. Supine radiograph in a middle-aged man 5 days after resection of an abdominal aortic aneurysm. A large abscess gas collection is in the left lower abdomen *(arrows)*. Surgery revealed a necrotic perforated sigmoid colon related to occlusion of the mesenteric arteries.

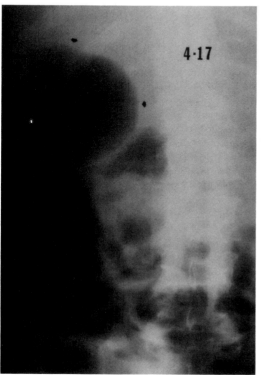

FIG 4–9.
Intra-abdominal abscess. A large homogeneous gas collection *(arrows)* is demonstrated in the right upper quadrant. Note the absence of fecal material and mucosal folds. At surgery an intra-abdominal abscess due to a perforation at an ileocolic anastomosis was found.

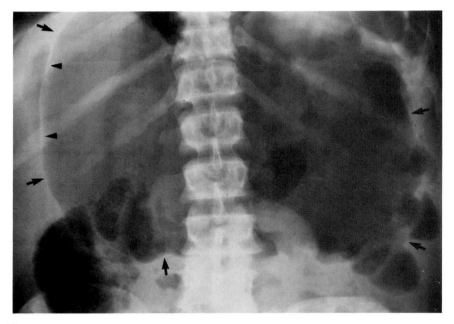

FIG 4–10.
Large upper abdominal abscess. Supine radiograph in a 52-year-old man with abdominal pain and sepsis. A large gas collection extends from the left subdiaphragmatic region across the midline *(arrows)*. Falci-

form ligament marked by *arrowheads*. At surgery a large abscess due to a perforated gastric ulcer was found in the anterior upper abdomen.

pericolic gutter. Conversely, pelvic abscesses may extend into the upper abdomen via the same pathways. When the patient is supine, Morrison's pouch is the most dependent portion of the peritoneal space; when the patient is upright, the prerectal space is the most dependent. Fluid dynamics favor the collection of pus in these areas.

The radiographic appearance of gas in an abscess may be subtle.[1–3] Differentiation from intraluminal gas may be difficult, especially because many patients with an abdominal abscess have multiple loops of gas-filled bowel due to an associated ileus. The bubbly mottled gas of an abscess may mimic stool in the colon (Fig 4–8). Abscess gas also may be homogeneous, a characteristic less commonly emphasized in the radiologic literature.[18, 19] This homogeneous gas collection can mimic normal or dilated bowel (Figs 4–9 and 4–10). The lack of any mucosal pattern or stool in this type of abscess sometimes can be recognized radiographically. Normal bowel usually contains some recognizable mucosa or intestinal content. Examination with a water-soluble contrast agent, administered either orally or rectally, is effective in confirming that a homogeneous collection of gas is extraluminal.[12]

With the development of the newer imaging methods the value of conventional radiographic techniques sometimes is neglected. Connell et al.[4] reported that more than two thirds of upper abdominal abscesses can be diagnosed with conventional films. Adding a contrast study of the gastrointestinal tract increases the accuracy of the conventional radiographic techniques when diagnosing abscesses in the left upper quadrant.[4] These authors point out that it is easy to overlook abnormal collections of gas in the left upper quadrant because both the stomach and splenic flexure normally contain gas. In addition to confirming an abnormal gas collection, contrast examinations of the gastrointestinal tract usually are the most reliable preoperative method for documenting anastomotic leaks or perforations responsible for an abscess.[1, 2]

The presence of a large amount of extraluminal gas over the liver is suggested in Figure 4–1 by the radiolucency over the liver and the thin line representing the falciform ligament. The change in orientation of the T tube to a V configuration suggests that the tube has been dislodged from the common duct and raises the possibility of bile leak. However, the abnormal position of the T tube and the

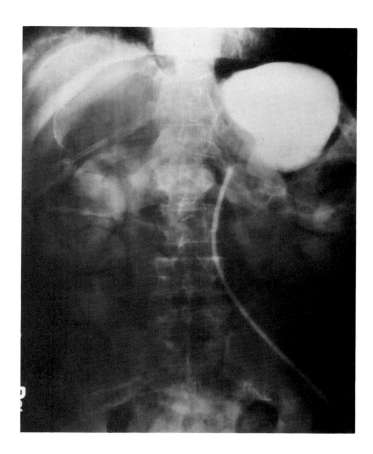

FIG 4–11.
(Same patient as in Fig 4–1) Follow-up supine radiograph taken after 1 day demonstrates contrast medium in the stomach after injection through the gastrostomy tube. An intra-abdominal abscess due to breakdown of the gastrostomy was suspected. Note the change in position of the T tube, indicating that it is outside the common duct. The film also demonstrates radiolucency over the liver due to an abscess. Surgery revealed a large abscess and biloma, both caused by the leak in the common bile duct that resulted from dislodgement of the T tube.

abnormal gas collection were not recognized. The next day a water-soluble contrast medium was injected through the gastrostomy tube because the physicians thought the sepsis was related to a leak from the gastrostomy site (Fig 4–11). On this radiograph the abnormal position of the T tube was noted and a more localized gas collection is apparent. A T tube cholangiogram demonstrated that the tube was out of the common duct. Surgery revealed a large upper abdominal abscess that was due to a leak of bile from the common duct. The abscess was drained and the T tube replaced; the patient subsequently recovered.

This case emphasizes the importance of the plain film in the detection of extraluminal abdominal gas and stresses some radiographic signs useful in diagnosing pneumoperitoneum and abdominal abscess.

REFERENCES

1. Rice RP, Thompson WM, Gedgaudas RK: The diagnosis and significance of extraluminal gas in the abdomen. *Radiol Clin North Am* 1982; 20:819–837.
2. Rice RP: The plain film of the abdomen, in Traveras JM, Ferrucci JT (eds): *Radiology: Diagnosis-Imaging-Intervention*, vol 4. Philadelphia, JB Lippincott Co, 1986, pp 1–21.

3. Mindelzun R: Abnormal gas collections, in McCort JJ (ed): *Abdominal Radiology.* Baltimore, Williams & Wilkins Co, 1981, pp 181–252.

4. Connell TR, Stephens DH, Carlson HC, et al: Upper abdominal abscess: A continuing and deadly problem. *AJR* 1980; 134:759–765.

5. Miller RE, Nelson SW: The roentgenologic demonstration of tiny amounts of free intraperitoneal gas: Experimental and clinical studies. *AJR* 1971; 112:574–584.

6. Nelson SW: Extraluminal gas collections due to disease of the gastrointestinal tract. *AJR* 1972; 115:225–248.

7. Miller RE, Mellins HZ: The radiological evaluation of intraperitoneal gas (pneumoperitoneum). *CRC Crit Rev Diagn Imaging* 1973; 4:61–85.

8. Fataar S, Schulman A: Subphrenic abscess: The radiologic approach. *Clin Radiol* 1981; 32:147–156.

9. Woodards S, Kelvin FM, Rice RP, et al: Pancreatic abscess: Importance of conventional radiology. *AJR* 1981; 136:871–878.

10. Menuck L, Siemers PT: Pneumoperitoneum: Importance of right upper quadrant features. *AJR* 1976; 127:753–756.

11. Felson B, Wiot JF: Another look at pneumoperitoneum. *Semin Roentgenol* 1973; 8: 437–443.

12. Weiner CI, Diaconig JN, Dennis JM: The "inverted V": A new sign of pneumoperitoneum. *Radiology* 1973; 107:47–48.

13. Paster S, Brogdon BG: Roentgenographic diagnosis of pneumoperitoneum. *JAMA* 1976; 235:1264–1267.

14. Thompson WM, Seigler HF, Rice RP: Ileocolonic perforation. A complication following renal transplantation. *AJR* 1975; 125:723–730.

15. Thompson WM, Meyers W, Seigler HF, et al: Gastrointestinal complications of renal transplantation. *Semin Roentgenol* 1978; 13: 319–328.

16. Meyers MA: Radiologic features of the spread and localization of extraperitoneal gas and their relationship to its source: An anatomical approach. *Radiology* 1974; 111:17–26.

17. Meyers MA: *Dynamic Radiology of the Abdomen: Normal and Pathologic Anatomy,* ed 2. New York, Springer-Verlag, 1976.

18. Masters SJ, Rice RP: The homogeneous density of gas in the diagnosis of intra-abdominal abscess. *Surg Gynecol Obstet* 1974; 139: 370–375.

19. Halvorsen RA, Jones MA, Rice RP, et al: Anterior left subphrenic abscess: Characteristic plain film and CT appearance. *AJR* 1982; 139:283–289.

CHAPTER 5

Portal Venous Versus Bile Duct Gas

William M. Thompson, M.D.

Case Presentation

A 46-year-old woman was admitted with abdominal pain of 6 hours' duration. She had a mildly elevated temperature and, on physical examination, had diffuse abdominal tenderness without rebound. Her white blood cell count was 10,000 cells/cm^3; other laboratory findings were normal. A plain film of the abdomen was ordered (Fig 5-1). What are the findings? What is the differential diagnosis?

DISCUSSION

Figure 5-1 demonstrates an abnormal branching tubular gas-filled structure superimposed on the liver. The location and orientation of the gas are strongly suggestive of air in either the bile ducts or portal vein. What radiographic findings are used to differentiate the two? Why is it important to make this differentiation?

Gas in the bile ducts usually is central and limited to the larger biliary radicles around the porta hepatis (Figs 5-2 and 5-3). This distribution probably is secondary to the centripetal direction of bile flow.[1-6] In contrast, portal venous gas is characterized by multiple small tubular lucencies in the periphery of the liver (Figs 5-4 to 5-6).[1, 2, 7-21] The gas collections are thin, moderately well delineated, and usually show branching. Typically they extend to the liver capsule, whereas biliary gas does not extend closer than 2 cm from the edge of the liver. Because portal vein gas has a high carbon dioxide content, it is highly soluble and likely to be absorbed by the circulation. Persistent visualization suggests persistent production. A left lateral decubi-

tus radiograph can help define the centrifugal air distribution and is useful for detecting free intraperitoneal air.

The differentiation of biliary from portal venous gas is important because of the different causes of the gas. In adults, air in the biliary system usually is of relatively benign origin (Table 5-1),[1-6] whereas air in the portal venous system usually has grave prognostic significance, a sign of imminent death (Table 5-2).[1, 2, 14] More than 90% of patients with portal venous gas die of the underlying disease.[14]

The most common cause of air in the biliary tree is previous surgery, usually a sphincterotomy, choledochoenterostomy, or cholecystenterostomy. Pathologic communication between the biliary system and gastrointestinal tract is due most commonly (approximately 90%) to erosion of a gallstone into the intestine.[1, 21] In most patients there is gas within the gallbladder but not the common bile duct, because the cystic duct usually is obstructed from long-standing inflammation. Occasionally gas passes from the gallbladder through a patent cystic duct into the bile ducts.[2] In fewer than 6% of pa-

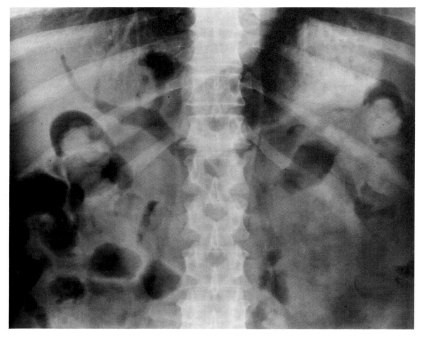

FIG 5–1.
Supine radiograph of upper abdomen. What is the abnormal finding? What does it represent, and what significance does it have?

FIG 5–2.
Radiograph of right upper quadrant demonstrating gas-filled tubular structure *(arrow),* which is the common bile duct. Note the absence of gas in the periphery of the liver. The patient had undergone a choledochoduodenostomy.

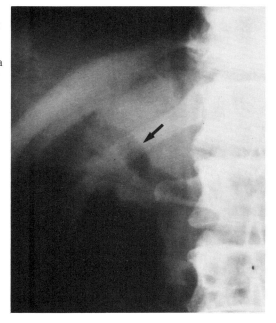

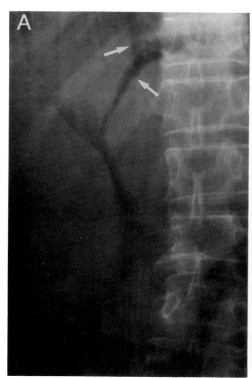 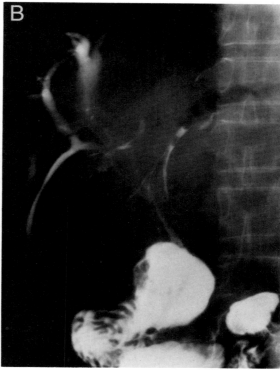

FIG 5–3.
Air in bile ducts. **A,** radiograph demonstrating branching tubular structure in right upper quadrant. Note some extension of gas into the periphery of the liver, especially over the left lobe *(arrows).* **B** (same patient as in **A**), upper gastrointestinal series demonstrates barium filling bile ducts through a choledochoduodenostomy.

tients the gas in the bile ducts is due to perforation of a peptic ulcer in the common duct,[4] and in approximately 4% it is secondary to malignancy or trauma. Malignant tumors in the gallbladder, duodenum, and colon can produce air in the bile ducts by directly extending into the contiguous structure and producing a fistula between the biliary system and the gastrointestinal tract (Fig 5–7). Rarely, pneumobilia is seen, with incompetence of the sphincter of Oddi (Fig 5–8), and can be due to a patulous sphincter in the elderly, anomalous duct insertion, chronic atrophic pancreatitis, or the passage of stones.[1, 2] Ascending cholangitis secondary to a gas-forming organism produces sufficient gas to be radiographically visible on rare occasions.[6] Other rare causes of biliary tree air include inflammatory disorders with significant scarring in the duodenal wall. Severe pancreatitis can disrupt the sphincter. In Crohn's disease, reflux can occur from a fistula or through a damaged ampulla of Vater.[5]

In strongyloidiasis, scarring in the periampullary region can produce incompetence of the sphincter of Oddi. Gas in the biliary tree can be caused by infestation of *Clonorchis sinensis* or *Ascaris lumbricoides*. The parasitic fluke *Clonorchis,* acquired by the ingestion of raw freshwater fish, migrates into the biliary system from the duodenum, where it may exist for years and produce an inflammatory reaction; this predisposes to stone formation, obstruction, secondary bacterial infection, and scarring. *Ascaris* invades the bile ducts in a similar fashion, and the migration of the worms through the sphincter disrupts its function, leading to reflux of air into the bile ducts. Emphysematous cholecystitis can be associated with gas in the bile ducts.[3] The presence of bile duct air suggests that the cystic duct is patent, allowing gas to escape from the gallbladder lumen. Rarely, anomalous insertion of the common ducts into a duodenal diverticulum allows gas to enter the bile ducts.[1, 2] Finally,

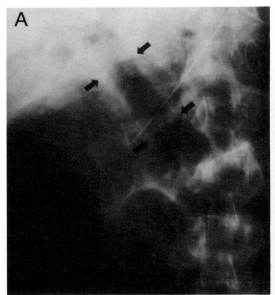

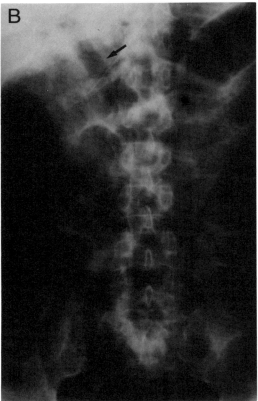

FIG 5–4.
Portal vein gas. **A,** coned view of the right upper quadrant demonstrating gas in central portal vein *(arrows)*. **B,** abdominal radiograph showing portal vein gas *(arrow)* and pneumatosis in small bowel. At surgery, the small bowel was infarcted.

spontaneous reflux of air from the duodenum into the pancreatic or common bile duct can occur without a specific duodenal or pancreatobiliary process.

The exact mechanism responsible for portal venous gas is unknown. Two theories have been proposed to explain the presence of portal venous gas in adults with acute abdominal disease. Sussman and Senturia[9] suggest that the bowel dilates extensively, causing the mucosa to tear and allowing gas to enter the portal venous system. Necrosis of the bowel wall with invasion of gas-forming organisms into the bowel and mesenteric veins is the other postulate. Both of these processes have been reported.[14, 21] The high incidence of bacteremia and bowel distention in patients with portal venous gas and bowel necrosis supports both explanations.

In infants the most common cause of portal venous gas is necrotizing enterocolitis, even though portal vein gas develops in only 30% of neonates with necrotizing enterocolitis. Of many causes of portal vein gas in adults, the most common is ischemic bowel disease.[1, 2, 8, 10–12] Most patients have symptoms and severe sepsis, and in the majority there is radiographic demonstration of distended bowel and pneumatosis (see Fig 5–5). Many reported causes of portal vein gas are not associated with ischemic bowel disease, [13, 14, 16, 18–20] and most of these are associated with non-life-threatening diseases or abnormalities. These patients do not have significant symptoms and the portal vein gas is discovered incidentally. Thus, if portal vein gas is recognized on an abdominal radiograph, it is important to correlate the finding immediately with the patient's history and clinical findings. In the absence of significant clinical symptoms or laboratory abnormalities suggesting ischemic enteritis, a careful search should be made to determine the cause of the gas so that it can be treated appropriately.

In the case presented, the abnormal gas noted in Figure 5–1 has a primarily central location in the porta hepatis, suggesting that it is in the bile ducts.

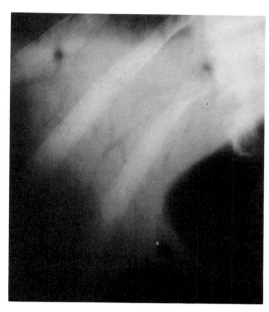

FIG 5–5.
Portal venous gas. Radiograph of the right upper quadrant in a patient with severe intestinal ischemia demonstrating gas in the peripheral branches of the portal vein.

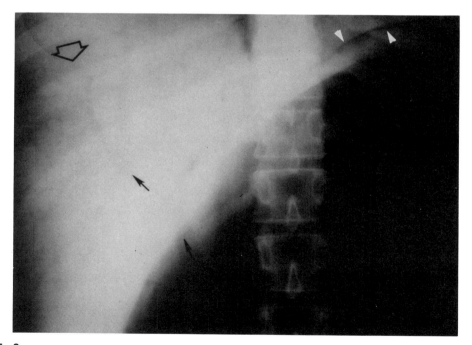

FIG 5–6.
Portal venous gas. Radiograph of the upper abdomen in a young woman with acute leukemia and marked gastric distention. There is both central *(arrows)* and peripheral *(open arrow)* portal venous gas. The patient also has emphysematous gastritis due to ischemic necrosis of the stomach and small bowel. Note gas in gastric wall *(arrowheads).*

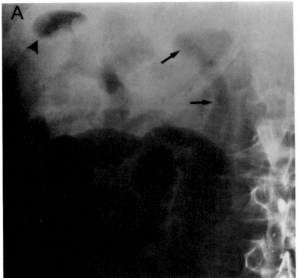

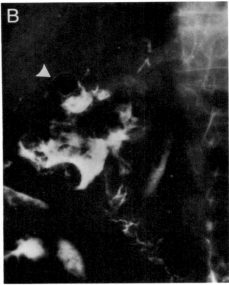

FIG 5-7.
Biliary air. **A,** supine radiograph demonstrating gas in the gallbladder *(arrowhead)* and bile ducts *(arrows).* **B,** post-evacuation radiograph from a barium enema study demonstrating a large carcinoma of the hepatic flexure that invaded the gallbladder *(arrowhead).* Note barium in the bile ducts.

FIG 5-8.
Biliary air. Upright spot film from an oral cholecystogram demonstrating gas in the gallbladder and bile ducts. Both were filled with multiple tiny stones. It was presumed that these stones were spontaneously passing through the sphincter of Oddi, permitting air to enter the biliary system.

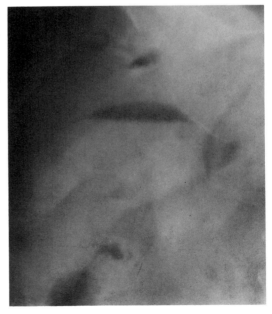

TABLE 5–1.

Reported Causes of Gas in the Biliary System

Common
    Surgery
        Sphincterotomy
        Choledochoduodenostomy
        Cholecystoduodenostomy
        Cholecystojejunostomy
    Gallstone erosion
Uncommon
    Perforated ulcer
    Neoplastic disease:
        Primary lesion in gallbladder, colon,
            duodenum, pancreas
    Trauma
    Passage of common duct stone
    Pancreatitis
    Crohn's disease
    Strongyloidiasis
    Clonorchis sinensis infestation
    Ascaris lumbricoides infestation
    Ascending cholangitis
    Emphysematous cholecystitis
    Incompetent sphincter of Oddi
    Anomalous insertion of common bile duct into
        a duodenal diverticulum
    Idiopathic

TABLE 5–2.

Causes of Portal Venous Gas

Common
    Adults: Ischemic bowel
    Infants: Necrotizing enterocolitis
Uncommon
    Infants:
        Umbilical vein catheterization
        Neonatal gastroenteritis
        Erythroblastosis fetalis
        Surgery
    Adults
        Barium enema
        Diverticulitis
        Inflammatory bowel disease
        Corrosive ingestion
        Gastric distention
        Diabetic coma
        Hemorrhagic pancreatitis
        Pelvic and intra-abdominal abscess
        Pneumatosis intestinalis (benign form)
        Hydrogen peroxide enema
        Perforated gastric ulcer into mesenteric vein
        Mechanical bowel obstruction with ischemia
        Necrotic colon cancer
        Emphysematous cholecystitis
        Jugular vein catheterization

However, the gas-filled tube is approximately 2.5 to 3 cm wide, and the orientation of the branches off the cephalad position of the main gas-filled structure is not characteristic of bile ducts. The configuration of the gas is much more compatible with the portal vein, which is the correct diagnosis. Thus, although the location of the gas is an important criterion for differentiating biliary from portal vein gas (central versus peripheral), the configuration of the gas is just as important. In this case the configuration of the gas was more critical than the location.

The patient had mild sepsis and lower abdominal pain and was taken to surgery after computed tomography (CT) confirmed the presence of portal vein gas and demonstrated gas in the superior mesenteric vein without revealing any specific abnormalities other than a small amount of fluid in the pelvis. At surgery a small area of sigmoid diverticulitis due to perforation from a bay leaf was found. The patient recovered after surgical resection of the diverticulitis. A repeat CT scan revealed that the previous portal vein gas had been absorbed; however, the portal and superior mesenteric veins were thrombosed, although the patient had no symptoms.

REFERENCES

1. McNulty JG: *Radiology of the Liver.* Philadelphia, WB Saunders Co, 1977, pp 54–60.
2. Mindelzun RE: Abnormal gas collections, in McCort JJ (ed): *Abdominal Radiology.* Baltimore, Williams & Wilkins Co, 1981, pp 181–252.
3. Harley WD, Kirkpatrick RH, Ferrucci JT: Gas in the bile ducts (pneumobilia). *AJR* 1978; 131:661–663.
4. Hoppenstein JM, Medoza B, Watne AL: Choledochoduodenal fistula due to perforating duodenal ulcer disease. *Ann Surg* 1971; 173: 145–147.
5. Legge DA, Carlson HC, Judd ES: Roentgenologic features of regional enteritis of the upper gastrointestinal tract. *AJR* 1970; 110: 355–360.
6. Wastie ML, Cunningham GE: Roentgenologic findings in recurrent pyogenic cholangitis. *AJR* 1973; 119:71–76.
7. Wolfe JN, Evans WA: Gas in the portal veins of the liver in infants. A roentgenographic demonstration with postmortem anatomical correlation. *AJR* 1955; 74:486–489.
8. Barrett AF: Gas in the portal vein. Diagnostic

value in intestinal gangrene. *Clin Radiol* 1962; 13:92–95.

9. Sussman N, Senturia HR: Gas embolization of the portal venous system. *AJR* 1960; 83: 847–850.

10. Wiot JF, Felson B: Gas in the portal venous system. *AJR* 1961; 86:220–229.

11. Sisk PB: Gas in the portal system. *Radiology* 1961; 77:103–106.

12. Rigler LG, Pogue WL: Roentgen signs of intestinal necrosis. *AJR* 1965; 94:402–409.

13. Fink DW, Boyden FM: Gas in the portal veins. A report of two cases due to ingestion of corrosive substance. *Radiology* 1966; 87:741–743.

14. Graham NG: Gas in the portal vein in association with a pelvic abscess. *Br Med J* 1967; 3:288.

15. Paciulli J, Jacobson G: Survival following roentgenographic demonstration of gas in the hepatic portal venous system. *AJR* 1967; 99:629–631.

16. Schmidt AG: Portal vein gas due to administration of fluids via the umbilical vein. *Radiology* 1967; 88:293–294.

17. Swaim TJ, Gerald B: Hepatic portal venous gas in infants without subsequent death. *Radiology* 1970; 94:343–345.

18. Kees CJ, Hester CL Jr: Portal vein gas following barium enema examination. *Radiology* 1972; 102:525–526.

19. Graham GA, Bernstein RB, Gronner AT: Gas in the portal and inferior mesenteric veins caused by diverticulitis of the sigmoid colon. Report of a case with survival. *Radiology* 1975; 114:601–602.

20. Gold RP, Seaman WB: Splenic flexure carcinoma as a source of hepatic portal venous gas. *Radiology* 1977; 122:329–330.

21. Lebman PR, Patten MT, et al: Hepatic portal vein gas in adults: Etiology, pathophysiology and clinical significance. *Ann Surg* 1978; 187:281–287.

CHAPTER 6

Pneumatosis Intestinalis

Howard J. Ansel, M.D.

Case Presentation

This 60-year-old man with known atrial fibrillation had acute abdominal pain with bloody diarrhea followed by abdominal distention; he appeared acutely ill. A view of the abdomen is shown in Figure 6–1. What are the findings, and what is their significance? What is the differential diagnosis?

DISCUSSION

A plain abdominal radiograph shows a linear gas collection within the bowel wall and a branching gas pattern within the liver (Fig 6–1). Mural bowel air (pneumatosis intestinalis) has many causes (Table 6–1). It is considered primary or idiopathic in 15% of cases and secondary to an underlying condition that causes loss of intestinal integrity or increased intraluminal pressure in the remaining cases. The distribution of gas may be cystic or linear.[1] In the cystic type, cysts usually are seen in the left colon, with the rectum spared (Fig 6–2,A and B). The cysts vary in size, are lined by endothelium, and contain nitrogen.[2] In most cases they are associated with a benign process and are asymptomatic or cause only mild nonspecific symptoms. They may spontaneously resolve.[3] When the cysts are symptomatic, the administration of oxygen by mask is beneficial in resolving them.[4]

In the adult, the major concern is that pneumatosis indicates bowel infarction[5] (Fig 6–3,A and B). With bowel necrosis there is loss of intestinal mucosal integrity and dissection of gas into the bowel wall. Pneumatosis was reported in 16% of patients with irreversible bowel infarction.[6] The gas may follow the portal venous system to the liver and be seen in a branching pattern in the right

upper quadrant. In contrast to biliary air, which is located centrally, portal air is distributed peripherally. The presence of pneumatosis and portal air associated with a clinical picture of abdominal catastrophe is an ominous sign. Bowel necrosis may lead to perforation, with subsequent peritonitis and death.

Not all forms of linear pneumatosis are as ominous as the type seen in bowel infarction. Pneumatosis may appear in patients with partial or complete bowel obstruction.[7] Distention of the bowel associated with increased intraluminal pressure may disrupt the integrity of the bowel wall and allow gas to dissect into the wall. After the obstruction is relieved, the pneumatosis usually disappears.

Pneumatosis also may be seen after surgical procedures, including jejunal bypass[8] and bowel resection with anastomosis.

Bowel distention from air insufflation at the time of endoscopy may cause gas to dissect into the bowel wall. Endoscopic biopsies are another source of intramural air (Fig 6–4).[9]

Colonic diverticular disease causing partial bowel obstruction also may lead to the dissection of gas into the bowel wall. At one time, the most common cause of pneumatosis was peptic ulcer disease with pyloric stenosis and gastric outlet obstruction.[10] In these cases pneumatosis involving the right colon

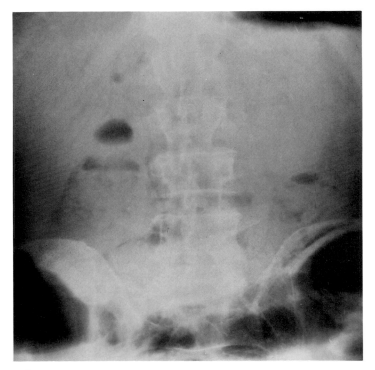

FIG 6–1.
Upright view of the abdomen in a 60-year-old man with abdominal pain
and distention fails to reveal free air. What are the radiographic findings?

TABLE 6–1.

Causes of Pneumatosis Intestinalis

Mesenteric vascular occlusive disease
Acute necrotizing enterocolitis
Pulmonary disease with pneumomediastinum
Caustic ingestion
Iatrogenic trauma (endoscopy, biopsy)
Peptic ulcer disease, pyloric strictures, gastric outlet
   obstruction
Intestinal obstruction
Collagen vascular disease (especially scleroderma)
Phlegmonous gastritis
Postsurgical anastomosis
Abdominal trauma
Chronic enteritis and colitis
Perforated colonic diverticulum
Whipple's disease
Intestinal parasites
Steroid treatment
Leukemia
Idiopathic

predominated.[11] Collagen vascular disease, especially scleroderma with pseudo-obstruction involving the small bowel, may be associated with chronic bowel distention, pneumatosis, and chronic pneumoperitoneum.[12] Other collagen diseases associated with vasculitis may lead to bowel ischemia and subsequent pneumatosis.

In infants, necrotizing enterocolitis, a disease of uncertain cause in premature infants, may be associated with pneumatosis and portal venous air[7] (Fig 6–5). Obstructive causes of pneumatosis in the infant include Hirschsprung's disease, meconium plug syndrome, and anal atresia.

Inflammatory conditions of the bowel, including regional enteritis, appendicitis, chronic colitis, and intestinal parasites, rarely cause pneumatosis.[13] Patients receiving steroid therapy for conditions such as collagen vascular disease and leukemias may have pneumatosis.[14] The pneumatosis appears benign, and whether it is the result of the steroid therapy or the underlying condition has yet to be determined.

Cystic pneumatosis often occurs in patients with chronic lung disease. The pneumatosis likely results from the rupture of alveoli into the mediastinum during episodes of coughing and vomiting; a pneumomediastinum results. The gas then dissects along the aorta and retroperitoneal vessels in the bowel wall.[15]

Other conditions are unlikely to be confused

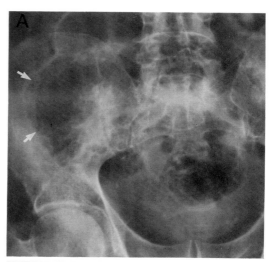

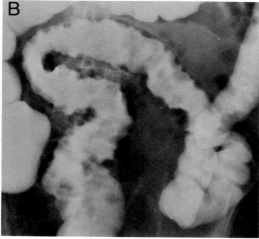

FIG 6–2.

A, cystic collections of gas *(arrows)* are noted along the distribution of the sigmoid colon on this plain film of the abdomen. **B,** (same patient as in **A**), film from a barium contrast study demonstrates multiple polypoid-like filling defects along the sigmoid colon. Close observation shows these defects to contain gas. As the colon fills, gas cysts in the wall tend to efface and flatten.

with linear pneumatosis. On the plain film, air-filled colonic diverticula may be mistaken for cystic pneumatosis (Fig 6–6,A and B). In the barium-filled bowel, air cysts may be mistaken for polyps, thumbprinting, colitis cystica profunda, lymphosarcoma, and metastases. The realization that the filling defects contain gas eliminates these diagnoses.[11]

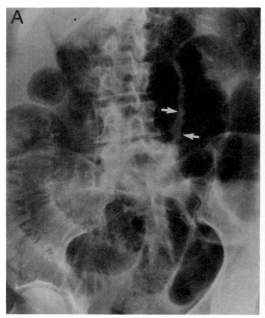 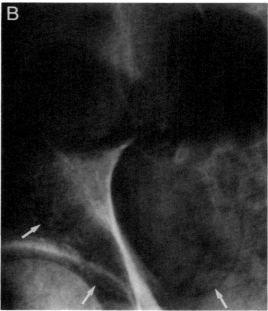

FIG 6–3.
Linear pneumatosis associated with bowel infarct. **A,** in this patient with extensive small bowel infarction, air outlines the bowel wall of fluid-filled small bowel loops in the right lower quadrant. More proximal small bowel loops in the left upper quadrant show ev- idence of fold thickening *(arrows),* an indication of bowel wall edema or hemorrhage. **B,** coned view of the right lower quadrant shows air outlining the wall of the cecum. The right colon and ileum are infarcted.

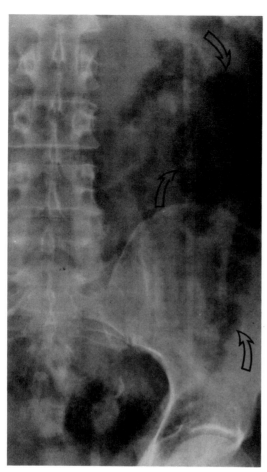

FIG 6–4.
Extensive pneumatosis *(arrows)* is present in the left colon after endoscopic biopsy of a sigmoid polyp. The patient had no symptoms. The pneumatosis resolved after several days.

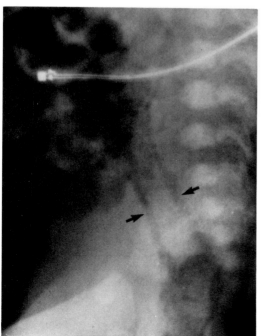

FIG 6–5.
Lateral view in a premature infant with necrotizing enterocolitis demonstrates pneumatosis involving the rectosigmoid colon *(arrows).* No air was seen within the portal venous system at this time.

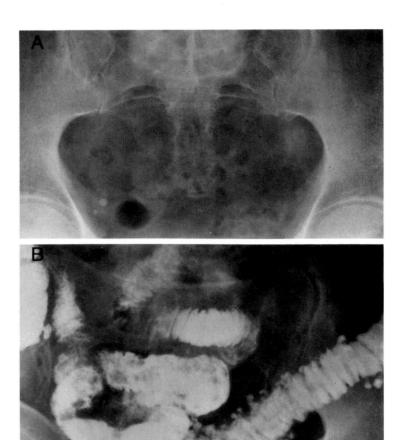

FIG 6–6.
A, multiple air-filled cystic densities are noted in the pelvic region, most likely within the sigmoid colon. The findings suggest pneumatosis. **B,** films from a barium contrast study demonstrate air within numerous sigmoid diverticula, simulating the appearance of pneumatosis.

In the case presented, the presence of air in the bowel wall and portal venous system within the liver in association with the patient's clinical history of pain and bloody diarrhea led to the diagnosis of bowel infarction. The patient died shortly after these films were obtained.

REFERENCES

1. Meyers MA, Ghahremani GG, Clements JL Jr, et al: Pneumatosis intestinalis. *Gastrointestinal Radiol* 1977; 2:91–106.
2. Langston CS: Other colonic disorders, in Dreyfuss JR, Janower ML (eds): *Radiology of the Colon.* Baltimore, Williams & Wilkins Co, 1980, pp 546–553.
3. Block C: The natural history of pneumatosis coli. *Radiology* 1977; 123:311–314.
4. Kelvin FM, Gardiner R: *Clinical Imaging of the Colon and Rectum,* ed 2. New York, Raven Press, 1987, pp 439–443.
5. Rigler LG, Pogue WL: Roentgen signs of intestinal necrosis. *Am J Roentgenol Radium Ther* 1965; 94:402–409.
6. Scott JR, Miller WT, Urso M, et al: Acute mesenteric infarction. *Am J Roentgenol Radium Ther* 1971; 113:269–279.
7. Schmidt AG: Intramural gas proximal to obstructing carcinoma. *Radiology* 1968; 91:785.
8. Wandtke J, Skucas J, Spataro R, et al: Pneumatosis intestinalis as a complication of jejunoileal bypass. *Am J Roentgenol Radium Ther* 1977; 129:601–604.

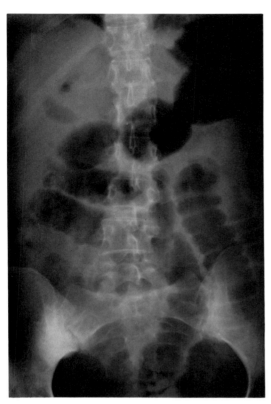

FIG 7–4.
Gallstone "ileus." Distended small bowel loops with minimal colon gas indicate small bowel obstruction. Note gas in the biliary system. The gallstone that caused the bowel obstruction is not visualized.

struction with an incompetent ileocecal valve may mimic generalized ileus. Demonstration of gas in the rectum on prone or right lateral decubitus views excludes complete colonic obstruction but does not rule out even a high-grade partial colonic obstruction, because some gas may pass into the rectum despite the occlusion. A localized small bowel ileus also can mimic either a partial or early complete small bowel obstruction (Fig 7–5).

Frequent vomiting can decompress loops of bowel which otherwise might have been distended. This is one of the reasons why a relatively gasless abdomen should always be viewed with suspicion. A suctioning alimentary tube can create a similar gasless pattern (Fig 7–6,A and B), which may be misleading. In this example the bowel gas pattern appears normal, but subsequent injection of barium through the tube confirmed the clinical suspicion of a small bowel obstruction. Last, fluid-filled loops

often are difficult to appreciate on plain films, and their presence may create an erroneous impression of a gas pattern.

Fluid-filled Loops

Large quantities of fluid-filled loops of small bowel generally suggest mechanical obstruction rather than adynamic ileus.[7] First described by Frimann-Dahl[8] as a "pseudotumor," they were initially believed to be pathognomonic for bowel strangulation. However, fluid-filled loops can be found with simple obstruction without bowel ischemia.[9, 10] Fluid-filled loops must be recognized as such, because they can mimic an abdominal or pelvic mass. At times the fluid-filled loops have a subtle but recognizable longitudinal contour and a lobulated margin that can help to identify them as fluid-filled intestine. At other times, however, there is a perfectly smooth border, mimicking a true abdominal or pelvic mass (Fig 7–7,A and B).[6, 7, 9, 10]

The detection of fluid-filled loops by plain film methods may be unreliable, especially if no gas is visible in the obstructed loop.[9] Occasionally, if there is a small amount of gas within the fluid-filled loop, erect or decubitus views allow the gas to separate into a series of tiny bubbles trapped beneath the valvulae conniventes, or the "string of beads sign."[11] Sometimes small amounts of gas can be seen rising to the surface of fluid-filled loops in a supine patient. These appear as a row of thin parallel radiolucencies, or the "positive stretch sign," and reliably indicate small bowel distention.[9, 12] With the advent of ultrasound and computed tomographic scanning, the accurate detection of fluid-filled bowel loops does not depend on plain film methods alone and should be less of a diagnostic dilemma than in the past. In fact, ultrasonography should be one of the first studies ordered when fluid-filled bowel loops are suspected on a plain film of the abdomen. Ultrasonography showed a "soft tissue pelvic mass" to be distended fluid-filled small bowel loops in a patient with a history of cervical carcinoma, previous surgery, and small bowel obstruction (see Fig 7–7,A and B).

Air-fluid Levels

Controversy concerning the presence, number, length, and significance of air-fluid levels in the bowel continues. In the past, the mere presence of air-fluid levels in the bowel was believed to be abnormal.[13] The heights and lengths of air-fluid levels

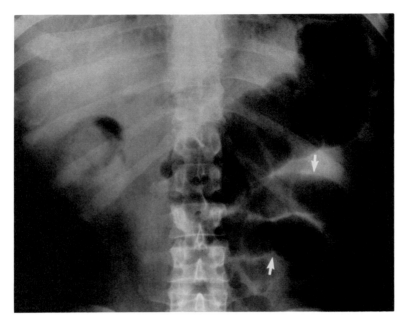

FIG 7–5.
Pancreatitis causing localized small bowel ileus. Notice gas in two loops of distended small bowel *(arrows)* in the left mid-abdomen and gas in the slightly distended distal transverse colon. Irritation from the adjacent inflammation caused regional bowel atony.

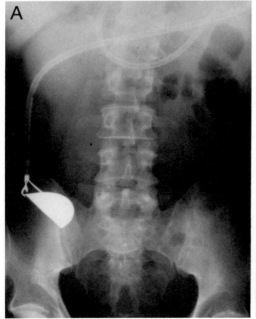 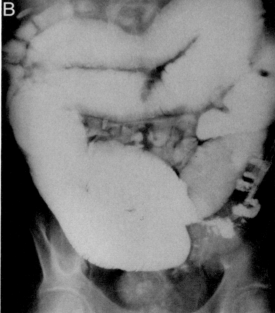

FIG 7–6.
A, misleading gas pattern secondary to a long intestinal tube. "Normal" appearance of the bowel gas pattern due to decompression from a long intestinal tube is misleading in a patient with symptoms of small bowel obstruction, **B,** small bowel enteroclysis. Barium fills distended small bowel loops, confirming a small bowel obstruction, which was decompressed by the intestinal tube. Contrast material in nondistended colon indicates an incomplete occlusion.

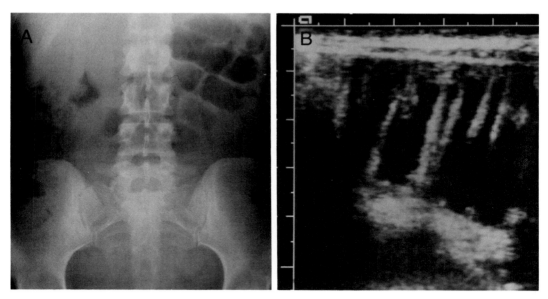

FIG 7–7.
A, fluid-filled small bowel loops mimic a pelvic mass. An apparent soft tissue mass in the pelvis was caused by distended fluid-filled loops of small bowel in this patient who had a surgically proved small bowel obstruction. A few gas-filled small bowel loops in the left upper quadrant are equivocally distended. **B,** fluid-filled small bowel. Ultrasound scan confirms that the apparent soft tissue mass is due to abnormally distended fluid-filled small bowel loops. Note the plicae circulares extending across the bowel lumen.

were thought to be useful in distinguishing between small bowel obstruction and ileus.[11–13] More recently, air-fluid levels at various heights have been documented as normal in small and large bowel, with rather long fluid levels occurring normally in the large bowel.[14] However, when several air-fluid levels are detected in definitely distended small bowel loops, abnormal stasis of gastrointestinal contents should be suspected. Differentiation between small bowel obstruction and adynamic ileus, however, is not reliable based on further characterization of the air-fluid levels.[6]

In summary, air-fluid levels may be of little help in diagnosis, and may be misleading in certain cases (Fig 7–8). Often an upright film is ordered to demonstrate air-fluid levels. In the majority of cases this view adds little information; in one study, the upright abdominal film increased the accuracy of diagnosing small bowel obstruction by only 5% and was of little help in delineating the site of obstruction.[15.]

Serial Examination

Serial films often are the key to unraveling confusing gas patterns. Progressive dilation of prox-

imal small bowel with decreasing gas distally occurs with small bowel obstruction, whereas there is usually little change in generalized bowel distention with adynamic ileus. Significant history can aid in the diagnosis. Figure 7–9 demonstrates gas in the distended small bowel with a relative lack of gas in the large bowel, although gas is present in the rectum. After obtaining the history of a recent subtotal colectomy with ileoproctectomy, and with little change on follow-up films, the clinician confidently diagnosed postoperative ileus.

Contrast Examination

A contrast examination may be useful in differentiating small bowel obstruction from adynamic ileus in atypical cases. More important, the small bowel contrast study may demonstrate and characterize the site of obstruction. If there is any possibility of a colon obstruction, a barium enema should be given prior to the oral small bowel examination. Barium sulfate suspension, rather than water-soluble contrast material, is the preferred agent. Contrary to popular concern, there is no risk of converting a partial small bowel obstruction to complete small bowel obstruction with the use of barium sulfate.[16]

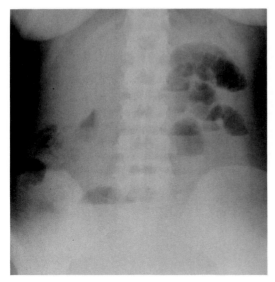

FIG 7–8.
Air-fluid levels. Multiple air-fluid levels are present. Their widths seem to indicate that the small bowel loops are normal in caliber. At surgery, this patient had a high-grade small bowel obstruction.

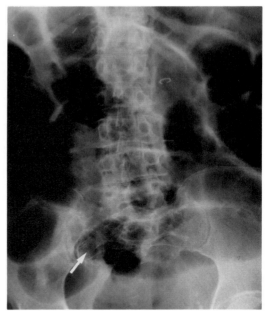

FIG 7–9.
Postoperative ileus. There is generalized small bowel distention with gas in the distal colon in this patient who had a subtotal colectomy and ileoproctectomy. Note the staple lines *(arrow)* medial to the right sacroiliac joint.

Because of the significant amount of fluid in the small bowel, the barium sulfate suspension does not thicken or harden. Water-soluble contrast should be avoided in the workup of small bowel obstruction. It will become diluted because of its hypertonicity, films will be nondiagnostic, and more important, the patient's fluid balance may be adversely affected.

Bowel Strangulation

Because mortality with bowel strangulation is 2 to 15 times higher than with simple obstruction, diagnosis must be timely and accurate. Bowel strangulation can be extremely difficult to detect. Several signs suggest strangulated bowel, but none are pathognomonic. Predominance of fluid-filled loops with long air-fluid levels, paucity of abdominal gas, effacement of small bowel folds, and the appearance of a small bowel loop folded on itself ("coffee bean sign") have been associated with bowel strangulation.[6, 8, 9, 11, 12, 17] However, these signs are neither sensitive, frequent, nor specific.[10, 12] Rigidity of bowel contour, narrowing of the bowel lumen, findings indicating bowel wall edema, and pneumatosis intestinalis are more useful signs that indicate gangrene, but these may not be present even in severe ischemia. The only sign that may be significant for differentiating a closed loop small bowel obstruction complicated by strangulation from a simple small bowel obstruction is reduced activity and fixation of the bowel loops on serial films.[10] However, inasmuch as simple obstruction is much more frequent than strangulating obstruction, strangulated bowel eventually will be diagnosed in only a minority of patients with decreased bowel activity.[10] Because radiologic findings and clinical and laboratory data all may be nonspecific, a high index of suspicion and a low threshold for surgical intervention should be maintained whenever bowel strangulation is a viable diagnostic option.

Case Discussion

In the case presented (see Fig 7–1,A and B), there is uniform dilation of large bowel and small bowel in a pattern consistent with generalized ileus rather than small bowel obstruction. Although causes of overall bowel distention are many (Table 7–1), there are coarsened interstitial structures at both long bases (see Fig 7–1,B) in this patient.

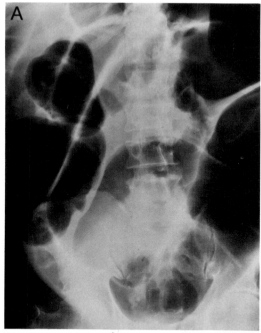

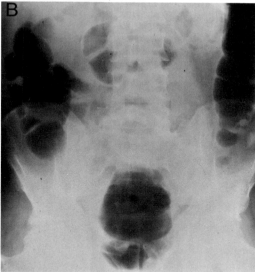

FIG 8−3.
A, supine film reveals severe gaseous distention of the colon and dilation of the small intestine. **B,** prone film permits colonic gas to move into the rectum, excluding complete distal colonic obstruction.

ill-advised because the barium can become impacted above the obstruction[3]; however, recent animal studies suggest that this may not be so great a risk as previously thought.[4]

Radiographic characteristics of a large bowel

obstruction include gaseous colonic distention with a transition point from dilated to normal caliber. Small intestinal dilation also can be seen if the ileocecal valve is incompetent. Left-sided obstruction is more common than right; however, distal colonic obstruction is often more difficult to characterize precisely. The transition point is usually easier to define when located in the right colon.[1, 2] Typically, the clinical presentation of colonic obstruction is more subacute than is small intestinal obstruction; therefore symptomatology may not help in differentiating colonic obstruction from colonic ileus.

The many causes of colonic obstruction[1, 2] include those within the differential diagnosis for stricture of the sigmoid colon, which have been discussed. In brief, malignant processes such as adenocarcinoma, lymphoma, and metastatic deposits must be considered, as well as inflammatory diseases, diverticulitis, infectious and noninfectious colitides, ischemia, and rarer conditions such as postradiation stricture, extrinsic mass effect (Fig 8−4), retractile mesenteritis, and adhesions. All of these processes can affect any segment of the colon or rectum; however, ischemia is rare in the rectum because of its rich collateral arterial supply.

When gaseous distention of the colon is seen in an adult, the differential diagnosis for colonic obstruction must be expanded beyond these considerations. Volvulus, torsion of the colon on a long, mobile mesentery, of either the cecum or the sigmoid colon, can produce complete colonic obstruction.[5] Cecal volvulus is related in part to incomplete rotation and fixation of the mid-gut, but may require an inciting secondary factor, such as colonic ileus, for presentation. Classically, the gas-filled cecum is displaced toward the left upper quadrant, but can be situated elsewhere in the abdomen. Consequently a contrast enema can be diagnostic, demonstrating a tapered beak of contrast directed at the stenosis (Fig 8−5). A cecal bascule also can produce proximal colonic obstruction.[6] In this condition, the cecum folds so that it is situated anterior to the ascending colon. Sigmoid volvulus produces a closed-loop obstruction as well as colonic obstruction. It is typically characterized by a very dilated, often featureless, U-shaped loop of bowel arising out of the pelvis and extending a variable extent into the abdomen. Contrast enema, as in cecal volvulus, shows a complete obstruction to flow of contrast medium, with a beaklike configuration.

External, or rarely internal, hernias can cause colonic obstruction.[1, 2, 7] External hernias can be seen in inguinal, femoral, umbilical, parasagittal,

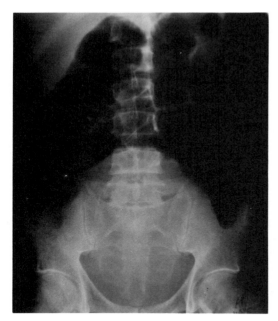

FIG 8–4.
Distal colonic obstruction due to extrinsic compression by a distended urinary bladder.

diaphragmatic, or incisional locations. Internal hernias are most common at the foramen of Winslow.

Although large bowel obstruction from intussusception is more common in children than in adults, colocolonic intussusceptions are more common in adults.[1, 2] A colonic lesion acting as a lead point for the intussusception is characteristic in the adult. Fluoroscopic reduction of intussusception with a barium enema is less successful in adults than in children. Plain films can suggest a proximal colonic obstruction and may show a soft tissue mass at the site of the intussusception. Contrast examinations may outline a filling defect (the intussusception) within the colonic lumen or outline the intussusception with its coiled-spring appearance. Computed tomography also can be of value in the diagnosis of intussusception, demonstrating a targetlike mass with eccentric areas of low density or a stratified pattern of alternating soft tissue and low density.[8]

Hirschsprung's disease, aganglionosis of the colon, is uncommonly detected in adults, but is a potential cause of large bowel obstruction.[9] This condition is characterized by loss of the ganglion cells of the myenteric plexus in the narrowed, distal transition zone. Although contrast enema defines the anatomy, confirmation of the diagnosis is made by rectal biopsy.

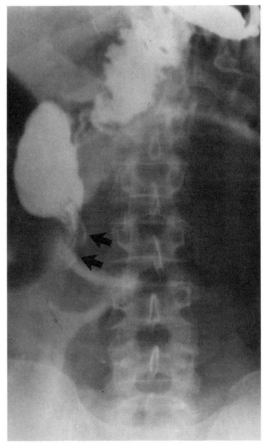

FIG 8–5.
Cecal volvulus is documented on barium enema study. Massive cecal distention is present. A tapered narrowing of the barium column is seen at the point of torsion *(arrows)*.

Fecal impaction occurs in a variety of clinical settings, including debilitation, narcotic abuse, and psychogenic anal dysfunction. It also can cause colonic obstruction.[1, 2]

Colonic ileus also occurs in a variety of clinical settings, including postoperative and postanesthetic conditions, chemotherapy, acute abdominal and pulmonary infections, and electrolyte and metabolic disorders, including diabetes mellitus[10–15] (Fig 8–6). Severe involvement of the colon in progressive systemic sclerosis with smooth-muscle dysfunction also can result in massive colonic distention.[16] When severe, such gaseous colonic distention can be difficult to differentiate from colonic obstruction and is denoted as "pseudo-obstruction" of

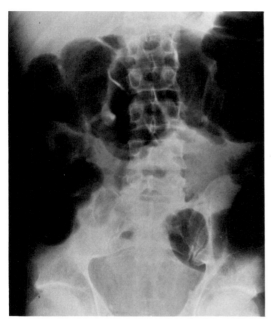

FIG 8–6.
Colonic ileus in a patient receiving psychotropic medication.

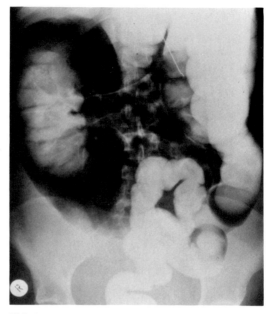

FIG 8–7.
Contrast enema excludes distal colonic obstruction. Massive cecal distention is seen.

the colon, or Ogilvie's syndrome. As with colonic obstruction, the massive dilation of the large bowel, particularly the cecum ("cecal ileus"), predisposes to perforation.[17] Therefore, even though an anatomic obstruction is not identified, aggressive decompressive measures should be undertaken when the cecal diameter exceeds 10 cm. If standard nasogastric and rectal decompression tubes are not effective in decompressing the colon, sigmoidoscopy or colonoscopy with suctioning of the intestinal gas may be required.[18, 19] Occasionally operative decompression, or cecostomy, is required. Percutaneous needle or catheter decompression of the massively dilated cecum also can be performed.[20, 21]

In our patient, there was concern about colonic obstruction with its associated risks of overdistention, ischemia, and perforation of the bowel. In this setting, possible causes for large bowel obstruction include ischemic stenosis, extrinsic mass effect, volvulus, and intussusception. Right lateral decubitus and prone films were not obtained in this patient. However, a contrast enema was performed. No evidence of colonic obstruction was found, indicating that the cause of the gaseous distention of the large bowel and small intestine was severe colonic

ileus (Fig 8–7). Mass effect in the pelvis was due to the presence of a urinoma.

In summary, massive gaseous distention of the colon presents a limited differential diagnosis of colonic obstruction or ileus. However, both conditions have a great number of causes, and these must be kept in mind after differentiation between obstruction and ileus has been made.

REFERENCES

1. Dreyfuss JR, Janower ML: *Radiology of the Colon.* Baltimore, Williams & Wilkins Co, 1980.
2. Marshak RH, Lindner AE, Maklansky D: *Radiology of the Colon.* Philadelphia, WB Saunders Co, 1980.
3. Frimann-Dahl J: The administration of barium orally in acute obstruction: Advantages and risks. *Acta Radiol* 1954; 42:285–295.
4. Grossman RI, Miller WT, Dann RW: Oral barium sulfate in partial large-bowel obstruction. *Radiology* 1980; 136:327–331.
5. Kerry RJ, Lee F, Ransom HK: Roentgenologic examination in the diagnosis and treatment of colon volvulus. *Am J Roentgenol* 1971; 113:343–348.

6. Bobroff LM, Messinger NH, Subbarao K, et al: The cecal bascule. *Am J Roentgenol* 1972; 115:249–252.

7. Javors BR, Bryk D: Colonic obstruction within inguinal hernia. J Can Assoc Radiol 1981; 32:162–163.

8. Iko BO, Teal JS, Siram SM, et al: Computed tomography of adult colonic intussusception: Clinical and experimental studies. *Am J Roentgenol* 1984; 143:769–772.

9. Mindelzun RE, Hicks SM: Adult Hirschsprung disease: Radiographic findings. *Radiology* 1986; 160:623–625.

10. Atherton LD, Leib ES, Kay MD: Toxic megacolon associated with methotrexate therapy. *Gastroenterology* 1984; 86:1583–1588.

11. Bryk D, Soong KY: Colonic ileus and its differential roentgen diagnosis. *Am J Roentgenol* 1967; 101:329–337.

12. Bullock PR, Thomas WEG: Acute pseudo-obstruction of the colon. Ann R Coll Surg Engl 1984; 66:327–330.

13. Clayman RV, Reddy P, Nivatvongs S: Acute pseudo-obstruction of the colon: A serious consequence of urologic surgery. *J Urol* 1981; 126:415–417.

14. Heer M, Pirovino M, Buhler H, et al: Diabetic megacolon—A rare late complication. *Radiologe* 1983; 23:233–235.

15. Walker JL, Walling AK: Ogilvie's syndrome in orthopaedic patients. *Orthop Rev* 1985; 14:493–496.

16. Battle WM, Snape WJ, Wright S, et al: Abnormal colonic motility in progressive systemic sclerosis. *Ann Intern Med* 1981; 94:749–752.

17. Johnson CD, Rice RP, Kelvin FM, et al: The radiologic evaluation of gross cecal distention: Emphasis on cecal ileus. *Am J Roentgenol* 1985; 145:1211–1217.

18. Lelcuk S, Ratan J, Klausner JM: Endoscopic decompression of acute colonic obstruction: Avoiding staged surgery. *Ann Surg* 1986; 203:292–294.

19. Sirazl KK, Agha FP, Strodal WE, et al: Nonobstructive colonic dilatation: Radiologic findings in 50 patients following colonoscopic treatment. *J Can Assoc Radiol* 1984; 35:116–119.

20. Casola G, Withers C, van Sonnenberg E, et al: Percutaneous cecostomy for decompression of the massively distended cecum. *Radiology* 1986; 158:793–794.

21. Crass JR, Simmons RL, Frick MP, et al: Percutaneous decompression of the colon using CT guidance in Ogilvie syndrome. *Am J Roentgenol* 1985; 144:475–476.

CHAPTER 9

Gross Cecal Distention

C. Daniel Johnson, M.D.

Case Presentation

A 71-year-old man with rheumatoid arthritis complained of bloating, abdominal pain, and nausea 5 days after surgical revision of total hip arthroplasty. The patient was not ambulating and remained supine in bed. An abdominal plain film was ordered to evaluate the abdominal complaints (Fig 9–1). What are the differential diagnosis and likely diagnosis? What important clinical information should be relayed to the primary physician?

DISCUSSION

The diagnostic approach to various abdominal gas patterns requires differentiation of small bowel gas from colonic gas. Colonic gas usually lies in a picture frame distribution surrounding smaller caliber small bowel loops. The ascending colon normally is positioned in the right flank, and the descending colon in the left flank, just medial to the properitoneal fat. The hepatic flexure, transverse colon, and splenic flexure are found immediately below the hepatic shadow, stomach bubble, and spleen, respectively. The sigmoid colon is variable in location but commonly spans the left mid-pelvis, joining the vertically oriented rectum. Identification of haustral markings confirms colonic location. Haustral folds may or may not extend completely across the colonic lumen, usually indent the colonic surface, and are spaced asymmetrically. Retained fecal debris in the colon has a mottled or bubbly appearance. Small bowel valvulae conniventes are usually recognizable only in the jejunum, as regular closely spaced folds that do not indent the bowel contour. The ileum is normally featureless, with few identifiable folds.

When colonic gas is identified, the distribution and amount of gas must be assessed. Normally a small to moderate amount of gas is present in non-distended colon. Supine and upright abdominal films commonly demonstrate gas predominantly in the anterior transverse colon. Air-fluid levels may be normal in the right colon on upright films. Gaseous distention of the colon usually is due to either mechanical obstruction or adynamic ileus[1, 2] (Table 9–1), commonly dilating the cecum early and to a greater extent than the remainder of the colon. A redundant cecal mesentery is present in 15% of the population,[3] allowing the cecum to rotate into the mid-abdomen with colonic distention.

Figure 9–1, demonstrates gas throughout most of the colon, as would be expected in colonic ileus, but the cecum is dilated out of proportion to the remainder of the colon and has rotated into the mid-abdomen (secondary to a redundant cecal mesentery). Medial rotation of the cecum often can be confirmed by locating small bowel loops lateral to the cecum, and an inferolaterally oriented ileocecal valve. This subtype of colonic ileus is referred to as cecal ileus, in which a dilated mobile cecum has rotated medially and anteriorly. This is a common clinical entity in patients with the triad of colonic ileus, mobile cecum, and prolonged recumbency

TABLE 9–1.
Differential Diagnosis of Gross Cecal Distention

Mechanical obstruction
  Nonvolvulus
    Primary adenocarcinoma
    Diverticulitis
    Metastasis
    Fecal impaction
  Volvulus
    Cecal volvulus
Ileus
  Adynamic ileus
    Small and large bowel ileus
    Colonic ileus
    Cecal ileus

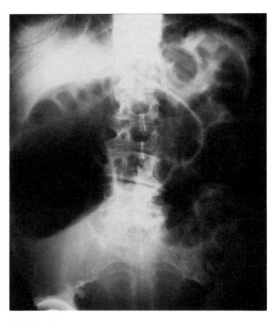

FIG 9–1.
Plain supine abdominal radiograph demonstrating gas throughout most of the colon, with disproportionate dilation of the medially rotated cecum.

(usually postoperative or intensive care patients).[4] The anteromedially placed cecum acts as a reservoir that progressively distends as gas from the small bowel empties into the colon. Emptying does not occur, because of the concurrent ileus and patient immobility. A competent ileocecal valve also may contribute to progressive cecal distention. Gross cecal distention greater than 8 to 10 cm is important because cecal perforation can occur, resulting in peritonitis and even death in some patients.[5] It is believed that high intraluminal cecal pressure decreases venous return, with subsequent ischemia, gangrene, and eventual perforation. Cecal perforation occurs in up to 20% of patients with untreated cecal ileus; death occurs in 80% of patients with perforation. The duration of cecal distention is a better predictor of impending perforation than actual cecal size. Cecal perforation usually occurs only if the cecum remains dilated for 2 or 3 days or longer. After it reaches at least 9 cm in diameter, there does not seem to be any correlation between cecal size and tendency to perforate.[4] Early treatment is usually conservative and includes use of nasogastric suction, cathartics, and rectal tubes. If these measures are not successful within a few days, aggressive decompression using either colonoscopy or surgically placed cecostomy tubes is warranted. Detection of perforation is unreliable on the basis of findings on the abdominal plain film because neither prompt decompression of the cecum nor cecal pneumatosis is commonly visible on plain films.[4] Clinicians caring for patients with cecal ileus should be alerted to the serious nature of this entity and potential for perforation if prompt decompression does not result with conservative therapy.

There is no doubt that in many patients a grossly dilated cecum has been diagnosed as cecal bascule when in fact it was cecal ileus. Bascule originally was used to describe a mechanically obstructed ascending colon in which the cecum was folded anteriorly over the ascending colon, with the posterior cecal surface facing anteriorly.[6] Various degrees of obstruction were reported to occur at the site of bend related to adhesive bands or a flap valve. Contrast enema studies in cecal ileus show no anatomic obstruction, but slow cecal filling is commonly observed due to high intraluminal pressure. Cecal ileus is common among patients without a history of prior surgery, and adhesions causing colonic fixation are found only rarely at surgical exploration.[4] Because the cecum is neither folded on itself nor anatomically obstructed, the term cecal ileus is preferred to bascule because it more adequately describes a dilated, anteromedially displaced cecum in the setting of colonic ileus. Contrast enema studies may be used to exclude mechanical obstruction in this condition, but if the radiographic findings (Table 9–2) and clinical history are typical, no further diagnostic test is necessary. A high-volume contrast enema could unnecessarily increase cecal size and intraluminal pressure.

Other differential considerations in this case include usual colonic ileus, mechanical colonic obstruction, and cecal volvulus. Usual colonic ileus (Fig 9–2) is differentiated from cecal ileus by a normally positioned cecum in the right lower quadrant. Gas is usually present uniformly throughout the colon, without disproportionate cecal distention. Associated gas in the small bowel and stomach is frequently seen but is not necessary for diagnosis. Standard supine abdominal films may demonstrate air only in small bowel and transverse colon, raising the possibility of a distal mechanical obstruction. Usually knowledge of the clinical history will resolve this issue. If a distal mechanical obstruction is to be excluded, the use of decubitus and prone films often will shift gas into the ascending and descending colon and rectum. Inconclusive plain film findings may be supplemented by a contrast enema study to exclude an obstruction. Usually contrast material does not need to be refluxed beyond the splenic flexure or that point at which a solid colonic air column is seen on the abdominal plain films. This limited examination prevents unnecessary dilation of an already distended cecum and is more expeditious and comfortable for the patient. Cecal perforation can occur in colonic ileus with gross cecal distention. The risk of perforation in colonic ileus, as in cecal ileus, depends on the duration of cecal distention rather than actual cecal size[4]; perforation occurs less commonly than in cecal ileus, because the normally positioned cecum empties gas more readily into the distal colon. If conservative measures are not successful within 2 or 3 days, emergency colonoscopic or surgical decompression may be necessary.

Nonvolvulus mechanical colonic obstruction (Fig 9–3) often can be diagnosed from findings on abdominal plain films. Usually the colon is dilated to the level of obstruction, with retained air and fecal debris in the proximal colon. Incompetence of the ileocecal valve allows air to reflux into the small bowel, which may have a variable amount of gas-

eous distention. Colonic obstruction of more than a few days' duration may be recognized by bowel wall (haustral) thickening and a granular appearance to the retained liquid stool.[7] Air-fluid levels are common in both acute and subacute obstruction. Gross cecal dilation in mechanical colonic obstruction most commonly occurs in patients with competent ileocecal valves. Small bowel contents may continue to be advanced into the colon despite the distal obstruction, often requiring urgent surgical decompression of the dilated cecum to prevent perforation. Determining the exact cause of obstruction (usually primary adenocarcinoma, metastasis, diverticulitis, or fecal impaction) by barium enema examination may be difficult if obstruction is complete. Refluxing a small amount of contrast medium beyond the lesion may allow better assessment of lesion length, surface characteristics, and mucosal integrity. If barium is used, only a small amount of contrast material should be refluxed proximal to a high-grade obstruction to prevent barium concretion and subsequent impaction.

Cecal volvulus (Fig 9–4) is an uncommon cause of gross cecal distention, characterized by the dilated cecum projecting from the right lower quad-

TABLE 9–2.
Radiographic Findings in Cecal Ileus

Continuous gas column in colon (as expected in
  colonic ileus)
Dilated cecum >9 cm
Anteromedially positioned cecum
    Small bowel lateral to cecum
    Inferolaterally positioned ileocecal valve
Cecal dilation greater than remainder of colon
No anatomic obstruction with contrast enema

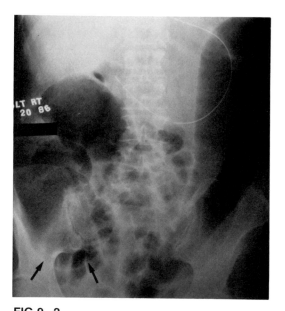

FIG 9–2.
Colonic ileus. Gaseous distention in a continuous uniform distribution throughout the colon. The cecum *(arrows)* is normally positioned in the right lower quadrant and not dilated out of proportion to the rest of the colon.

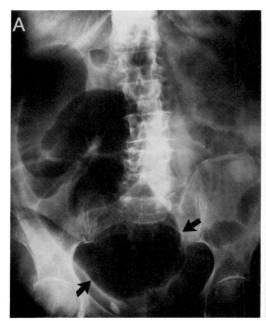
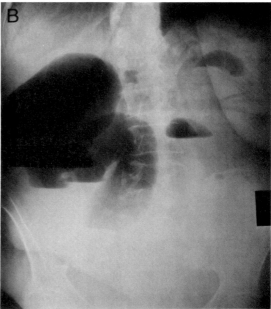

FIG 9–3.
Nonvolvulus mechanical colonic obstruction. **A,** supine abdominal radiograph demonstrates gaseous distention of a normally positioned cecum *(arrows)*, with colonic dilation to the midtransverse colon. **B,** upright abdominal radiograph demonstrates multiple air-fluid levels in the dilated proximal colonic loops. At surgery an incarcerated loop of transverse colon was found secondary to an incisional hernia.

rant into the mid-abdomen or left upper quadrant.[8] Air-fluid levels often are seen within the obstructed colonic loop on the upright abdominal film, with little or no gas in colon distal to the level of the colonic obstruction. Usually small bowel gaseous distention is present. Contrast enemas demonstrate

beaking of the ascending colon at the site of mechanical twist. Conservative treatment is rarely helpful, and emergency surgery is necessary to prevent cecal perforation.

Sigmoid volvulus (Fig 9–5) usually does not result in gross cecal distention. The obstructed

FIG 9–4.
Cecal volvulus. Supine abdominal radiograph demonstrates a dilated mobile cecum in the right mid-abdomen *(arrows)*. No other colonic gas is seen distal to the cecum. Multiple dilated small bowel loops are seen in the left and lower abdomen. Cecal volvulus was surgically confirmed.

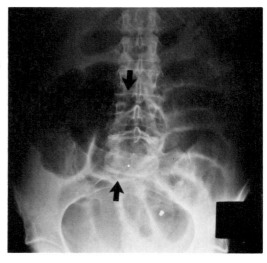

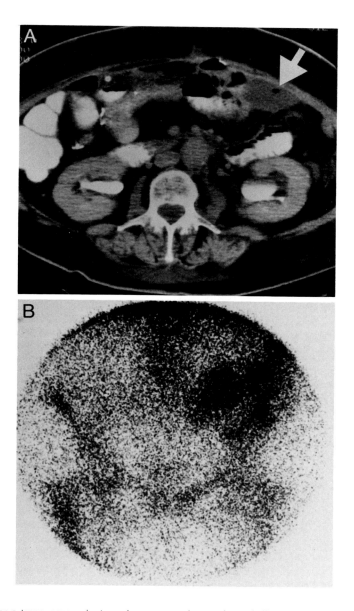

FIG 10–2.
Fourteen days after a transverse colectomy because of colon carcinoma, this patient became febrile. **A,** computed tomography (CT) demonstrates gas within a fluid collection in the left lower quadrant of the abdomen *(arrow).* **B,** anterior view of indium leukocyte scan consistent with abscess in abnormal area seen on CT scan.

tient is, within a broad range, similar to that with CT.

Gallium 67 is a cyclotron-produced agent. Although large radiopharmacies may keep supplies on hand, usually it must be ordered from a central supplier, resulting in a 24-hour lag time before injection; an additional 6 to 24 hours is needed to obtain accurate images. Gallium scanning therefore is not suitable for the acutely ill patient in whom an immediate diagnosis is required.

An extensive review of the literature in 1979 showed the sensitivity for detecting abdominal infections to be 95% to 100%, with specificity of 89% to 100%.[12] Recent work suggests that the sensitivity and specificity of gallium scintigraphy may be lower than that of US or CT.[13–16] False positive findings

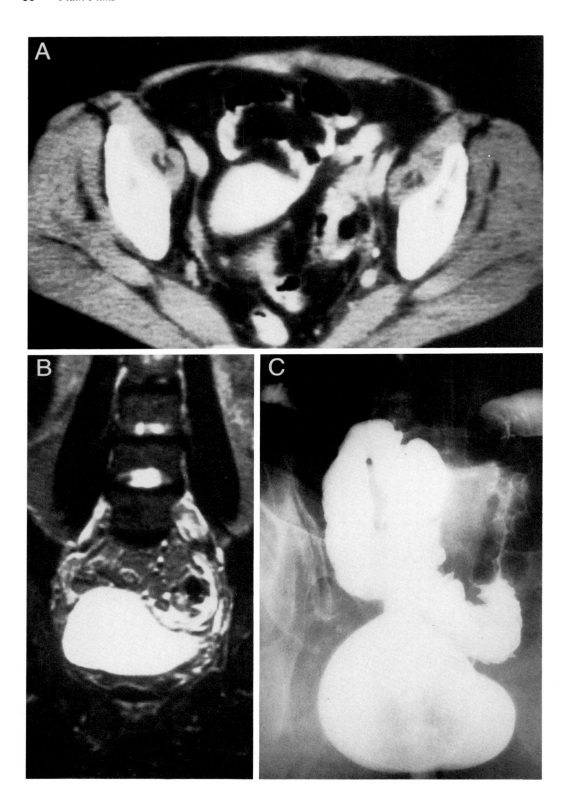

can result from the normal excretion of gallium into the bowel or genitourinary tract or from uptake in recent surgical sites and neoplasms. False negative findings have been reported in anaerobic abscesses[17] and can result from confusing an abscess with normal bowel excretion.

Gallium scintigraphy is not considered the method of first choice for ruling out abdominal abscess because of the time required for the study and the possibility of confusing the normal excretion by bowel as an abscess.

Indium 111 White Blood Cell Scintigraphy

Indium 111–labeled white cell scintigraphy primarily offers specificity in the workup of abscesses (Fig 10–4). Time and care are necessary for an adequate examination. Blood is drawn from the patient, the leukocytes are separated and labeled with indium 111 oxine, and the cells are reinjected. The preparation of labeled cells is exacting and requires a careful and dedicated technologist. Necessary equipment includes a sterile laminar flow hood and clinical centrifuge. Central radiopharmacies in large cities often offer this service, but it is not universally available. Indium 111 is a cyclotron-produced agent with a 3-day half-life. Small centers may not keep a supply of indium 111 oxine on hand; hence there can be a 24-hour delay time for ordering the agent in addition to the 2 hours needed for preparation of the white cells. Imaging is performed at least 4 to 8 hours after injection, and 24-hour images are routinely obtained. Therefore this test is not desirable for the acutely ill patient in whom an immediate diagnosis is required.

The cost of the indium 111 white cell scan is usually higher than that for gallium scintigraphy and lower than that for an abdominal CT scan. The radiation dose to the spleen and liver may be slightly more than that with CT, but the total body dose is similar.

Relatively good sensitivity and specificity have been reported for white cell scintigraphy.[3, 4, 14–16, 18–21] False positive findings result from accessory spleens, swallowed granulocytes in the gastrointestinal tract, gastrointestinal bleeding, bowel infarction, inflammatory bowel disease, and hematomas.[22, 23] False negative findings can occur around the liver, but the use of a subsequent liver-spleen sulfur colloid examination can improve accuracy.[24, 25] Indium 111–labeled leukocytes are not taken up by sterile surgical wounds or sterile fluid collections and are not excreted by the bowel,[26] and therefore are an ideal agent to rule out infection in the postoperative patient. Unsuspected extra-abdominal sites of infection occasionally are detected by labeled leukocytes because the total body is routinely studied[24] (see Fig 10–3).

Diagnostic Approach in the Patient With Sepsis

Diagnosis in the patient with sepsis must begin with a careful history and physical examination. Appropriate laboratory studies are important in choosing the appropriate imaging method. Plain films are inexpensive, rapid, and often prove helpful in localizing intra-abdominal disease. If findings on plain films are normal, the clinical data dictate the next examination of choice. If there is evidence of hepatic or pelvic abnormality, US is considered the examination of first choice at many centers. Computed tomography is used by most centers as the first test to screen for abscesses in the remainder of the abdomen. In the postoperative patient in whom the bowel cannot be opacified with oral contrast material and who may have intra-abdominal fluid and gas collections, indium 111–labeled white blood cell scintigraphy is the procedure of choice if the patient's condition allows the lengthy examination. These guidelines are general; a diagnostic workup must always be tailored to the individual patient, the available instrumentation, and the local technical expertise.

SUMMARY

Indium 111 white blood cell study in our patient detected the abscess that had been missed on both CT and US examination (see Fig 10–1). On retrospective review, the CT examination showed

---

FIG 10–3.
Imaging studies in a 46-year-old woman with fever. **A,** pelvic computed tomography demonstrates a subtle area of stranding of pericolonic fat. **B,** coronal magnetic resonance imaging of the pelvis performed with T2 contrast weighting (TR = 2,500, TE 80 msec) demonstrates marked elongation of T2 within the fat around the sigmoid colon, consistent with edematous change. **C,** barium enema demonstrates findings of diverticulitis.

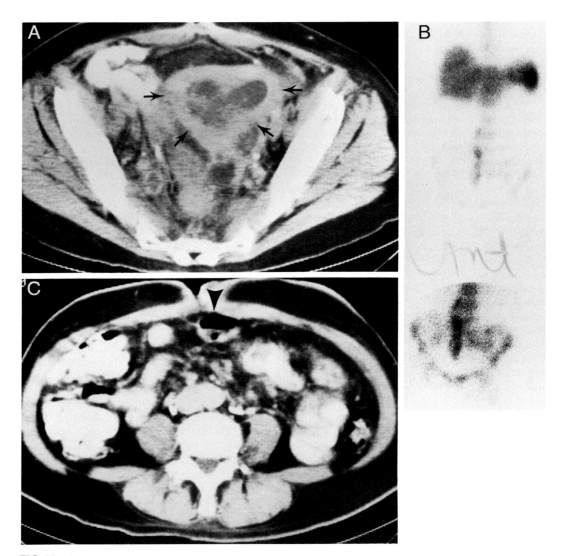

FIG 10–4.
Febrile patient after colectomy because of colon carcinoma. **A,** computed tomography (CT) of the pelvis demonstrates a large fluid-filled mass in the midline extending to the left *(arrows)*. Needle aspiration demonstrated pus and a drainage catheter was placed, but the patient remained febrile. **B,** indium leukocyte scan obtained 8 days later revealed an abnormal accumulation of leukocytes in the midline of the abdomen and pelvis. **C,** retrospective review of the previous CT scan showed a fluid collection that contained air immediately behind the incision site *(arrowhead)* corresponding to a "hot spot" on the indium study. Pus was evacuated and the patient's temperature returned to normal.

thickening of the rectus sheath on the left. A surgical wound and drainage site were present along the left lateral portion of the abdomen. It was not appreciated until after the white blood cell scan that the patient had myositis in this compartment. Other imaging tests detected abnormalities that did not represent the abscess, and only after indium 111 scintigraphy showed accumulation of white blood cells in the rectus sheath was the correct diagnosis of rectus sheath abscess made.

REFERENCES

1. Korobkin M, Callen PW, Filly RA, et al: Comparison of computed tomography, ultra-

sonography, and gallium-67 scanning in the evaluation of suspected abdominal abscess. *Radiology* 1978; 129:89–93.

2. Halber MD, Daffner RH, Morgan CL, et al: Intraabdominal abscess: Current concepts in radiologic evaluation. *Am J Roentgenol* 1979; 133:9–13.

3. Knochel JQ, Koehler PR, Lee TG, et al: Diagnosis of abdominal abscess with computed tomography, ultrasound and 111-In leukocyte scans. *Radiology* 1980; 137:425–432.

4. Carroll B, Silverman PM, Godwin DA, et al: Ultrasonography and indium-111 white blood cell scanning for the detection of intra-abdominal abscesses. *Radiology* 1981; 140:155–160.

5. Moir C, Robins RE: Role of ultrasonography, gallium scanning, and computed tomography in the diagnosis of intra-abdominal abscess. *Am J Surg* 1982; 143:582–585.

6. Wicks JD, Silver TM, Bree RL: Gray scale features of hematomas: An ultrasonic spectrum. *AJR* 1978; 133:977–980.

7. Baker ME, Blinder RA, Rice RP: Diagnostic imaging of abdominal fluid collections and abscesses. *CRC Crit Rev Diagn Imaging* 1986; 26:233–278.

8. Whitley NO, Shatney CH: Diagnosis of abdominal abscesses in patients with major trauma: The use of computed tomography. *Radiology* 1983; 147:179–183.

9. Neff CC, Simeone JF, Ferrucci JT, et al: The occurrence of fluid collections following routine abdominal surgical procedures: Sonographic survey in asymptomatic postoperative patients. *Radiology* 1983; 146:463–466.

10. Gerzof SG, Robbins AH, Birkett DH, et al: Percutaneous catheter drainage of abdominal abscesses guided by ultrasound and computed tomography. *Am J Roentgenol* 1979; 133:1–8.

11. Wall SD, Fisher MR, Amparo EG, et al: Magnetic resonance imaging in the evaluation of abscesses. *Am J Roentgenol* 1985; 144:1217–1221.

12. Biello DR, Levitt RG, Melson GL: The roles of gallium-67 scintigraphy, ultrasonography, and computed tomography in the detection of abdominal abscesses. *Semin Nucl Med* 1979; 9:58–65.

13. Lisbona R, Cassoff J, Angtuaco E, et al: Comparative accuracy and complementary use of 67-Ga-citrate imaging and ultrasound in the diagnosis of abdominal infections. *Clin Nucl Med* 1979; 4:108–110.

14. Sfakianakis GN, Al-Sheikh W, Heal A, et al: The sensitivity, specificity and accuracy of In-111-wbc and Ga-67 scintigraphy in a population with acute and chronic infections. *J Nucl Med* 1982; 23:P65.

15. Sfakianakis GN, Al-Sheikh W, Heal A, et al: Comparisons of scintigraphy with In-111 leukocytes and Ga-67 in the diagnosis of occult sepsis. *J Nucl Med* 1982; 23:618–626.

16. Sfakianakis GN, Al-Sheikh W, Spoliansky G, et al: Correlation of In-111-leukocyte (In-wbc) and gallium-67 (Ga-67) scintigraphy with transmission computed tomography (CT), ultrasonography (US) and plane radiography (R) in the diagnosis of focal infection. *J Nucl Med* 1983; 24:P38.

17. Holland RD, Gooneratne NS, West TE, et al: Gallium-67 scintigraphy in abdominal anaerobic abscesses. *Clin Nucl Med* 1980; 5:393–396.

18. McDougall IR, Baumert JE, Lantieri RL: Evaluation of 111-In leukocytes whole body scanning. *Am J Roentgenol* 1979; 133:849–854.

19. Coleman RE, Black RE, Welch DM, et al: Indium-111 labeled leukocytes in the evaluation of suspected abdominal abscesses. *Am J Surg* 1980; 139:99–104.

20. Peters AM, Saverymuttu SH, Reavy HJ, et al: Imaging of inflammation with indium-111 tropolonate labeled leukocytes. *J Nucl Med* 1983; 24:39–44.

21. Seabold JE, Wilson DG, Leiberman LM, et al: Unsuspected extra-abdominal sites of infection: Scintigraphic detection with indium-111-labeled leukocytes. *Radiology* 1984; 151:213–217.

22. McAfee JG, Samin A: In-111 labeled leukocytes: A review of problems in image interpretation. *Radiology* 1985; 155:221–229.

23. Coleman RE, Welch D: Possible pitfalls with clinical imaging of indium-111 leukocytes: Concise communication. *J Nucl Med* 1980; 21:122–125.

24. Rovekamp MH, van Royen EA, Reinders Folmer SCC, et al: Diagnosis of upper-abdominal infection by In-111 labeled leukocytes with Tc-99m colloid subtraction technique. *J Nucl Med* 1983; 24:212–216.

25. Datz FL, Luers P, Baker WJ, et al: Improved detection of upper abdominal abscesses by combination of 99m-Tc sulfur colloid and 111-In leukocyte scanning. *Am J Roentgenol* 1985; 144:319–323.

26. Abdel-Nabi H, Hinkel GH, Olson JO: Nonmigration of indium–111-labeled leukocytes into healing sterile incisions in rats. *J Nucl Med Allied Sci* 1984; 28:99–101.

PART II

Esophagus

CHAPTER 11

Examining the Patient With Dysphagia

Bronwyn Jones, M.B., B.S.
Martin W. Donner, M.D.

Case Presentation

A 56-year-old man complained of food sticking in his throat and the sensation of constantly having to clear his throat. How would you examine this patient? What do the radiographs in Fig 11–1 obtained during a barium esophagogram demonstrate?

DISCUSSION

Examining the pharynx is not a routine procedure for most radiologists. Unless symptoms or physical findings suggest disease above the suprasternal notch, the routine barium esophagogram usually includes only the thoracic esophagus. Accurate interpretation requires an understanding of the anatomy and physiology of the normal swallow (Fig 11–2).[1–5] The many muscles involved in swallowing contract far too rapidly for the human eye to perceive a subtle abnormality. Dynamic imaging with slow motion, freeze-frame, and back-up modes (videofluoroscopy or cineradiography) is essential for frame-by-frame analysis of individual swallows necessary to understand a complex motility disturbance.[6]

The pharynx participates in speech, airway maintenance, respiration, and swallowing. Respiration is automatically suspended during swallowing and resumes after swallowing with an obligatory inspiration. The airway is protected by a combination of elevation and closure of the larynx and tilting of the epiglottis, which deflects food into the lateral food channels.[7] Comprehensive evaluation therefore should include not only the pharynx and esophagus but the entire swallowing apparatus: mouth, tongue, palate, and larynx. During swallowing, pharynx and larynx rise and descend in a pistonlike fashion. Restriction of this movement (e.g., from scarring after neck surgery or because of cervical spondylosis) may result in swallowing difficulties.

TECHNIQUE

A preliminary soft tissue lateral film may provide important information about the surrounding structures such as the cervical spine and the relationship of the hyoid to the mandible. Atrophy of the tongue or prevertebral tissues may be seen as well.

During the study, the patient's head must be straight to allow appreciation of subtle asymmetry. Tilting or rotation of the head results in asymmetric passage of the bolus into one of the lateral food channels, creating pseudotumors and resultant misinterpretation. If necessary, the head may be posi-

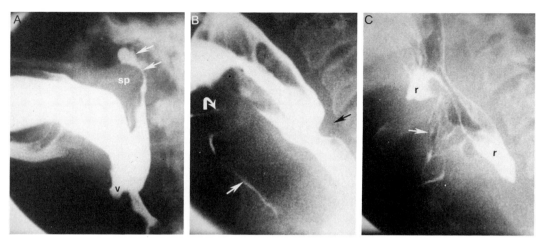

FIG 11–1.

Selected freeze-frame prints from a cinepharyngoesophagogram (obtained with a 16 mm film at 24 frames per second) demonstrate multiple abnormalities. **A,** nasal regurgitation *(arrows)* behind the incompletely elevated soft palate *(sp).* There is no evidence of Passavant's cushion. Compare this with the normal film (Fig 11–2,A). The bolus is in the proximal pharynx, with contrast material ballooning the valleculae *(v)* and partially distending the piriform sinus. **B,** incomplete opening of the cricopharyngeus *(black arrow)* and some contrast in the larynx *(curved arrow)* and down the anterior wall of the trachea *(white arrow).* There is no evidence of a peristaltic wave posteriorly. **C,** after the bolus has passed, there is retention of contrast material in the valleculae and piriform sinuses *(r)* and in the larynx *(arrow).* Retention results in the potential for overflow aspiration. Retention was responsible for the patient's symptom of throat clearing.

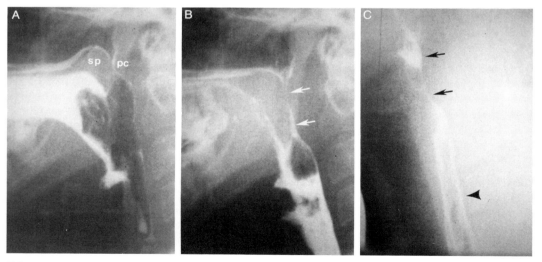

FIG 11–2.

Selected freeze-frame prints from a normal cinepharyngoesophagram. **A,** as a bolus is thrown to the back of the mouth, the soft palate *(sp)* elevates to a right angle to appose a converging portion of the posterior pharyngeal wall, Passavant's cushion *(pc).* This prevents nasal regurgitation. **B,** as the bolus passes the larynx, the peristaltic wave propels it further. This can be observed as a progressive anterior movement of the posterior pharyngeal wall *(arrows).* **C,** progressive contraction of the pharyngeal constrictors *(arrows)* propels the bolus onward. The cricopharyngeal region *(arrowhead)* is completely open to accept bolus passage.

tioned manually with the lead-gloved hand. Alteration in head posture, however, may be a compensatory maneuver to improve swallowing.[8] Patients with dysphagia often flex the head during swallowing; in this position the pharynx and larynx do not have so far to rise for safe swallowing. Patients with tongue weakness may actively hyperextend the neck during swallowing, decanting the bolus from the mouth into the pharynx using gravity rather than active tongue contraction.

Observation of the soft palate and vocal cord movement is included in the examination (see Fig 11–2,A).[9] Soft palate movement is observed during both speech (a good word to observe is "candy") and swallowing. Soft palate function can be diminished during speech and normal during swallowing, and vice versa.

Frontal and lateral views of several swallows of contrast material should be observed. The lateral view usually is recommended initially, because many aspects of pharyngeal function, such as tongue and palate movement, epiglottic tilt, and laryngeal closure and elevation, as well as laryngeal entry of bolus, the pharyngeal stripping wave, and the cricopharyngeal muscle are best observed in this position. Two sequences should be observed, the first higher to include the dorsum of the tongue, the soft palate, and the proximal stripping wave (see Fig 11–2,A and B); the second centered slightly more distally to view the distal stripping wave, epiglottic movement, and cricopharyngeal relaxation (see Fig 11–2,C). If aspiration is suspected clinically, it is wise to watch the first swallow centered over the larynx. Collimation is important to decrease radiation and improve contrast and resolution. In the obese patient an oblique view may be necessary for adequate visualization of the cricopharyngeal muscle, which otherwise may be obscured by the shoulders.

In the frontal position it is important that the patient's chin be tilted upward slightly; otherwise the mandible will be projected over the pharynx. Excessive hyperextension, however, will project the occiput over the pharynx. It is also more difficult to swallow in the hyperextended position, even for a normal person. The frontal position is most helpful in evaluating symmetry of pharyngeal distention and contraction. Lateral pharyngeal pouches may be appreciated only on this view. Insufflation (Valsalva maneuver) is important to demonstrate symmetry during distention. Oblique views are seldom helpful in functional evaluation of the pharynx but may be vital in demonstrating subtle structural disease.

Double-contrast spot films of the pharynx with high-density barium should be taken to delineate structural disease. All studies should include a single-contrast study for motility and a double contrast examination for structure.[6, 10]

A suggested series is as follows.

1. Erect lateral (with heavy-density barium):
   a. Observe soft palate movement with speech.
   b. Observe tongue movement as the bolus is ingested.
   c. Record one swallow centered high for tongue, soft palate, and proximal pharynx.
   d. Record a second swallow centered lower to include larynx, distal pharynx, and cervical esophagus.
   e. Spot film of the barium-coated pharynx at rest and during phonation of a prolonged "eee."
   f. Optional oblique view through the shoulders.
2. Upright frontal (with heavy-density barium) for view of the pharynx:
   a. Observe vocal cord movement.
   b. Record two swallows for distended pharyngeal views.
   c. Two spot films of the barium-coated air-filled pharynx, one at rest and one during insufflation.
3. Upright left posterior oblique (with heavy-density barium) for air contrast views of the esophagus.
4. Prone oblique (with thin barium) for esophageal peristalsis and drinking views:
   a. Observe a single swallow for the primary stripping wave.
   b. Spot films during rapid drinking for distended esophageal views.
   c. Optional mucosal relief view.
5. Check for gastroesophageal reflux.
6. Upright left posterior oblique for view of the stomach:
   a. Spot film of the gastric fundus.
   b. Check for delayed gastric emptying.

The examination should be tailored to each patient. Depending on symptoms, additional maneuvers may be indicated, including swallowing in different positions (supine, prone, head extended), rapid repetitive swallowing, use of a solid bolus, or use of acidified or chilled barium.[11]

A solid bolus (barium marshmallow, barium bread, or Wolf tablet) should be given if a subtle stricture or solid-induced spasm is suspected or if a liquid barium esophagogram in a patient with solid food dysphagia is normal.[12] A solid bolus, however, should be given with caution, if at all, if pharyngeal decompensation (especially laryngeal penetration) is seen with liquid barium swallow.

NORMAL SWALLOW

Comprehensive reviews of swallowing are available.[1, 5, 7] Swallowing involves a complex series of events, with sensory innervation from the glossopharyngeal (IX) and vagus (X) nerves, mediated centrally in the "swallowing center" (thought to be situated in the brain stem), and accomplished peripherally by sequential contraction of muscles innervated by the trigeminal (V), facial (VII), vagus (X), and hypoglossal (XII) nerves. The extrinsic support muscles of the pharynx are innervated through cranial nerve XI (accessory) and cervical nerves I through III.

The oral phase of swallowing is under voluntary control of the cerebral cortex. After the bolus leaves the mouth, however, swallowing becomes a reflex, no longer under voluntary control.

The bolus is masticated in the mouth in preparation for swallowing and is then propelled into the oropharynx by an upward, posterior tongue thrust. While the bolus is in the mouth, leakage into the oropharynx is prevented by apposition of soft palate to tongue. Leakage prior to swallowing may result in laryngeal penetration, because the entrance to the larynx is open between swallows.

As the bolus enters the oropharynx, the soft palate elevates to a right angle and apposes Passavant's cushion, an anteriorly converging portion of the posterior pharyngeal wall. Nasopharyngeal regurgitation is thus prevented. Sequential contraction of the superior, middle, and inferior constrictor muscles propels the bolus onward, the pharyngeal stripping wave being seen as a progressive anterior movement of the posterior pharyngeal wall. The pharyngeal stripping wave may be impaired by intrinsic weakness of the pharyngeal musculature or by extrinsic disease (such as cervical spondylosis or retropharyngeal fibrosis). Incomplete emptying of the pharynx results in retention of contrast material in the valleculae and piriform sinuses after swallowing (with the potential for overflow aspiration).

Laryngeal penetration during bolus passage is prevented by elevation and closure of the larynx and tilting of the epiglottis, which both covers the entrance to the larynx and deflects food into the lateral food channels. The relative contribution of larynx and epiglottis to the prevention of laryngeal penetration is difficult to assess, but certainly laryngeal competence can prevent aspiration after epiglottectomy. Competence of laryngeal elevation and closure can be assessed by observation of apposition of hyoid to mandible and the absence of air in the ventricle, with the appearance of the conus.

The upper esophageal sphincter, normally closed between swallows, must relax to allow unimpeded bolus passage. Although the "sphincter" as measured by manometry consists of a 2 to 3 cm long high-pressure zone, radiographic evaluation of the pharyngoesophageal region is directed toward the cricopharyngeal muscle. The diameter of the cricopharyngeal area during bolus passage should be approximately the same as that of the lumen of the cervical esophagus; any narrowing or posterior indentation on the barium column suggests cricopharyngeal dysfunction. Indentation may be seen in some asymptomatic individuals, especially with increasing age.[13, 14] In the extreme, a prominent horizontal posterior indentation, also referred to as a "hypopharyngeal bar," may be seen. This appearance has been compared to esophageal achalasia (cricopharyngeal achalasia).

The cricopharyngeal muscle, however, may not only fail to relax but may open late or incompletely or may close early. Because cricopharyngeal opening depends in part on pharyngeal contraction, a prominent cricopharyngeal muscle may be seen with pharyngeal paresis, subsequent to bulbar poliomyelitis, in bulbar palsy, and in some patients with esophageal disease. Failure of coordination between pharyngeal contraction and cricopharyngeal opening may be a contributing factor in the development of Zenker's diverticulum and lateral pharyngeal pouches.

ANALYSIS OF SWALLOWING

Because swallowing is so complex, there are many opportunities for decompensation (misswallowing) to occur. The normal swallow should completely empty the pharynx of liquid barium; there should be no oral leakage, nasal regurgitation, laryngeal penetration, or aspiration. There should be no significant luminal narrowing at the level of the cricopharyngeal muscle.

By careful analysis of dynamic recordings, the radiologist can determine how an abnormality has occurred. Basic to this discussion is the ability to recognize certain abnormal radiographic findings, such as leakage, nasal regurgitation, penetration or aspiration, and retention. In reviewing the examination, slow motion, back-up, and freeze-frame modes are important. With these techniques the movement of individual structures can be analyzed, first in isolation and subsequently in combination with others.

Individual factors requiring analysis include:

1. Head and neck posture (at rest, during swallow).
2. Mouth and tongue coordination (poor bolus control, abnormal movement).
3. Tongue-palate competence (leakage).
4. Palate-pharyngeal wall coordination (speech, nasal regurgitation).
5. Pharyngeal constrictors (posterior wave, squeeze, retention).
6. Epiglottis (upright during swallow, laryngeal penetration).
7. Laryngeal elevation and closure (laryngeal penetration or aspiration).
8. Cricopharyngeal opening (indentation on bolus posteriorly in lateral position, narrowing of the pharyngoesophageal segment on the frontal view).

Why do we need detailed analysis of the dynamic study of all structures participating in deglutition? What can we do with this information? This analysis establishes the degree of abnormality and the structures involved in the disease process. It can establish how the patient handles feeding and the circumstances of decompensation or whether the patient has bolus-specific dysphagia. Such information is important to the speech and language pathologist (therapist trained in treatment of dysphagia) to permit swallowing reeducation.

SUMMARY

The cinepharyngoesophagogram in our patient revealed that incomplete opening of the cricopha-ryngeal muscle (upper esophageal sphincter), with retention of barium in the valleculae and piriform sinuses, was causing the sensation of constantly having to clear his throat. Careful performance and analysis of swallowing function provided the diagnosis in this patient.

REFERENCES

1. Donner MW, Bosma JF, Robertson DL: Anatomy and physiology of the pharynx. *Gastrointest Radiol* 1985; 10:196–212.
2. Bosma JF, Donner MW, Tanaka E, et al: Anatomy of the pharynx, pertinent to swallowing. *Dysphagia* 1986; 1:23–33.
3. Curtis DJ: Radiographic anatomy of the pharynx. *Dysphagia* 1986; 1:51–62.
4. Rubesin SE, Jessurun J, Robertson D, et al: Lines of the pharynx. *Radiographics* 1987; 7:217–237.
5. Miller AJ: Neurophysiological basis of swallowing. *Dysphagia* 1986; 1:91–100.
6. Jones B, Kramer SS, Donner MW: Dynamic imaging of the pharynx. *Gastrointest Radiol* 1985; 10:213–224.
7. Curtis DJ: Laryngeal dynamics. *CRC Crit Rev Diagn Imaging* 1982; 19:29–80.
8. Buchholz DW, Bosma JF, Donner MW: Adaptation, compensation and decompensation of the pharyngeal swallow. *Gastrointest Radiol* 1985; 10:235–240.
9. Rubesin SE, Jones B, Donner MW: Radiology of the adult soft palate. *Dysphagia* 1987; 2:8–17.
10. Ekberg O, Nylander G: Double-contrast examination of the pharynx. *Gastrointest Radiol* 1985; 10:263–272.
11. Donner MW, Silbiger ML, Hookman R, et al: Acid-barium swallows in the radiographic evaluation of clinical esophagitis. *Radiology* 1966; 87:220–225.
12. Curtis DJ, Cruess DF, Willgress ER: Normal solid bolus swallowing: Erect position. *Dysphagia* 1986; 1:63–67.
13. Ekberg O, Nylander B: Dysfunction of the cricopharyngeal muscle. *Radiology* 1982; 143:481–486.
14. Curtis DJ, Cruess DF, Berg T: The cricopharyngeal muscle: A videorecording review. *AJR* 1984; 142:497–500.

CHAPTER 12

Post-Laryngectomy Dysphagia

Dennis M. Balfe, M.D.

Case Presentation

A 76-year-old man who had undergone total laryngopharyngectomy 11 weeks previously returned to his otolaryngologist complaining of dysphagia. Prior to the surgical procedure he had received a full course of radiation therapy for supraglottic epidermoid cancer. Physical examination revealed only woody edema of the neck; the neopharynx appeared normal. Barium pharyngography was performed (Fig 12–1). What is the differential diagnosis? What radiologic tests may be useful in this clinical setting?

DISCUSSION

Most patients treated with total laryngectomy because of epidermoid carcinoma of the larynx recover uneventfully, and many have no further clinical problems related to the epidermoid primary lesion.[1] However, up to one sixth of the laryngectomy population ultimately develop dysphagia and return for reevaluation.[2]

The problems in accurately assessing postlaryngectomy complications are formidable. The spectrum of potential problems is wide (Table 12–1) and the contribution of physical examination is relatively small. For example, many patients have woody induration of the neck, which may reflect radiation-induced edema, postsurgical fibrosis, or submucosal recurrence of epidermoid cancer. Moreover, even such apparently direct diagnostic maneuvers as laryngoscopy and biopsy may fail to produce an answer; nodal or soft tissue recurrences may elude superficial mucosal biopsy.[2]

Not infrequently, therefore, the otolaryngolo-

gist calls on the radiologist for assistance. Barium pharyngography and cross-sectional imaging techniques, computed tomography (CT), magnetic resonance imaging (MRI), and rarely ultrasonography (US) are useful in limiting the differential diagnosis. The pharyngogram obtained in the case presented certainly is a reasonable initial study.

A confident diagnosis of an abnormality requires a working knowledge of the normal pharyngographic appearance of the neopharynx. The surgeon, after removing the entire laryngeal skeleton and with it the anterior surface of the hypopharynx, closes the residual pharyngeal mucosa using a nasogastric tube as a stent. The superior margin of the line of closure is fixed to the tongue base. Whenever possible, the inferior constrictor and cricopharyngeal muscles are incorporated into the second layer of closure. If insufficient mucosal surface remains for the surgeon to produce a tube of adequate luminal diameter, myocutaneous grafts may be used to provide greater epidermoid tissue surface.

Accordingly, on radiographs the neopharynx

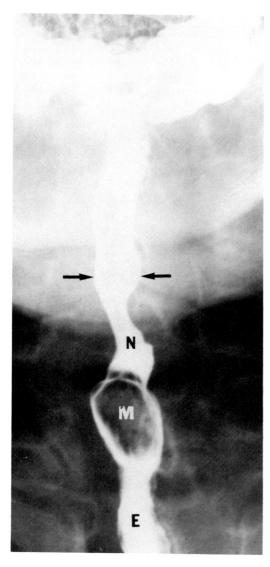

FIG 12–1.
Anteroposterior film from a pharyngogram in a patient with dysphagia after total laryngectomy. The normal neopharynx *(N)* is a midline smooth tube *(arrows)*. At the junction between the neopharynx and the cervical esophagus *(E)*, a small round mass *(M)* projects into the lumen but does not obstruct the passage of barium. (See text for pathologic diagnosis.)

appears as a simple cylinder extending from the oropharynx and base of the tongue to the cervical esophagus. In the frontal projection (Fig 12–2,A), tapering of the sides of the neopharynx may be observed. A pouch of variable size may be seen on the anterosuperior surface of the neopharynx in the lateral projection (Fig 12–2,B). This pouch is located at the site of fixation of the neopharynx to the tongue base.

The radiographic finding in the case presented is a smooth oval fixed filling defect located at the junction of the surgically created food passage, or neopharynx, with the cervical esophagus. There is

slight narrowing of the neopharynx immediately above the mass, but barium passes quickly through the narrowed area, around the filling defect, and fills the distal esophagus. Some conditions listed in the differential diagnosis (see Table 12–1) can be readily eliminated, but a number of pathologic processes remain to be considered.

In any patient who has undergone therapy for a malignant lesion, persistent, recurrent, or second primary neoplasms must be considered. Patients particularly likely to experience laryngectomy failure due to residual tumor include those with highly aggressive tumors (pyriform sinus and hypopharyn-

TABLE 12–1.

Spectrum of Pathologic Conditions Producing Dysphagia After Laryngectomy

Condition	Time Since Primary Treatment
Neoplasm—metastatic or persistent*	
Stomal	Months
Pharyngeal	Months
Esophageal	Months
Neoplasm—second primary lesion	
Pharyngeal	>2 years
Esophageal	>2 years
Inflammatory	
Abscess	Postoperative
Fistula	Postoperative
Stitch granuloma	Weeks
Ulcer	Weeks after radiation
Stricture	Months
Mechanical	
Cricopharyngeal	Weeks
Nasopharyngeal reflux	Anytime
Hair growth	Months
Blom-Singer prosthesis pressure erosions	Anytime
Esophageal abnormality unrelated to surgery	
Primary motility defects	Anytime
Reflux esophagitis	Anytime
Distal strictures	Anytime

*Persistent disease tends to become clinically apparent within a few months; metastatic deposits tend to occur somewhat later.

geal cancers, in particular), cancers with histologically "pushing" margins, or evidence of tumor at the margin of surgical resection and those in whom surgical salvage was performed because previous therapy failed (as in this patient).[3]

The selection of a radiologic method most sensitive in detecting recurrent carcinoma depends greatly on the anatomic site of tumor. Mucosal cancer is best detected by pharyngography,[4] whereas extramucosal (nodal, parastomal, or soft tissue) disease is more effectively imaged with CT or MRI.[5, 6] The time interval between laryngectomy and dysphagia is a helpful guideline. A new primary cancer generally requires many months to develop to a size that produces symptoms; untreated extramucosal disease may occur within weeks to a few months of laryngectomy.

Barium examination in a patient with persistent mucosal disease demonstrates a mass with irregular borders and usually ulceration as well (Fig 12–3). Findings in patients with extramucosal recurrence are due to extrinsic deviation of the neopharynx away from its usual midline location (Fig 12–4).

Computed tomography accurately displays the relationship of recurrent tumor to the carotid sheath, the spinal accessory nerve, and the tracheostoma. If salvage therapy is feasible, these areas are important to surgical planning.[7] Contrast-enhanced CT may demonstrate nodal metastases as large peripherally enhancing masses, frequently displaying central low attenuation due to tumor necrosis.[8] Extranodal soft tissue recurrence is particularly likely to occur near the tracheostoma[3] (Fig 12–5,A) but may be seen anywhere in the neck, extending laterally from the original primary site. Computed tomography demonstrates these lesions as ill-defined infiltrative soft tissue masses that obscure perivascular fat planes, blurring the boundaries of intrinsic neck muscle (Fig 12–5,B). Because modest swelling and edematous infiltration of the neck is a normal response to surgery or radiation, small soft tissue cancers may be difficult to detect.

Magnetic resonance imaging displays anatomy similarly to CT but with less spatial resolution (Figs 12–6 and 12–7). Its major advantage in this clinical setting lies in its ability to detect small tumors within a field of edema or fibrosis.[9] Experience with MRI in this specific region remains limited and

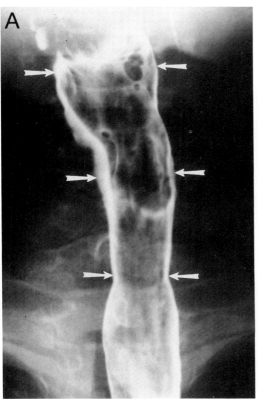

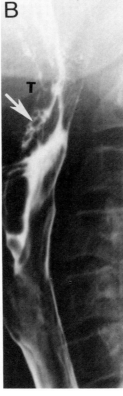

FIG 12-2.
Normal neopharynx. Air contrast views in an asymptomatic volunteer. **A,** anteroposterior view shows a featureless cylindrical structure (the neopharynx) extending from the oropharynx to the cervical esophagus. There is gentle tapering of the lumen as it proceeds inferiorly and very slight deviation of the neopharynx from right to left. **B,** lateral view shows a small outpouching *(arrow)* on the anterior wall of the neopharynx at its junction with the tongue base *(T)*. The prevertebral space is of normal thickness.

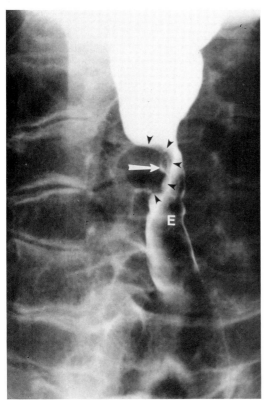

FIG 12-3.
Mucosal recurrence 18 months after laryngectomy in a patient whose primary cancer originated in the pyriform sinus. Anteroposterior film from a pharyngogram shows a mucosal lesion *(arrowheads)* with central ulceration *(arrow)* arising just proximal to the cervical esophagus *(E)*. Biopsy findings confirmed mucosal recurrence.

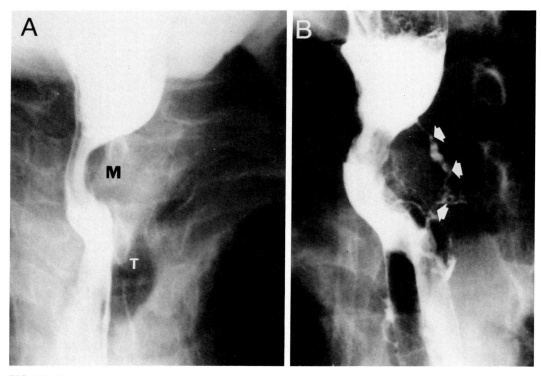

FIG 12–4.
Peristomal recurrence 7 months after total laryngectomy. **A,** anteroposterior view of a pharyngogram obtained when the patient first complained of dysphagia. The distal neopharyngeal lumen is swept to the right of midline by an extrinsic mass *(M)* arising immediately cephalad to the tracheostoma *(T)*. Direct laryngoscopy showed normal mucosa; biopsy studies returned no diagnosis. **B,** six weeks later the patient complained of sudden onset of choking with meals. Repeat pharyngogram shows pharyngotracheal fistula *(arrows)* coursing through a necrotic peristomal recurrence.

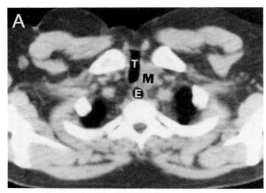

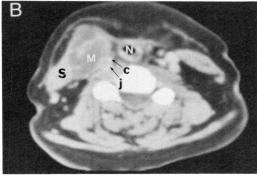

FIG 12–5.
Computed tomography scan of soft tissue recurrence. **A,** peristomal recurrent neoplasm *(M)* frequently arises in this location, lateral to the tracheostoma *(T)* and anterior to the cervical esophagus *(E)*. **B,** an infiltrating low attenuation mass *(M)* expands the anterior portion of the sternocleidomastoid muscle *(S)* and partially obscures the fat plane anterolateral to the carotid sheath. *N* = neopharynx; *c* = carotid sheath; *j* = jugular vein.

largely anecdotal. MRI can confidently predict the presence of fibrosis; however, posttherapy edema can mimic the signal characteristics of recurrent tumor.[9]

Second primary epidermoid carcinomas most frequently occur in the pharynx, but esophageal carcinomas also occur quite regularly[10]; they may be heralded by relatively innocuous symptoms of dysphagia, mimicking pharyngeal disease. An esophagram is therefore warranted in any patient who develops swallowing difficulties after laryngectomy[11] (Figs 12–8 and 12–9).

Inflammatory processes occur as both early and late complications of pharyngeal surgery. In the immediate postoperative period fistulas are a frequent cause of dysphagia. The point in the suture line subjected to the greatest stress is the superior margin, which closes the anterior neopharynx and attaches it to the tongue base. Anterior protrusion of the tongue is capable of producing suture dehiscence[12] (Fig 12–10). Sinus tracts arising from this site typically dissect anterolaterally and are seen as pharyngocutaneous fistulas. If radical neck dissection has

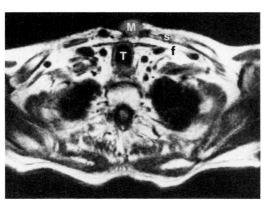

FIG 12–6.
Magnetic resonance imaging of peristomal recurrence. A mass *(M)* of signal intensity intermediate between fat *(f)* and sternocleidomastoid muscle *(s)* is shown on the anterior surface of the chest wall immediately to the left of the tracheostoma *(T)*.

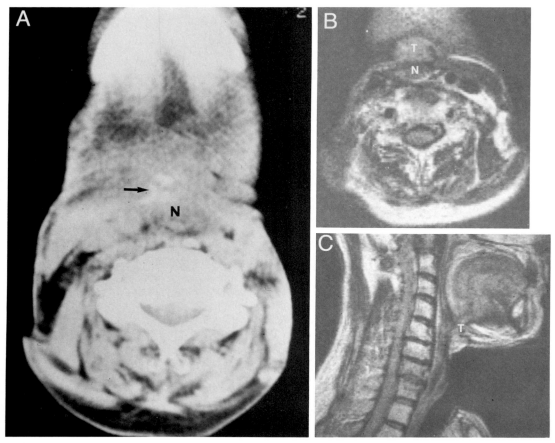

FIG 12–7.
Soft tissue recurrence. **A,** computed tomography scan obtained through the floor of the mouth in a patient with submental soft tissue swelling after total laryngectomy. Note calcification *(arrow)* immediately anterior to the neopharynx *(N);* an ill-defined soft tissue mass surrounds this calcification. **B,** axial mag- netic resonance imaging (MRI) at the same level shows a well-defined medium intensity tumor *(T)* located in the tissues adjacent to the floor of the mouth. *N* = neopharynx. **C,** sagittal midline MRI shows recurrent tumor *(T)* arising in the submental region.

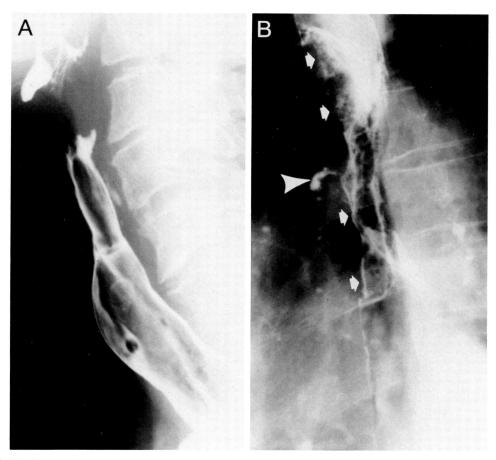

FIG 12–8.
Second primary cancer of the esophagus. **A,** pharyngogram in a patient complaining of dysphagia 30 months after total laryngectomy. The neopharynx is normal. **B,** film of the thoracic esophagus obtained during the same examination shows a bulky epidermoid carcinoma *(arrows)* with central ulceration *(arrowhead).*

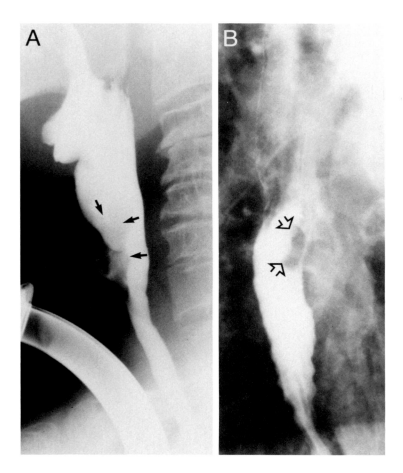

FIG 12–9.
Recurrent and second primary carcinomas. **A,** pharyngogram obtained in a patient complaining of dysphagia 24 months after total laryngectomy. A soft tissue mass *(arrows)* is fixed to the anterior wall of the neopharynx. This mass proved to be a soft tissue recurrence of the pharyngeal primary. **B,** film of the esophagus from the same examination. A 2 cm smooth nodule *(arrows)* is present on the anterior esophageal wall. Biopsy tissue showed epidermoid carcinoma; it was not clear to the pathologists whether this was a mucosal primary lesion or a lymphatic metastasis that had eroded through the mucosa.

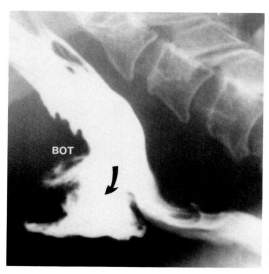

FIG 12–10.
Pharyngogram obtained 2 weeks after total laryngectomy shows an anterior sinus tract *(arrow)* arising from the suture line near the base of the tongue *(BOT)*. The tract ends blindly within the subcutaneous tissues of the neck.

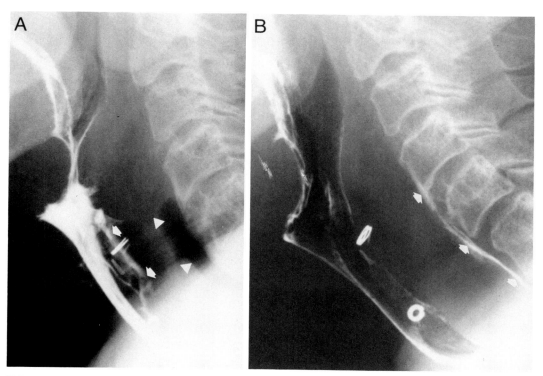

FIG 12–11.
A free myocutaneous thigh graft was constructed to repair a long neopharyngeal stricture. **A,** pharyngogram obtained on the third postoperative day shows a long sinus tract *(arrows)* that extends inferiorly and posteriorly into the prevertebral space; note air *(arrowheads)* within the superior part of this collection. **B,** 8 weeks later a pharyngogram showed healing of the sinus tract. Residual barium *(arrows)* persists in the prevertebral space.

been performed, the fistula usually extends to that side. Abscesses may be detected as a complication of such fistula tracts or may arise de novo in the soft tissues of the neck. Clinically these complications are not difficult to diagnose; barium pharyngography is useful in identifying the site of a fistula (Fig 12–11). The full extent of an abscess can be determined by CT or US examination.[13]

Later postoperative complications may be clinically much more problematic. Strictures can arise or progress months after the original therapy. Short weblike narrowings are often observed at the lower end of the surgical margin (Fig 12–12); despite their innocuous appearance, they may be symptomatic and difficult to treat. If repeated bougienage fails, surgical reconstruction may offer symptomatic relief. Long, smoothly tapered narrowings generally occur in patients who have undergone both surgical

and radiation therapy[2, 4, 11] (Fig 12–13). They, too, may be difficult to treat; restricturing after dilation is the rule, not the exception. A short weblike stricture with a proximally impacted bolus would be a reasonable diagnosis in the case presented. However, in such circumstances complete obstruction of the neopharynx would be expected; instead, there is no appreciable interference by the mass to passage of contrast material.

Ulceration of neopharyngeal mucosa is unusual; the single case seen in our files resulted from radiation-induced necrosis of the anterior pharyngeal mucosa (Fig 12–14).

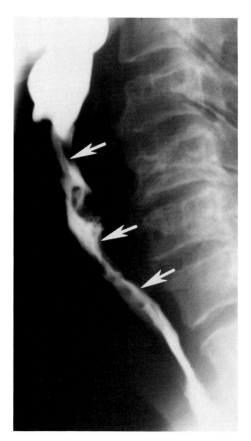

FIG 12–13.
Long neopharyngeal stricture *(arrows)* producing dysphagia in a patient 8 months after laryngectomy. The operative procedure was performed after full-course radiation therapy to the original pharyngeal cancer. Repeated bougienage failed to relieve the dysphagia, necessitating reconstructive surgery. Specimen showed radiation effect and diffuse fibrosis.

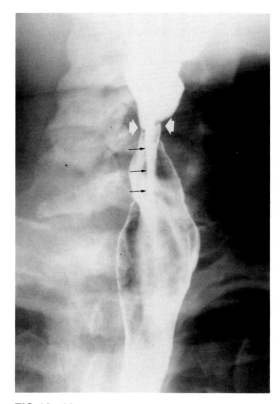

FIG 12–12.
Short neopharyngeal stricture arising in a patient 6 months after laryngectomy. A thin web *(white arrows)* narrows the distal neopharyngeal lumen, producing a jet of contrast material *(black arrows)* during forceful swallowing.

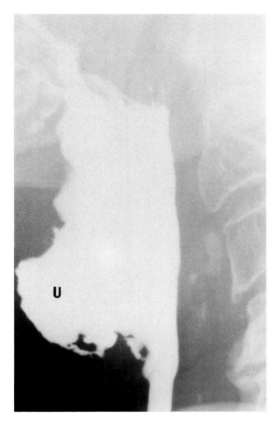

FIG 12–14.
Neopharyngeal ulceration *(U)* occurred in a patient who received postoperative radiation after total laryngectomy. The entire anterior wall of the neopharynx was necrotic.

Foreign body granulomas (induced by suture material) have clinical and radiologic features identical to those of the case presented. They arise within weeks to months of surgery, cause relatively mild clinical symptoms, and produce smooth mucosal filling defects related to the line of surgical closure.

Strictly mechanical (noninflammatory) factors may produce post-laryngectomy dysphagia. Because the removal of the laryngeal skeleton deprives the cricopharyngeal muscle of an anterior insertion, a portion of the inferior constrictor mechanism retracts to form a soft tissue bulge posterior to the neopharynx[12, 14] (Fig 12–15,A). In some patients this cricopharyngeal impression is quite striking and no doubt contributes to partial pharyngeal outlet obstruction (Fig 12–15,B). In most patients the cricopharyngeal mass retains some motility; thus demonstration of a changeable posterior mass on videotaped fluoroscopy reliably differentiates the muscle from a posterior recurrent cancer.[4]

Nasopharyngeal reflux is often multifactorial. A degree of pharyngeal obstruction (e.g., distal stricture or cricopharyngeal spasm) certainly contributes to the problem. Bolus formation and propulsion by the tongue is frequently ineffective in laryngectomized patients, particularly when the original surgical resection included a portion of the tongue base. Finally, incompetence or incoordination of the soft palate is always present, allowing swallowed material to enter the nasopharynx. Pharyngography is the critical imaging procedure and is helpful in analyzing which factor is dominant in producing reflux (Fig 12–16).

Two rare mechanical abnormalities are capable of producing dysphagia: (1) Pharyngeal reconstructions are sometimes accomplished using pedicles of the pectoralis major, which are rotated with the skin attached to close the neck defect. In these patients the neopharyngeal surface is hair bearing. Pharyngeal hirsutism can produce the sensation of a retained food bolus.[15] (2) In laryngectomized patients who are unable to master the air swallowing and regurgitation techniques required to develop esophageal speech, small pharyngoesophageal fistulas can be surgically created. These are fitted with bullet-

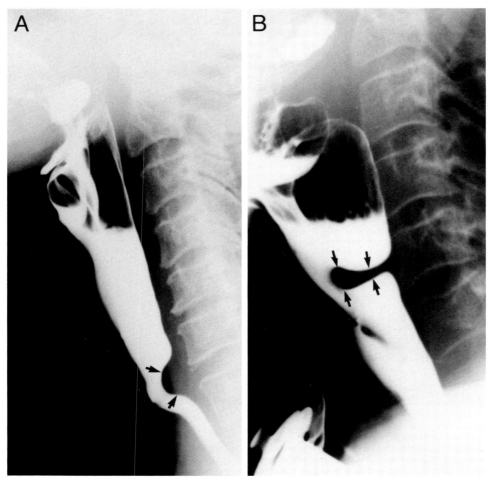

FIG 12–15.
Cricopharyngeal impressions. **A,** asymptomatic patient examined 18 months after total laryngectomy. A cricopharyngeal impression *(arrow)* is present on the posterior wall of the neopharynx. **B,** patient with dysphagia and inability to learn esophageal speech 12 months after total laryngectomy. A duck bill-shaped cricopharyngeal indentation *(arrows)* almost completely traverses the contrast column in mid-swallow. The patient's symptoms resolved after myotomy.

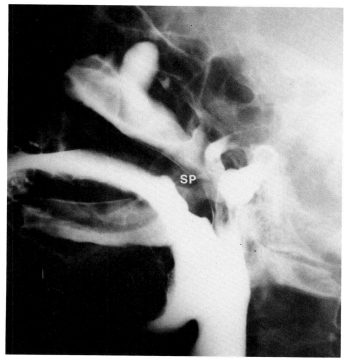

FIG 12–16.
Nasopharyngeal reflux in this patient was due to combined factors: the soft palate *(SP)* failed to provide a barrier by opposing Passavant's ridge; global glossal paresis resulted in ineffective propulsion of a bolus into the pharynx; and there was a neopharyngeal stricture (not shown).

shaped one-way valves that prevent passage of material from the pharynx to the airway. Ill-fitting valves produce ulcerations on the posterior surface of the neopharynx by direct pressure erosion[16] (Fig 12–17). Both of these conditions are easily diagnosed by pharyngography.

Finally, it should be remembered that a patient who has undergone total laryngectomy is almost always in the age group in which esophageal disorders unrelated to the pharyngeal process are common. Thus reflux esophagitis, distal esophageal stricture, and primary motility disorders should always be evaluated by complete esophagography.[11]

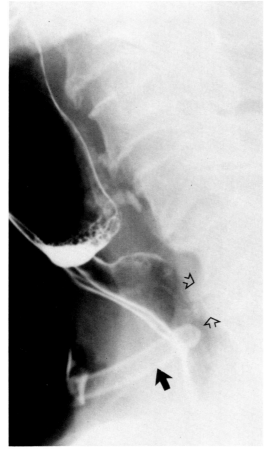

FIG 12–17.
A Blom-Singer prosthesis *(arrow)* in this patient with dysphagia repeatedly encountered a portion of the posterior neopharyngeal wall, which was more anterior than usual because of the large anterior vertebral spur *(open arrows)*, producing pressure erosions.

TABLE 12–2.

Radiologic Evaluation in Patients With Post-Laryngectomy Dysphagia: Clinical Indications

Pharyngography
    Mucosal cancer recurrence
    Second primary lesion in pharynx or esophagus
    Fistula
    Ulcer
    Foreign body
    Stricture
    Dysmotility
Computed tomography
    Extramucosal cancer recurrence
    Abscess
Magnetic resonance imaging
    Differentiation of fibrosis from tumor

CONCLUSION

The pathologic diagnosis in the case presented (see Fig 12–1) was foreign body granuloma produced by suture material. Endoscopic resection rendered the patient asymptomatic, and he has had no recurrence or further dysphagia.

A host of pathologic conditions can produce post-laryngectomy dysphagia. Radiologic evaluation can be useful in accurately assessing the nature and extent of the disease (Table 12–2).

REFERENCES

1. Ogura JH, Bello JA: Laryngectomy and radical neck dissection for carcinoma of the larynx. *Laryngoscope* 1952; 62:1–52.
2. Jung TTK, Adams GL: Dysphagia in laryngectomized patients. *Otolaryngol Head Neck Surg* 1980; 88:25–33.
3. Batsakis JG: *Tumors of the Head and Neck,* ed 2. Baltimore, Williams & Wilkins Co, 1979, pp 200–225.
4. Balfe DM, Koehler RE, Setzen M, et al: Barium examination of the esophagus after total laryngectomy. *Radiology* 1982; 143:501–508.
5. DiSantis DJ, Balfe DM, Hayden RE, et al: The neck after total laryngectomy: CT study. *Radiology* 1984; 153:713–717.
6. Som PM, Biller HF: Computed tomography of the neck in the postoperative patient: Radical neck dissection and the myocutaneous flap. *Radiology* 1983; 148:157–160.
7. Harnsberger HR, Mancuso AA, Muraki AS, et al: The upper aerodigestive tract and neck: CT

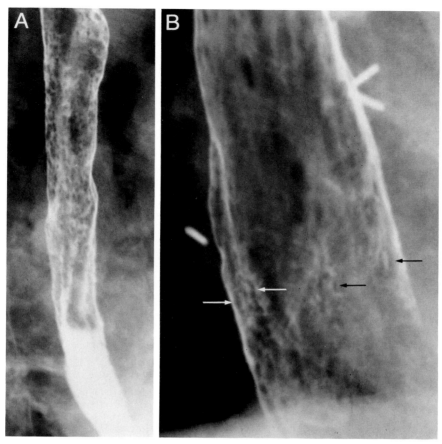

FIG 13–3.
A, diffuse, finely granular mucosa in the lower thoracic esophagus. Biopsy studies confirmed the radiographic diagnosis of reflux esophagitis. **B,** multiple small erosions *(arrows)* on a background of finely granular mucosa in the distal esophagus in a 54-year-old woman with gastroesophageal reflux after partial gastrectomy and gastrojejunostomy, now with biopsy-proved esophagitis.

esophagus"[4, 6, 7] (Fig 13–2,B). Hairlike projections of barium resembling ulcers actually represent barium burrowing under detached pseudomembranes[6] (see Fig 13–2,B). Esophageal motility is impaired.[6]

With chronic infection an esophageal stricture may develop, seen radiographically as a smooth, concentric, tapered narrowing of the mid- or lower esophagus. Esophageal narrowing due to inadequate distention may mimic a stricture.[11]

A definitive radiologic diagnosis of *Candida* esophagitis often obviates the need for endoscopy. The patient is empirically treated for *Candida* esophagitis, and follow-up examination in 2 weeks should show resolution of abnormal radiographic findings.

Ulcers

Reflux Esophagitis.— A few patients with reflux esophagitis have odynophagia as well as heartburn. Mild reflux esophagitis often appears radiographically as numerous 1 to 3 mm lucent elevations of the mucosal surface (Fig 13–3,A). This finely granular or nodular mucosal pattern is due to mucosal edema and inflammation.[9] Shallow ulcers or erosions are seen in approximately 10% of patients[9] (Fig 13–3,B). Other findings include a coarsely nodular mucosal pattern, smooth or scalloped thickened longitudinal folds greater than 3 mm wide, fixed transverse folds, a serrated luminal contour, and sentinel polyps.[9] Inflammatory exudates or pseudomembranes may be seen as focal plaquelike lesions.[12] Long-standing reflux esophagitis produces scarring, which may result in transverse folds, sacculation, or stricture; or in Barrett's esophagus. However, these chronic changes usually are not associated with odynophagia.

Viral Esophagitis.— Viral esophagitis is usually an opportunistic infection, occurring in patients immunocompromised by malignancy, debilitation, radiation therapy, steroids, or chemotherapy. The most common viral invader of the esophagus is herpes simplex type 1, a DNA core virus and a frequent inhabitant of adult salivary glands.[13] Occa-sionally cytomegalovirus or other viruses cause esophagitis.

The patient with herpes esophagitis has odynophagia, dysphagia, or less frequently upper gastrointestinal bleeding[13, 14]; most patients do not have associated mucocutaneous lesions.[14] Recovery is usually spontaneous without sequelae, in contrast to *Candida* esophagitis, which may progress to esophageal stricture or systemic dissemination.[14] Pathologically, a small herpetic vesicle progresses to a punched-out ulcer with raised margins.[13] Ulcers then coalesce and are covered by a white fibrinous exudate.

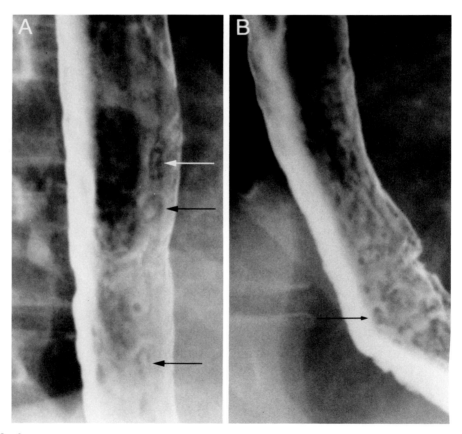

FIG 13–4.
Herpes esophagitis. **A,** this 47-year-old patient, 6 months after renal transplantation, has acute odynophagia. Focal ulcers *(arrows)* in the mid-esophagus are seen as small barium collections surrounded by radiolucent halos of edema. These erosions are typical for viral esophagitis, especially herpes. Biopsy and brush cytologic studies showed large epithelial cells with multinucleation and many intranuclear inclusions, compatible with herpes esophagitis. Culture was positive for herpes simplex type 1. **B,** the distal esophagus (same patient) shows irregular plaquelike lucencies *(arrow).* This region is not specific for herpes esophagitis and could represent any infectious esophagitis in an immunosuppressed patient.

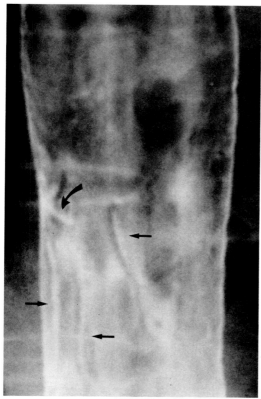

FIG 13–5.
Close-up of the mid-esophagus in a patient with drug (potassium chloride)–induced esophagitis shows several long longitudinal ulcers *(short arrows)* and a transversely oriented ulcer *(curved arrow).*

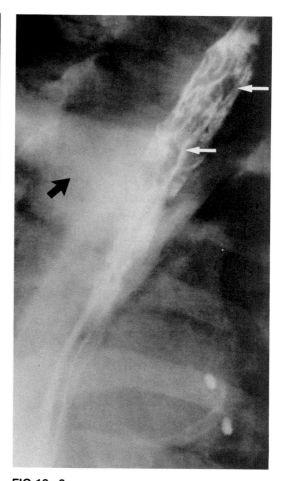

FIG 13–6.
Oblique spot film of the upper esophagus shows enlarged folds *(white arrows)* in the cervical and upper thoracic esophagus in a 67-year-old man with prostate carcinoma metastatic to the thoracic spine and clavicle recently treated with radiotherapy. Findings are characteristic of radiation edema. Note the dense bones due to blastic metastases *(black arrow).*

The early ulcers can be detected by double-contrast radiography as discrete, shallow punctate or stellate collections of barium surrounded by a radiolucent halo of edema[13, 14] (Fig 13–4,A). The ulcers are usually clustered in the mid- or distal esophagus on a background of normal smooth mucosa. With advanced herpetic infection, a shaggy mucosal contour and multiple nodular filling defects may be present, indistinguishable from advanced *Candida* esophagitis[13, 14] (Fig 13–4,B). The radiologist can only diagnose severe opportunistic esophagitis in these cases. In fact, concurrent infection with both *Candida* and herpesvirus is not uncommon.

Drug-Induced Esophagitis.—Numerous oral medications can induce esophagitis, some because of their acidic nature (e.g., tetracycline hydrochloride, ascorbic acid, iron sulfate) and others by a direct cytotoxic effect (e.g., potassium chloride, digoxin or digitoxin, quinidine).[15] Some drugs (e.g., emepronium bromide and alcohol) lower esophageal sphincter pressure, leading to reflux esophagitis. The typical clinical history is that of sudden odynophagia, dysphagia, or substernal pain occurring 1 to 8 hours after drug ingestion.[15] The medication is typically taken with little or no water immediately before lying down.[15] Diminished clearance of the drug leads to prolonged mucosal contact and esophagitis.

TABLE 13–2.
Radiographic Findings in Odynophagia

Finding	Clinical History	Diagnosis
Mucosal plaques	Immunocompromised host	*Candida* esophagitis
	Chronic pyrosis	Reflux esophagitis
	Asymptomatic	Glycogenic acanthosis
Discrete ulcers	Immunocompromised host	Viral esophagitis
	Radiation therapy	Radiation esophagitis
	Drug ingestion	Drug-induced esophagitis
	Food laceration	Traumatic esophagitis
	Caustic ingestion	Caustic esophagitis
	Pyrosis	Reflux esophagitis
	Systemic disorder	Crohn's disease, Behçet's disease

Radiographically, a focal cluster of shallow ulcers is present on a background of normal smooth esophageal mucosa[9, 15] (Fig 13–5). The ulcers are seen at the level of the aortic arch or in the distal esophagus, where transient delay of a bolus normally occurs. The diagnosis is made by combining the clinical history of drug ingestion with the radiographic findings. A repeat esophagram 7 to 10 days after cessation of drug therapy usually demonstrates healing of the ulcers. Furthermore, the patient should be instructed to drink water before, during, and after ingestion of medications to prevent recurrence of drug-induced esophagitis.

Radiation Esophagitis.— Irradiation of the mediastinum because of metastatic adenopathy, lymphoma, lung carcinoma, or thoracic spine metastases may lead to radiation esophagitis. The esophagus is relatively radioresistant, the threshold for esophagitis being 4,500 to 6,000 rads over 6 to 8 weeks. However, the combination of chemotherapy and radiation therapy greatly increases the risk of esophagitis.[16]

The patient with a history of radiation therapy and odynophagia may have esophageal ulceration, edema, or fistula formation. Shortly after radiotherapy the esophagram may demonstrate punctate barium collections due to focal ulceration or thick folds due to mucosal edema (Fig 13–6). The region of ulceration is confined to the radiotherapy portal. Between 4 and 12 weeks, peristalsis is abnormal in the region of the radiotherapy portal.[16] A radiation stricture may develop as early as 4 weeks, but most develop between 6 and 8 weeks after completion of radiotherapy.[16] The stricture is manifested radiographically by a focal area of narrowing with smooth tapered margins, ending at the inferior boundary of the radiation portal.[16] Fistulas may appear, especially in areas associated with extrinsic impression of the esophagus, as where carcinomas of the left mainstem bronchus cross the esophagus or mediastinal adenopathy impinges on the esophagus.

Differential Diagnosis

Mucosal Plaques

Small mucosal plaques or nodules are typical of *Candida* esophagitis, reflux esophagitis, and glycogenic acanthosis (Table 13–2). Coarse mucosal nodularity seen in reflux esophagitis may be confused with candidal plaques; however, the coarse nodules in reflux esophagitis have poorly defined borders, whereas candidal plaques are sharply circumscribed, etched with a white line of barium, and longitudinally oriented. A hiatal hernia and gastroesophageal reflux usually are seen with reflux esophagitis. Furthermore, reflux esophagitis is a chronic illness characterized by pyrosis, whereas *Candida* esophagitis has an acute onset and usually occurs in an immunocompromised host.

Plaquelike elevations may be seen in glycogenic acanthosis, a benign degenerative condition in which glycogen accumulates in the cytoplasm of hyperplastic squamous epithelial cells.[4] Uniform round elevations form focal plaques that are not as well demarcated as those seen with *Candida* esophagitis (Fig 13–7). Differentiation of glycogenic acanthosis plaques from candidal or reflux esophagitis plaques is facilitated by the clinical history, because glycogenic acanthosis usually is asymptomatic.

Discrete Ulcers

Small discrete esophageal ulcers are seen in a wide variety of illnesses (see Table 13–2). In the immunocompromised host small ulcers strongly suggest viral, especially herpetic, esophagitis. Occasionally an immunocompetent patient may have viral esophagitis. Aphthous ulcers also are seen occasionally in patients with Crohn's disease[17] or Behçet's disease. The aphthous ulcers are radiographically similar to those seen with herpetic esophagitis[10] or drug ingestion; however, a history of Crohn's disease or Behçet's disease suggests the correct diagnosis. A history of recent radiotherapy or of drug or caustic ingestion suggests the cause of the ulceration in these patients. The patient with reflux esophagitis and shallow ulcers generally has

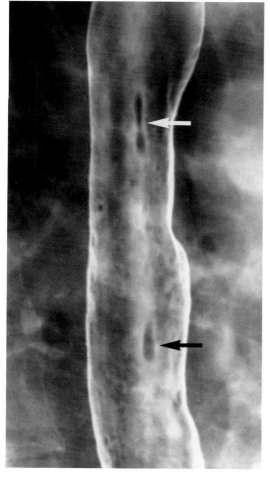

FIG 13–7.
In a 70-year-old man with epigastric pain, several plaquelike longitudinally oriented lucencies *(arrows)* and fine nodularity are seen in the mid-thoracic esophagus. Biopsy showed glycogenic acanthosis.

long-standing heartburn and usually radiographically demonstrable gastroesophageal reflux and hiatal hernia. The shallow ulcers of reflux esophagitis usually are distal, just above the gastroesophageal junction; the ulcers of radiotherapy are at the mediastinal level; and those of drug ingestion are at the level of the aortic arch or left atrium. The healthy adult with acute odynophagia and dysphagia associated with eating food with sharp margins ("taco tear") has a long longitudinal ulcer in the mid-esophagus.[18]

Cystic dilation of adnexal glands normally present in the submucosa may be demonstrated on an esophagram as barium-filled outpouchings extending from the esophageal lumen. This has been termed "intramural pseudodiverticulosis" because the dilated, barium-filled submucosal glands resemble 1 to 3 mm flask-shaped diverticula.[19] En face, the sacculations may be confused with discrete esophageal ulcers (Fig 13–8), but viewing the esophagus in several projections permits the diagnosis. In some patients, a smoothly tapered proximal esophageal stricture occurs in the area of the greatest number of outpouchings. Most patients with intramural pseudodiverticulosis complain of dysphagia. Approximately one third of patients are diabetic, and approximately one half have esophageal candidiasis. Esophagitis may be seen endoscopically in one half of patients, but the openings of the intramural sacculations are rarely seen.[19]

Masses
Some patients with carcinoma have odynophagia (Fig 13–9), usually associated with dysphagia. The radiographic diagnosis usually is obvious as an ulcerated mass (see Fig 13–9) or annular lesion. Rarely a large focal ulcer associated with mounds of edema due to *Candida* or tuberculosis mimics a small ulcerated carcinoma.[9]

Motility Disorder
Some patients with odynophagia have fluoroscopically detected motility disorders, such as achalasia or diffuse esophageal spasm.[20] The vigorous form of achalasia is more frequently associated with chest pain.[20] The primary esophageal stripping wave is absent and a beak-like narrowing is present at the gastroesophageal junction, due to impaired relaxation of the lower esophageal sphincter. Many tertiary waves may be seen, especially in the vigorous form of achalasia. In diffuse esophageal spasm, high-amplitude, repetitive and prolonged contrac-

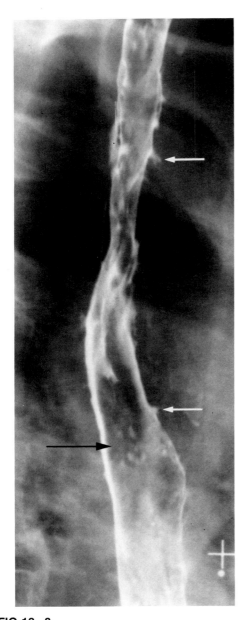

FIG 13–8.
Intramural pseudodiverticulosis with stricture in a patient with dysphagia and odynophagia. Punctate barium collections mimic ulcers *(black arrow);* these are the intramural sacculations seen en face. Barium collections projecting from the lumen *(white arrows)* indicate the true diagnosis of intramural pseudodiverticulosis. Diffuse narrowing above the level of the aortic arch indicates stricture formation.

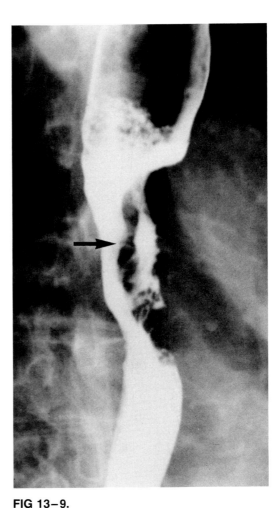

FIG 13–9.
Ulcerating squamous carcinoma of the esophagus in an elderly smoker with odynophagia. A large, polypoid mass projects into the lumen of the esophagus. An irregular barium collection *(arrow)* represents ulceration on the surface of the tumor.

tions of the esophagus are seen, sometimes causing sacculations or a corkscrew appearance.

Various forms of esophagitis may result in esophageal dysmotility, such as focal spasm or diminished amplitude of peristalsis. However, the presence of mucosal ulcers or plaques should suggest that esophagitis is the cause of the dysmotility.

CONCLUSION

In the case presented, Figure 13–1,A shows diffuse nodularity of the pharyngeal mucosa; Figure

13–1,B shows well-circumscribed plaques oriented longitudinally and separated by areas of normal intervening mucosa. In this patient with acute odynophagia, the findings are typical for *Candida* pharyngitis and esophagitis. Although intravenous drug abusers may be debilitated enough to have *Candida* esophagitis, the clinician should consider searching for an underlying immunologic disorder. In this case the radiologist suggested to the clinician that the patient was immunocompromised by acquired immune deficiency syndrome (AIDS) associated with intravenous drug abuse. A subsequent workup confirmed the radiologist's impression that the patient has AIDS.

The double-contrast esophagram is a valuable tool in the evaluation of odynophagia. A combination of the clinical history and radiographic findings suggests the cause for odynophagia in most patients.[4, 5] The esophagram therefore may lead to rapid diagnosis and therapy and obviate the need for endoscopy in many patients.

REFERENCES

1. Cattau EL, Castell DO: Symptoms of esophageal dysfunction, in Castell DO, Johnson LF (eds): *Esophageal Function in Health and Disease.* New York, Elsevier Biomedical, 1983, pp 31–43.
2. Ouyang A, Cohen S: Heartburn, regurgitation and dysphagia, in Berk JE (ed): *Bockus Gastroenterology,* ed 4. Philadelphia, WB Saunders Co, 1985, pp 59–63.
3. Creteur V, Thoeni RF, Federle MP, et al: The role of single and double contrast radiography in the diagnosis of reflux esophagitis. *Radiology* 1983; 147:71–75.
4. Levine MS, Macones AJ, Laufer I: *Candida* esophagitis: Accuracy of diagnosis. *Radiology* 1985; 154:581–587.
5. Vahey TN, Maglinte DDT, Chernish SM: State-of-the-art barium examination in opportunistic esophagitis. *Dig Dis Sci* 1986; 31:1192–1195.
6. Lewicki AM, Moore JP: Esophageal moniliasis. A review of common and less frequent characteristics. *AJR* 1975; 125:218–225.
7. Athey PA, Goldstein HM, Dodd GD: Radiologic spectrum of opportunistic infections of the upper gastrointestinal tract. *AJR* 1977; 129:419–424.
8. Gefter WB, Laufer I, Edell S, et al: Candidiasis in the obstructed esophagus. *Radiology* 1981; 138:25–28.
9. Levine MS: Radiology of esophagitis. *Contemp Diagn Radiol* 1985; 8:1–5.
10. Laufer I: Radiology of esophagitis. *Radiol Clin North Am* 1982; 20:687–699.
11. Roberts L, Gibbons R, Gibbons G, et al: Adult esophageal candidiasis: A radiographic spectrum. *Radiographics* 1987; 7:289–307.
12. Levine MS, Cajade AG, Herlinger H, et al: Pseudomembranes in reflux esophagitis. *Radiology* 1986; 159:43–45.
13. Shortsleeve MJ, Gavin GP, Gardner RC, et al: Herpetic esophagitis. *Radiology* 1981; 141:611–617.
14. Levine MS, Laufer I, Kressel HY, et al: Herpes esophagitis. *AJR* 1981; 136:863–866.
15. Creteur V, Laufer I, Kressel HY, et al: Drug-induced esophagitis detected by double-contrast radiography. *Radiology* 1983; 147:365–368.
16. Lepke RA, Libshitz HI: Radiation-induced injury of the esophagus. *Radiology* 1983; 148:375–378.
17. Gohel VK, Long BW, Richter G: Aphthous ulcers in the esophagus with Crohn colitis. *AJR* 1981; 137:872–873.
18. Hunter TB, Protell RL, Horsley WW: Food laceration of the esophagus: The taco tear. *AJR* 1983; 140:503–504.
19. Meshkinpour H: Esophageal diverticula, in Berk JE (ed): *Bockus Gastroenterology.* Philadelphia, WB Saunders Co, 1985, pp 809–814.
20. Cohen S: Motor disorders of the esophagus. *N Engl J Med* 1979; 301:184–192.

CHAPTER 14

Esophageal Strictures

David W. Gelfand, M.D.
Yu Men Chen, M.D.
David J. Ott, M.D.

Case Presentation

A 41-year-old white man was admitted to the hospital after a 5-month history of constant nonradiating back pain. He obtained no relief from antacids or physical maneuvering. The patient was referred to the rheumatology service, where degenerative arthritis of the thoracic spine was diagnosed. However, laboratory tests revealed hypochromic microcytic anemia. As part of the workup to determine the source of blood loss, an upper gastrointestinal series was performed (Fig 14–1). What are the findings? What action should be taken?

DISCUSSION

Although reflux esophagitis is the most common cause of esophageal strictures, they can result from a variety of pathologic processes. The radiologic examination is usually the first study performed in these patients and often produces findings characteristic of the individual pathologic condition. Awareness of the causes of esophageal strictures and their radiographic appearances is thus important for accurate initial evaluation. Causes of esophageal strictures include congenital abnormalities, reflux esophagitis, infectious esophagitis, and esophageal neoplasms, among others (Table 14–1).

Congenital esophageal stricture is usually associated with tracheal esophageal fistula or extremely rarely with esophageal atresia or esophageal duplication.[1] Strictures are seen in approximately 20% of children and adults after tracheoesophageal fistula repair (Fig 14–2), most commonly in the mid-portion of the thoracic esophagus.[2, 3] Multiple congenital webs and stenoses also have been reported but are rare.[4]

By far the most common cause of esophageal stricture is reflux esophagitis. The stricture is the direct result of the inflammatory process and usually develops after repeated episodes of esophagitis. Onset of stricture may be preceded by development of a lower esophageal ring or web, and evolution of lower esophageal rings into esophageal strictures has been documented.[5] The characteristic radiographic appearance is that of a narrowing of variable length located at or just above the esophagogastric junction (Fig 14–3). Esophageal stricture due to reflux esophagitis is invariably associated with hiatal hernia.

Barrett's syndrome is increasingly thought to develop in a background of reflux esophagitis.[6–8] Frequently the initial symptom, among other findings of reflux esophagitis, is stricture of the middle or distal third of the esophagus. Barrett's syndrome now is believed to be the result of chronic ulceration due to gastroesophageal reflux disease. The more

The resulting prolonged retention of the drug in the esophagus is thought to produce direct mucosal injury. Mucosal edema and superficial ulceration are the typical endoscopic and radiologic findings.[34] The ulcers are most common in the region of the aortic arch, are often multiple, and are surrounded by normal mucosa. Esophageal stricture (Fig 14–8) is an infrequent result of medication-induced esophagitis.

Traumatic injury and subsequent stricture of the esophagus may be due to a variety of causes. However, it is most often iatrogenic and usually related to intubation, surgery, or endoscopy. The most common cause of posttraumatic esophageal stricture is the prolonged presence of a nasogastric

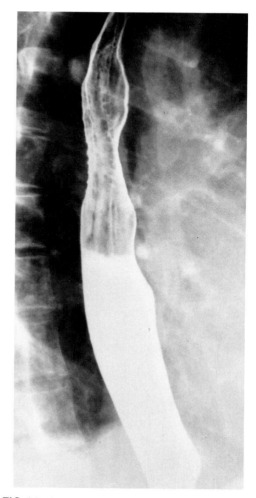

FIG 14–8.
Stricture of the esophagus at the level of the aortic arch due to "dry" ingestion of doxycycline in a patient with acne vulgaris.

tube, which may cause esophagitis and stricture due to direct injury or as a result of induced gastroesophageal reflux. Strictures have been reported after only several days of intubation, but most often after several weeks.[39, 40] Esophageal strictures induced by indwelling tubes are usually extensive and closely simulate strictures due to caustic ingestion.

CONCLUSION

Figure 14–1 shows an esophageal stricture and ulcer suggestive of Barrett's syndrome. Endoscopy

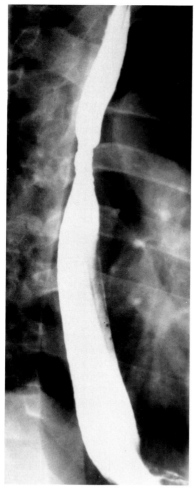

FIG 14–7.
Localized stricture of the mid-esophagus due to lye ingestion.

confirmed the diagnosis, and biopsy of the distal esophagus revealed columnar epithelium. The patient was treated symptomatically with magnesium hydroxide–aluminum hydroxide suspension (Maalox).

Two years later, the patient was readmitted to the hospital with a complaint of solid food dysphagia. Endoscopy showed a carcinoma of the distal esophagus that on biopsy proved to be an adenocarcinoma. The patient underwent resection of the distal esophagus with esophagogastrostomy, followed by radiation therapy and chemotherapy. Two years after surgery dysphagia again developed, and recurrent carcinoma at the esophagogastric anastomosis was diagnosed. After a course of chemotherapy the patient was lost to follow-up and is presumed to have died of carcinoma.

REFERENCES

1. Kwok-Liu JPY, Tuttle RJ: Duplication of the esophagus. *J Can Assoc Radiol* 1982; 33:281–282.
2. Dominguez R, Zarabi M, Oh KS, et al: Congenital esophageal stenosis. *Clin Radiol* 1985; 36:263–266.
3. Mares AJ, Bar-Ziv J, Lieberman A, et al: Congenital esophageal stenosis: Transendoscopic web incision. *J Clin Gastroenterol* 1986; 8:555–558.
4. Munitz HA, Ott DJ, Rocamora LR, et al: Multiple webs of the esophagus. *South Med J* 1983; 76:405–406.
5. Chen YM, Gelfand DW, Ott DJ, et al: Natural progression of the lower esophageal mucosal ring. *Gastrointest Radiol* 1987; 12:93–98.
6. Chen YM, Gelfand DW, Ott DJ, et al: Barrett esophagus as an extension of severe esophagitis: Analysis of radiologic signs in 29 cases. *AJR* 1985; 145:275–281.
7. Agha FP: Radiologic diagnosis of Barrett's esophagus: Critical analysis of 65 cases. *Gastrointest Radiol* 1986; 11:123–130.
8. Barrett NR: Chronic peptic ulcer of the oesophagus and oesophagitis. *Br J Surg* 1950; 38:175–182.
9. Robbins AH, Hermos JA, Schimmel EM, et al: The columnar-lined esophagus—Analysis of 26 cases. *Radiology* 1977; 123:1–7.
10. Allison PR, Johnstone AS: The oesophagus lined with gastric mucous membrane. *Thorax* 1953; 8:87–101.
11. Agha FP, Lee HH, Nostrant TT: Herpetic esophagitis: A diagnostic challenge in immunocompromised patients. *Am J Gastroenterol* 1986; 81:246–253.
12. Agha FP: Candidiasis-induced esophageal strictures. *Gastrointest Radiol* 1984; 9:283–286.
13. Gelter WB, Laufer I, Edell S, et al: Candidiasis in the obstructed esophagus. *Radiology* 1981; 138:25–28.
14. Ott DJ, Gelfand DW: Esophageal stricture secondary to candidiasis. *Gastrointest Radiol* 1978; 2:323–325.
15. Kroneke K, Cuadrado R: Esophageal stricture following esophagitis in a patient with herpes zoster: Case report. *Milit Med* 1984; 149:479–481.
16. Goldstein HM, Zornoza J, Hopens T: Intrinsic disease of the adult esophagus: Benign and malignant tumors. *Semin Roentgenol* 1981; 16:183–197.
17. Bosch A, Frias Z, Caldwell WL: Adenocarcinoma of the esophagus. *Cancer* 1979; 43:1557–1561.
18. Ghahremani GG, Gore RM, Breuer RI, et al: Esophageal manifestation of Crohn's disease. *Gastrointest Radiol* 1982; 7:199–203.
19. Cooper TW, Bauer EA: Epidermolysis bullosa: A review. *Pediatr Dermatol* 1984; 1:181–188.
20. Tishler JM, Han SY, Helman CA: Esophageal involvement in epidermolysis bullosa dystrophica. *AJR* 1983; 141:1283–1286.
21. Person JR, Rogers RS III: Bullous and cicatricial pemphigoid: Clinical, histopathologic, and immunopathologic correlations. *Mayo Clin Proc* 1977; 52:54–66.
22. Al-Kutoubi MA, Eliot C: Oesophageal involvement in benign mucous membrane pemphigoid. *Clin Radiol* 1984; 35:131–135.
23. Agha FP, Raji MR: Esophageal involvement in pemphigoid: Clinical and roentgen manifestations. *Gastrointest Radiol* 1982; 7:109–112.
24. Goldman LP, Weigert JM: Corrosive substance ingestion: A review. *Am J Gastroenterol* 1984; 79:85–90.
25. Chen YM, Ott DJ, Thompson JN, et al: Progressive radiographic appearance of caustic esophagitis. *South Med J* 1988; 81:724–729.
26. Gaudreault P, Parent M, McGuigan MA, et al: Predictability of esophageal injury from signs and symptoms: A study of caustic ingestion in 378 children. *Pediatrics* 1983; 71:767–770.
27. Kirsh MM, Ritter F: Caustic ingestion and subsequent damage to the oropharyngeal and digestive passages. *Ann Thorac Surg* 1976; 21:74–82.
28. Martel W: Radiologic features of esophagogastritis secondary to extremely caustic agents. *Radiology* 1972; 103:31–36.
29. Franken EA Jr: Caustic damage of the gastrointestinal tract: Roentgen features. *Am J Roentgenol* 1973; 118:77–85.

30. Boal DKB, Newburger PE, Teele RL: Esophagitis induced by combined radiation and adriamycin. *AJR* 1979; 132:567–570.
31. Lepke RA, Libshitz HI: Radiation-induced injury of the esophagus. *Radiology* 1983; 148:375–378.
32. Creteur V, Laufer I, Kressel HY, et al: Drug-induced esophagitis detected by double-contrast radiography. *Radiology* 1983; 147:365–368.
33. Teplick JG, Teplick SK, Ominsky SH, et al: Esophagitis caused by oral medication. *Radiology* 1980; 134:23–25.
34. Agha FP, Wilson JAP, Nostrand TT: Medication-induced esophagitis. *Gastrointest Radiol* 1986; 11:7–11.
35. Lambert JR, Newman A: Ulceration and stricture of the esophagus due to oral potassium chloride (slow release tablet) therapy. *Am J Gastroenterol* 1980; 73:508–511.
36. Mason SJ, O'Meara TF: Drug-induced esophagitis. *J Clin Gastroenterol* 1981; 3:115–120.
37. Ravich WJ, Kashima H, Donner MW: Drug-induced esophagitis simulating esophageal carcinoma. *Dysphagia* 1986; 1:13–18.
38. Daunt N, Brodribb TR, Dickey JD: Oesophageal ulceration due to doxycycline. *Br J Radiol* 1985; 58:1209–1211.
39. Banfield WJ, Hurwitz AL: Esophageal stricture associated with nasogastric intubation. *Arch Intern Med* 1974; 134:1083–1086.
40. Hafner CD, Wylie JH Jr, Brush BE: Complications of gastrointestinal intubation. *Arch Surg* 1961; 83:147–160.

CHAPTER 15

Polypoid Lesions of the Esophagus—Large and Small: A Clinical and Radiographic Approach

Seth N. Glick, M.D.

Case Presentation

A barium esophagogram in a middle-aged man showed an abnormality in the distal esophagus (Fig 15–1). What are the findings? What is the differential diagnosis?

DISCUSSION

"Polyp" is a generic term referring to any type of discrete protrusion into the lumen. The site of origin may be the mucosa or submucosa; the pathogenesis may be congenital, hyperplastic, inflammatory, or neoplastic. The radiographic principles regarding the detection and interpretation of polyps are basically similar to those for all of the hollow viscera of the gastrointestinal tract. The spectrum or frequency of pathologic entities and the clinical significance of these various lesions, however, varies with each organ.

Most polypoid lesions of the esophagus are detected incidentally as part of a routine upper gastrointestinal tract examination. When a lesion is large enough to compromise the lumen, dysphagia may occur. In general, malignant lesions are more likely to produce symptoms than are benign lesions of a similar size. Whether the radiologist uses a double-contrast technique, a single-contrast tech-

nique, or a multiphasic technique, the radiographic approach is the same. Polyps appear as barium rings when viewed en face and as semicircular lines arising from the esophageal walls when viewed in tangent on air contrast scans. With full-column and mucosal relief technique they appear as round or semicircular filling defects in the barium column, depending on the projection and the location of the polyp.

First the presence of artifacts must be excluded as a cause of the apparent lesion. Such artifacts may include air bubbles, undissolved adherent granules from recently administered gas-producing powders, kissing artifacts caused by approximation of two walls of the esophagus, extrinsic impressions from the aorta and left mainstem bronchus, and ring densities from the posterior elements of the thoracic spine superimposed on the air contrast esophagogram. All of these artifacts usually disappear when the patient is turned or swallows repeatedly.

In some situations a variably sized polypoid

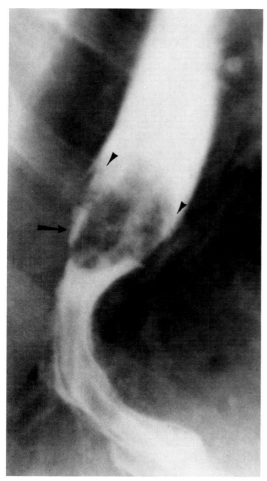

FIG 15–1.
Large lobulated filling defect *(arrow)* with nodular surface. Note the meniscoid configuration of the barium column above the lesion *(arrowheads)*, indicative of an intraluminal mass.

glucagon or gas-producing granules. After the foreign body has been eliminated, it is important to perform a follow-up examination to evaluate the esophagus for an underlying structural or functional disorder and to detect residual damage produced by the impacted material.

When it is determined that a true polyp or polypoid lesion is present, systematic analysis of the radiographic findings and the clinical information is performed to arrive at a diagnosis or limited differential diagnosis. In most situations a specific histologic diagnosis is impossible. However, based on the appropriate analytical process, a statistical probability can be suggested and a recommendation made as to whether the abnormality requires further investigation, such as endoscopy or other imaging procedures.

The most important feature is the size of the le-

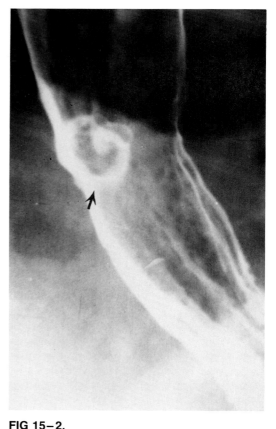

FIG 15–2.
Squamous papilloma. Lobulated 1 cm polyp in the distal esophagus *(arrow)*. The location and configuration are highly suggestive of the diagnosis, but malignancy might be difficult to exclude without biopsy.

filling defect may be produced by an ingested substance lodged in the esophagus (see Fig 15–1). This substance, usually a piece of meat, as in the case presented, usually can be diagnosed by the history, the completely intraluminal nature of the defect (i.e., barium forms a meniscoid configuration in all projections above it), and the typical locations. These locations represent points of physiologic delay, such as the thoracic inlet, the left mainstem bronchus, and the gastroesophageal junction. After the radiologist recognizes the true nature of the abnormality, an attempt may be made to dislodge the foreign body using pharmacologic agents such as

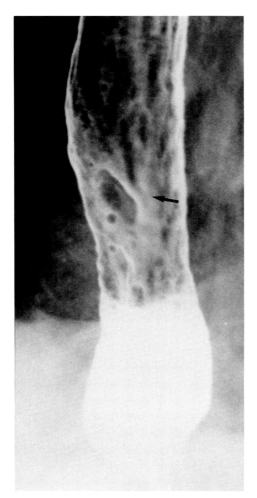

FIG 15–3.
Glycogenic acanthosis. Sessile plaque in distal esophagus *(arrow)* with numerous small surrounding nodules. The typical nodules of glycogenic acanthosis suggest the diagnosis, but endoscopy may be necessary for complete evaluation.

(i.e., previous head or neck carcinoma, Barrett's syndrome, previous lye ingestion), biopsy of all solitary excrescences in the esophagus is advisable. Nevertheless, almost all of the polyps in this size range represent either squamous papillomas or glycogenic plaques (Figs 15–2 and 15–3). Squamous papillomas are benign lobulated sessile lesions of surface epithelium; characteristically they are composed of fingerlike projections of tissue lined by increased numbers of squamous cells with cores of connective tissue containing small blood vessels.[2] They most commonly occur in the distal third of the esophagus, and half are multiple. The cause is un-

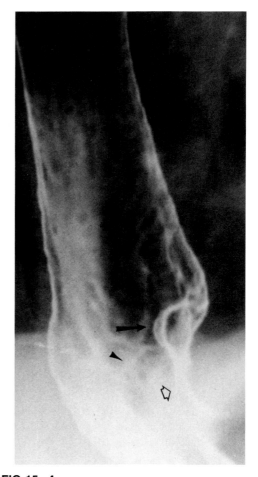

FIG 15–4.
Inflammatory polyp and fold. Smooth 8 mm polyp *(long arrow)* located just above the gastroesophageal Z line *(arrowhead),* with characteristic associated fold *(open arrow)* in a patient with radiographic and clinical reflux esophagitis.

sion. In most cases any polyp that is 1 cm or smaller can be considered of no clinical significance. Clinical significance indicates that the lesion is responsible for the symptoms, may be a precursor of malignancy, or actually may represent a malignancy. In one study of 4,100 consecutive barium examinations 22 incidental esophageal polyps were discovered.[1] Fourteen of these were smaller than 1 cm, and histologic analysis of the 9 that were biopsied proved that all were benign. In patients with a known predisposition to esophageal carcinoma

known, and there is no association with malignancy. Although considered rare, squamous papillomas constitute the majority of tiny esophageal polyps. Rarely they are larger than 1 cm, and giant papillomas have been reported.

Glycogenic acanthosis represents small white elevations in the esophagus that are usually smaller than 0.5 cm and are diffusely distributed.[3] There is no pathologic association with this process, and it is identified in about one third of the population. The nodule consists of hyperplastic and hypertrophied squamous epithelium; the vacuolated squamous cells are filled with glycogen. Glycogen plaques ranging from 0.5 to 2 cm usually can be distinguished by the presence of the more typical appearing glycogenic nodules throughout the esophagus. When these plaques are exceptionally large, biopsy may be indicated.

Although polyps smaller than 1 cm are rarely of clinical significance, they may be an indicator of another disease process. In one study a polyp occurring at the gastroesophageal junction and associated with an enlarged gastric fold was described as a sign of reflux esophagitis[4] (Fig 15–4). These polyps may represent localized gastritis, but the precise pathophysiologic relationship to reflux esophagitis remains obscure. There is no association of this polyp-fold complex with malignancy. A small polypoid carcinoma of the gastroesophageal junction may simulate this lesion, but the absence of the associated fold and the presence of lobulation or nodularity of the polyps should raise the suspicion of malignancy.

Submucosal tumors smaller than 1 cm commonly are identified on routine esophagography. However, it is extremely difficult to apply the radiographic criteria that distinguish mucosal from submucosal lesions for filling defects in this size range. When upper tract endoscopy is performed either to evaluate the esophageal lesion or for unrelated indications, such submucosal lesions often go undetected because of their minimal protrusion into the lumen and their normal overlying mucosa. Even when such lesions are visualized, endoscopic biopsy specimens are unrewarding, yielding only normal esophageal epithelium. Most of these polyps are presumed to be leiomyomas; benign smooth muscle tumors are the most common benign neoplasm of the esophagus, constituting over two thirds of all such lesions.[5, 6] However, lipomas are not uncommon and may be accurately assessed endoscopically (Fig 15–5). When this type of lesion is found, the endoscopist should consider the possibility of a soli-

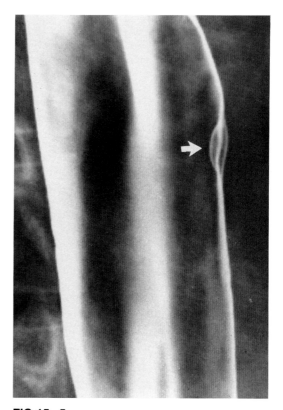

FIG 15–5.
Lipoma. Smooth-surfaced 1 cm filling defect *(arrow)* with obtuse transition with adjacent esophageal wall. This is most suggestive of a submucosal lesion but nonspecific for the histologic diagnosis.

tary varix. Prior knowledge may preclude a potentially hazardous biopsy procedure.

Polypoid lesions larger than 1 cm require closer scrutiny because of the possibility of a small malignancy. In actuality, diagnosis of small esophageal carcinomas as an incidental finding on routine esophagrams is extremely rare and symptoms of carcinoma of the esophagus rarely develop until the tumor has progressed to an advanced stage. An attempt should be made to demonstrate the filling defect en face and in tangent in order to assess the surface contour and the geometry of the interface between the polypoid lesion and the adjacent esophageal wall. As a rule, a submucosal tumor has a smooth surface and forms a right or obtuse angle at its proximal and distal margin with the normal esophagus (Fig 15–6). These features usually aid in distinguishing these lesions from tumors of epithelial origin. However, the converse is not true, because tumors (benign and malignant) arising from elements in the submucosal layer may have a considerable intraluminal growth pattern with a nodular and lobulated contour. Other potential pitfalls include the rare, entirely submucosal growth pattern of a squamous cell carcinoma[7] or an extrinsic lesion (i.e., lymph node; Fig 15–7) that impresses on the esophagus and simulates a submucosa mass. An estimation of the location of the "center" of the mass as being intramural may be helpful. However, submucosal masses such as leiomyomas may have a predominantly extramural growth pattern and appear extrinsic. Lobulation of the mass in association with a smooth surface may predict a leiomyoma (Fig 15–8). The approach to polypoid lesions larger than 1 cm may vary with the clinical background and the radiographic appearance on barium study. With larger lesions, particularly those more than 2 cm, management should be more aggressive. In most lesions larger than 1 or 2 cm with a characteristic submucosal appearance, endoscopy may be performed or a repeat barium study may be performed 6 months to 1 year later to assess any change in size or appearance.

If there is no change, the patient may be examined at intervals at the discretion of the referring physician. A similar protocol may be followed when initial endoscopic findings are negative or demonstrate a submucosal mass. In the case of apparent extramucosal lesions larger than 3 cm endoscopy should be performed, and if the extramucosal nature is confirmed, computed tomography of the chest should be performed to rule out the possibility of an intrinsic disease process (i.e., lymph nodes, carcinoma of the lung, aortic aneurysm), to assess the size of the lesion and its relationship to adjacent structures (for potential surgery), and to possibly obtain further information concerning the nature of the lesion. If the patient has a known primary malignancy, metastatic disease should be considered.[8] Carcinoma of the lung and breast are the tumors most frequently associated with esophageal metastases, but subdiaphragmatic tumors also may spread to the submucosa or periesophageal tissues by lymphatic or hematogenous routes.[8, 9]

Discrete mucosal polyps in the range of 1 to 4 cm are extremely unusual but, when they occur, usually represent carcinoma. A benign tumor arising from the submucosa may appear to have an intraluminal location and simulate a mucosal lesion. This is extremely characteristic for leiomyoma, but submucosal tumors such as granular cell myoblastoma and hemangioma demonstrate these morphologic features radiographically.[10, 11] Endoscopy usually clarifies the situation. Small malignant esophageal polyps tend to be of three morphologic types.[12, 13] Most common is the sessile plaque (Fig 15–9). These lesions appear as a smooth or lobulated flat

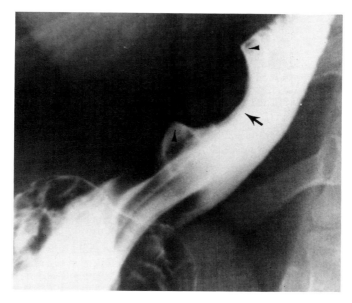

FIG 15–6.
Leiomyoma. Smooth-surfaced 3 cm polypoid filling defect in the distal esophagus *(arrow)* with character- istic submucosal transition with adjacent esophageal wall *(arrowheads).*

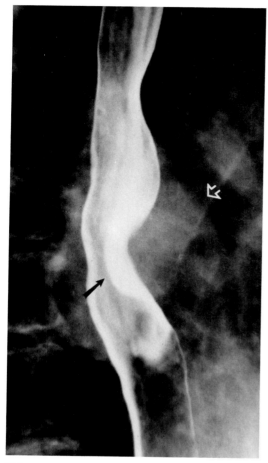

FIG 15–7.
Subcarinal lymph node (lymphoma) simulating submucosal esophageal mass. Smooth-surfaced filling defect in mid-esophagus *(black arrow)*. The peripheral soft tissue margin is outlined against the air-filled lung just under the left mainstem bronchus *(open arrow)*. Computed tomography may be necessary to determine the cause.

elevation of the mucosal contour when viewed in tangent. Areas of ulceration are often present. The margin of the tumor with the adjacent wall is an angle of 90 degrees or more. When demonstrated en face, they usually are oval and have a coarse surface. Unfortunately, in spite of their small size many of these extend beyond the submucosa or metastasize to the regional lymph nodes, thereby representing advanced carcinoma with its associated poor prognosis.

The second type of small "polypoid" carci-

noma appears as a broad-based lobulated contour defect viewed in tangent; however, when projected en face, it appears as a variably sized area of nodular granular mucosa rather than a discrete polypoid defect with definable contours. These most likely represent the earliest form of radiographically demonstrable esophageal carcinoma. However, because of their subtle nature they may be easily overlooked, particularly if the esophagus is only routinely radiographed in one projection. The least common small malignant esophageal polyp is the discrete sessile intraluminal polyp with normal surrounding mucosa (Fig 15–10). When smooth, such

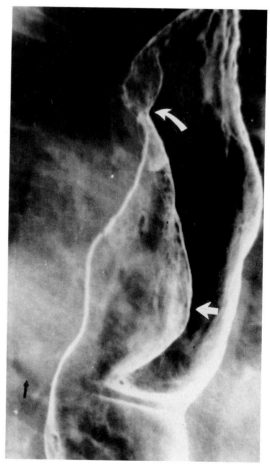

FIG 15–8.
Leiomyoma. This large, smooth-surfaced polypoid mass *(straight white arrow)* appears similar to the extrinsic mass in Figure 15–7, with air-filled lung defining the peripheral soft tissue margin *(black arrow)*. Lobulation *(curved arrow)* is typical of a leiomyoma.

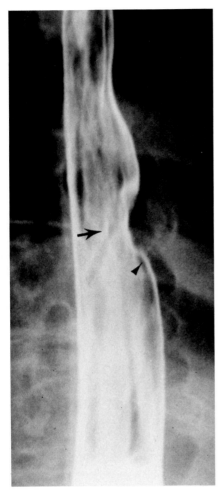

FIG 15–9.
Plaque carcinoma. Small flat plaque in mid-esophagus *(arrow)* with slightly uneven surface and elevation of the adjacent wall *(arrowhead)* due to infiltration. This should not be confused with the normal impression by the left mainstem bronchus.

cion may depend on the size of the polyp and the presence of symptoms. Rarely, other benign processes, including focal esophageal candidiasis, pseudomembranes associated with reflex esophagitis, and medication-induced esophagitis, produce a similar appearance.[15–17] Any esophageal mucosal protrusion larger than 1 cm warrants initial endoscopy and biopsy.

As the size of polypoid mucosal lesions increases the diagnostic specificity of the barium study significantly decreases. These lesions appear as large bulky intraluminal masses that expand the lumen and are markedly lobulated. The pathologic spectrum includes benign and malignant lesions arising in both the mucosa and submucosa. These tumors range from 3 cm to involve most of the length of the esophageal body. Very large lesions,

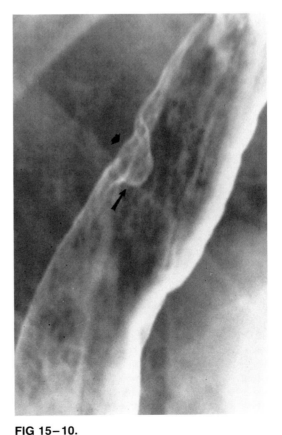

FIG 15–10.
Sessile malignant polyp. Nonuniform smooth filling defect *(long arrow)* with asymmetric shape and slightly lobular margin *(arrowhead)*. The typical transition features that distinguish a mucosal from a submucosal lesion are not present.

polyps may resemble a submucosal lesion. A detailed study with careful evaluation is necessary to search for any asymmetry or irregularity in the shape or surface contour. On the other hand, when the polyp is markedly lobulated it can be recognized easily as a mucosal lesion. In these cases, distinction from a larger squamous papilloma may be made histologically. A potential pitfall is the rare verrucous carcinoma, a slow-growing polypoid malignancy that is well differentiated and may appear benign on endoscopic biopsy.[14] The index of suspi-

particularly when smooth and soft, may be overlooked, the long lucent filling defect being mistaken for nonuniform flow of the barium column. The most common large polypoid tumor is the spindle cell carcinoma (Fig 15–11).[18] The spindle cell represents anaplastic transformation of the conventional squamous cell, which may be present but does not predominate. This tumor also has been referred to as pseudosarcoma but should not be confused with carcinosarcoma, which also typically produces a bulky, lumen-expanding esophageal polypoid mass but is much less common. Carcinosarcoma consists of typical squamous cell carcinoma mixed with sarcomatous elements including fibrosarcoma, chondrosarcoma, and osteosarcoma. Both entities have a

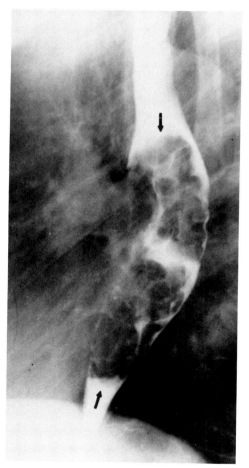

prognosis similar to that of the more common squamous cell carcinoma, and any of the malignant histologic components may metastasize. Biopsy results may vary depending on the portion of the lesion sampled. Squamous cell carcinoma rarely is seen as an intraluminal mass; only 2% of 129 squamous cell carcinomas had this appearance in one series.[18] Polypoid malignancies may be pedunculated, but the pedicle is rarely demonstrated on thecontrast study. Other malignant tumors that have a similar gross morphologic appearance include oat cell carcinoma, primary esophageal melanoma, verrucous carcinoma, and leiomyosarcoma.[14, 18–20] Although leiomyosarcoma arises from the submucosa, the majority of these tumors have a bulky lobulated appearance. Endoscopic biopsy frequently allows distinction among these entities, but their true nature often is revealed only at resection or autopsy. In most cases the distinction is academic because the underlying histologic findings do not affect therapy or prognosis.

Although the vast majority of large polypoid masses are malignant, a benign tumor may have this appearance. The most common example is a fibrovascular polyp, which typically arises in the proximal esophagus and, because of its long pedicle, may be regurgitated into the mouth or extend the entire length of the esophagus.[21] Malignancy is uncommon in the proximal esophagus, which may help in the differential diagnosis. Computed tomography might be diagnostic, considering the marked adipose component in this lesion. Benign intraluminal polypoid tumors less commonly include leiomyoma, lipoma, and giant squamous papillomas.[22] Resection of large tumors is usually necessary for diagnosis.

In summary, evaluation and management of polypoid esophageal lesions depends on a variety of factors, including size and radiographic appearance. In most cases the role of the radiologist is to detect and describe these lesions, sometimes observe them with interval examinations, and integrate the various imaging techniques in the management of malignant lesions.

FIG 15–11.
Spindle cell carcinoma. Large bulky nodular intraluminal polypoid filling defect *(arrows)*. This appearance is nonspecific, but statistically the most likely diagnosis is spindle cell carcinoma.

REFERENCES

1. Montesi A, Pesaresi A, Graziani L, et al: Small benign tumors of the esophagus: Radiologic diagnosis with double-contrast examination. *Gastrointest Radiol* 1983; 8: 207–212.

2. Colina F, Solis JA, Munoz MT: Squamous papilloma of the esophagus. *Am J Gastroenterol* 1980; 74:410–414.

3. Glick SN, Teplick SK, Goldstein J, et al: Glycogenic acanthosis of the esophagus. *AJR* 1982; 139:683–688.

4. Styles RA, Gibb PS, Tarshis A, et al: Esophagogastric polyps: Radiographic and endoscopic findings. *Radiology* 1985; 154:307–311.

5. Schmidt A, Lockwood K: Benign neoplasms of the esophagus. *Acta Chir Scand* 1967; 133:640–644.

6. Attah EB, Hajdu SI: Benign and malignant tumors of the esophagus at autopsy. *J Thorac Cardiovasc Surg* 1968; 55:396–404.

7. Engelman RM, Scialla AV: Carcinoma of the esophagus presenting radiographically as a benign lesion. *Dis Chest* 1968; 53:652–655.

8. Agha FP: Secondary neoplasms of the esophagus. *Gastrointest Radiol* 1987; 12:187–193.

9. Steiner H, Lammer J, Hackl A: Lymphatic metastases to the esophagus. *Gastrointest Radiol* 1984; 9:1–4.

10. Govani AF: Hemangiomas of the esophagus. *Gastrointest Radiol* 1982; 7:113–117.

11. Gershwind ME, Chiat H, Addei KA, et al: Granular cell tumors of the esophagus. *Gastrointest Radiol* 1978; 53:652–655.

12. Sako T, Sakai Y, Kajita A, et al: Radiographic microstructures of early esophageal carcinoma: Correlation of specimen radiography with pathologic findings and clinical radiography. *Gastrointest Radiol* 1986; 11:12–19.

13. Zornoza J, Lindell MM Jr: Radiologic evaluation of small esophageal carcinoma. *Gastrointest Radiol* 1980; 5:107–111.

14. Agha FP, Weatherbec, Sams JS: Verrucous carcinoma of the esophagus. *Am J Gastroenterol* 1984; 79:844–849.

15. Roberts L Jr, Gibbons R, Gibbons G, et al: Adult esophageal candidiasis: A radiographic spectrum. *Radiographics* 1987; 7:289–307.

16. Kikendall JW, Friedman AC, Morakinyo AO, et al: Pill induced esophageal injury. *Dig Dis Sci* 1983; 28:174–182.

17. Levine MS, Cajade AG, Herlinger H, et al: Pseudomembranes in reflux esophagitis. *Radiology* 1986; 159:43–45.

18. Olmstead WW, Lichtenstein JE, Hyams VJ: Polypoid epithelial malignancies of the esophagus. *AJR* 1983; 140:921–925.

19. Partyka EK, Sanowski RA, Kozarek RA: Endoscopic diagnosis of a giant esophageal leiomyosarcoma. *Am J Gastroenterol* 1981; 75:132–134.

20. Sostman HD, Keohanc MF, Lee CH, et al: Primary oesophageal melanocarcinoma. *Br J Radiol* 1980; 53:589–592.

21. Barki Y, Elias H, Tovi F, et al: A fibrovascular polyp of the oesophagus. *Br J Radiol* 1981; 54:142–144.

22. Walker JH: Giant papilloma of the thoracic esophagus. *AJR* 1978; 131:519–520.

CHAPTER 16

Chest Pain: Rule Out Hiatal Hernia, Gastroesophageal Reflux, Reflux Esophagitis

Matilde Nino-Murcia, M.D.
Gerald W. Friedland, M.D.

Case Presentation

A 69-year-old man was admitted to the hospital with acute chest pain. To differentiate a hiatal hernia with esophagitis from myocardial infarct, the clinicians ordered an esophagogram. An esophagogram obtained with the patient upright showed a semioval projection of barium at the lower end of the esophagus (Fig 16–1,A). A double-contrast esophagogram performed with the patient prone over a bolster showed no adjacent edema or mass and indicated that the projection was located at and below the A ring (Fig 16–1,B). What is the differential diagnosis? What is the diagnosis?

DISCUSSION

Radiologists frequently are asked to perform esophagograms to distinguish hiatal hernia with reflux esophagitis from myocardial infarction; however, such request is inappropriate. Acute myocardial infarction must be established positively by all the appropriate tests and should not be excluded by the finding of a hiatal hernia with esophagitis on an esophagogram. In our experience, a significant number of these patients have esophageal abnormalities, to which the pain is ascribed, and later die of myocardial infarct.*

Is a barium study the most appropriate examination to rule out reflux? Simply showing that gastroesophageal reflux exists does not mean, for example, that a patient has peptic esophagitis. Most

---

*Three friends of one of the authors went to the emergency room complaining of chest pain, and in each case the diagnosis of hiatal hernia was made. Two died at home a few hours later of myocardial infarct; a third had cardiac arrest and was resuscitated by his wife. He was mentally incompetent, however, and died later of another myocardial infarct.

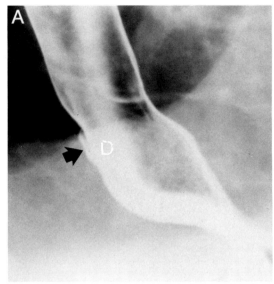

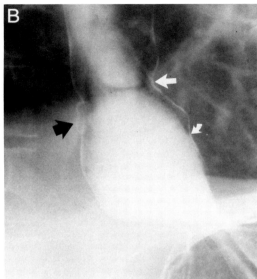

FIG 16–1.
A, esophagogram, upright view. Note semioval projection of barium at the lower end of the esophagus *(arrow).* **B,** double-contrast esophagogram performed with the patient prone over a bolster. The projection *(black arrow)* is located at and below the A ring *(straight white arrow).* The B ring formed in the region of the *curved white arrow.*

FIG 16–2.
Normal anatomy. Specimen of esophagus and stomach distended with barium. Note tubular esophagus *(T),* vestibule *(V),* and A ring *(arrowheads).* *Curved arrows* point to the margins of the hiatus.

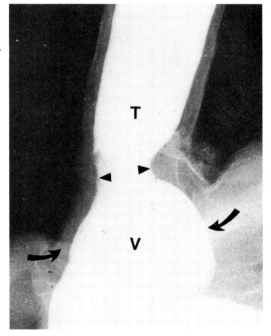

healthy persons have isolated episodes of gastroe-sophageal reflux[1]; those with reflux esophagitis may have more frequent episodes than normal.[1] If barium flows freely between the stomach and the esophagus, gastroesophageal reflux is likely. A barium study demonstrates this free reflux between the stomach and the esophagus in only 40% to 50% of patients with documented gastroesophageal reflux and reflux esophagitis.[1]

Various tests, such as the water siphon test, have been devised to induce reflux, but these are of little value. The 24-hour pH monitoring of the esophagus (Tuttle test) is a very good method for demonstrating reflux; another good method for showing and quantifying reflux is gastroesophageal scintigraphy.[2]

Is there evidence of a hiatal hernia in our patient? The lower end of the normal well-distended esophagus ordinarily is more distensible than the rest of the esophagus. This distensible area is called the vestibule (Fig 16–2).[3] Normally there is a con-

tractile, rounded muscular ring at the upper end of the vestibule, called the A ring (although other terms for this feature have been used).[3] The vestibule lies partially in the thorax, partially in the hiatus, and partially in the abdomen (Fig 16–3).[3]

Swallowing normally causes the vestibule to rise (Fig 16–4), and in persons older than 30 years as much as 2 cm of the stomach can temporarily protrude into the thorax.[3] The vestibule is normally pulled back into the abdomen at the end of swallowing, because it is attached to the hiatus by a strong fibroelastic membrane, the phrenoesophageal membrane,[3] described in greater detail below.

In the patient with hiatal hernia the hiatus is widened and the phrenoesophageal membrane is attenuated or may be almost entirely absent. Thus if any part of the stomach rises into the thorax it is not immediately pulled back. The lax membrane also allows a greater amount of the stomach to slide into the thorax than is normal.[3]

It is sometimes difficult to establish how much

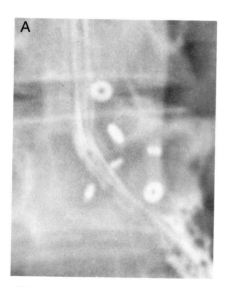
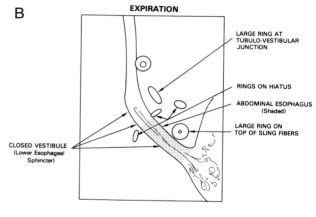
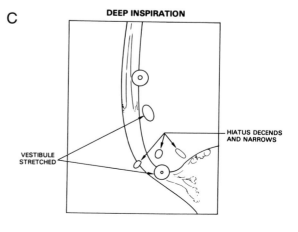

FIG 16–3.
Effect of respiration on position of the vestibule. **A,** three small tantalum rings on the hiatus; large tantalum rings on proximal and distal end of the vestibule and tubular esophagus. The vestibule lies partially in the thorax, partially in the hiatus, and partially in the abdomen. **B,** diagram of **A. C,** During deep inspiration the hiatus descends relative to the vestibule. (From Berridge FR, Friedland GW, Tagart REB: *Thorax* 1966; 21:499–510. Used by permission).

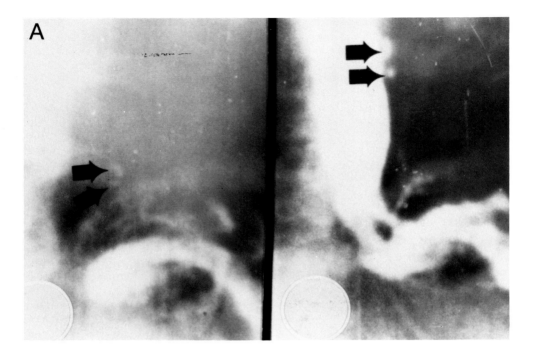

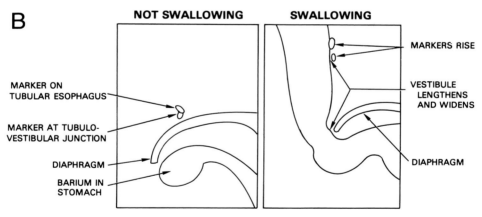

FIG 16–4.
Effect of swallowing. **A,** cine-esophagogram at rest and during swallowing. Note tantalum rings *(arrows)* on upper margin of vestibule and on esophagus above. **B,** diagram of **A.** The vestibule rises on swallowing.

stomach has ascended into the thorax. The stomach has multiple coarse, thick mucosal folds, so a herniated stomach may have thicker folds than a normal vestibule (Fig 16–5). The herniated stomach usually is much wider than the vestibule. Sometimes, however, it is not possible to distinguish gastric from vestibular mucosal folds, and the width of the herniated stomach may not exceed that of the nor-

mal vestibule. In these cases we rely on the B ring, which is a transverse mucosal fold at the upper end of the sling fibers of the stomach (the esophagogastric junction).[3] When the lower end of the vestibule is abnormally distended, as with a hiatal hernia, the B ring may appear as a thin ledgelike noncontractile narrowing (see Fig 16–5).[3]

Thus, if A and B rings are visible and the

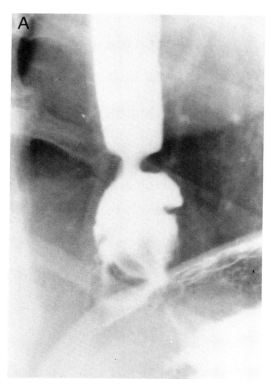

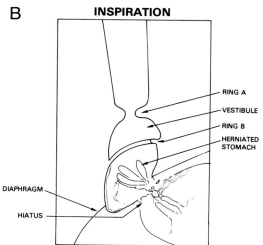

FIG 16–5.
Small, sliding hiatal hernia. **A,** esophagogram made with the patient lying prone over a bolster and swallowing barium. Film was exposed on inspiration. **B,** diagram of **A.** Note A and B rings, herniated pouch of stomach with thick gastric folds, and narrow hiatus. (From Friedland GW: *The causes of the various appearances normally seen at the lower end of the esophagus during a barium meal examination* (thesis). University of Pretoria, Republic of South Africa, 1967.)

pouch below the B ring is longer than 2 cm, the patient probably has a hiatal hernia.[3] On deep inspiration the hiatus narrows and compresses the herniated stomach, so it is possible to determine how much of the stomach has herniated into the thorax.[3] Sometimes areae gastricae are visible in the herniated pouch of the stomach, which aid in identification.

All of these features can be seen better if the patient swallows barium while lying prone over a bolster.[3] This increases the intra-abdominal pressure by about 5 to 10 mm Hg, which is far less than might be experienced in bending over to tie a shoelace, for example, so the pressure remains physiological.[4]

The sling fibers of the stomach are a thickening of the inner muscle layer of the stomach and are shaped like a horseshoe hooking around the notch between the lower edge of the vestibule and the fundus of the stomach.[3] The two arms run anteriorly and posteriorly toward the pylorus, parallel to the lesser curve of the stomach.[3] Sometimes these sling fibers create a notch, which is visible on an esophagogram between the distal end of the vestibule and the stomach when the patient has a sliding hiatal hernia (Fig 16–6).[3] It is important to recognize that the herniated stomach usually is pouch shaped, not stomach shaped. In most cases herniation occurs in

part of the fundus and part of the lesser curve of the stomach, which passes through the hiatus into the thorax. Because the hiatus compresses this herniated stomach, the portion that passes into the thorax resembles a pouch (see Fig 16–5).[3]

Our patient was 69 years old and examined prone over a bolster. No more than 1 to 2 cm of stomach was visualized in the thorax (see Fig 16–1), and this entire portion of the stomach immediately returned to the abdomen. Therefore the diagnosis of hiatal hernia was incorrect.

Does our patient have an ulcer in the distal esophagus as a result of reflux esophagitis? Protru-

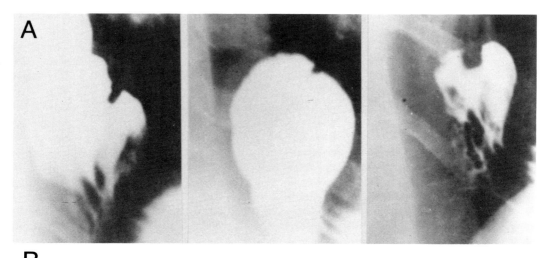

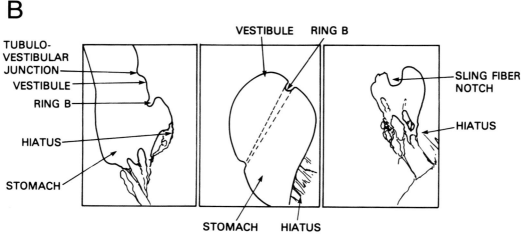

FIG 16–6.
A, hiatal hernia, showing sling fiber notch. The sling fibers lie immediately beneath the transverse mucosal fold (B ring) and become more prominent as the vestibule closes. **B,** diagram of **A.** (From Friedland GW: *The causes of the various appearances normally seen at the lower end of the esophagus during a barium meal examination* (thesis). University of Pretoria, Republic of South Africa, 1967.)

sions from the lumen of the distal esophagus are of two varieties: false or pseudoulcers and true ulcers.[5] Distinguishing between the two is important; if the patient does not have an ulcer, disastrous results may follow. A patient with chest pain may not receive treatment for a myocardial infarct; the clinicians, who should not rule out the diagnosis of myocardial infarct in this fashion, could be misled and the patient forced to undergo treatment for nonexistent ulcer, including procedures such as esophagoscopy.

Pseudoulcers occur in two locations: radiologically the vestibular pseudoulcer simulates a penetrating ulcer in the vestibule; the paravestibular pseudoulcer radiologically simulates a penetrating ulcer, at the A or B ring, at the A ring and extending above, or at the B ring and extending below.[5] There are two main types of pseudoulcer: Type 1 is a normal variation in which the results of endoscopy or autopsy are completely negative; in type 2 abnormalities found at endoscopy, surgery, or pathologic examination, such as an epiphrenic diverticulum, are not ulcers.[5]

Type 1 pseudoulcers have four features in common[5]: (1) they lie within the vestibule, or at the A ring and above, or at the B ring and below; (2) they are more readily visualized when the distal esophagus is well distended and are less prominent or disappear entirely when the esophagus empties; (3) they change size and shape with respiration; (4) they have no mucosal abnormality at endoscopy or autopsy that corresponds with the protrusion of barium seen on an esophagogram. Type 1 pseudoulcers can occur on either the right or left margins of the vestibule and may assume a variety of shapes. They are reproducible; they always look the same, even on two or three different studies obtained at different times.

The cause of type 1 pseudoulcer is not known, but there are two possibilities. Although the two layers of the muscularis propria of the esophagus (the inner transverse and outer longitudinal layers) lie more or less at right angles to each other in the middle of the esophagus, as they approach the vestibule the inner layer becomes more oblique, thins out, and separates.[6, 7] Thus type 1 pseudoulcers may consist of the bulging out of the mucosa in this area, as can happen in the pylorus in the torus defect.[8, 9]

Another possibility is that the phrenoesophageal membrane pulls out part of the wall of the esophagus on deep inspiration and on swallowing, causing a pseudoulcer.

The phrenoesophageal membrane is a tough, fibroelastic membrane that arises on the undersurface of the diaphragm and has two limbs. The upper limb passes through the hiatus and inserts into the esophagus more or less at the upper margin of the vestibule, in the region of the A ring, and does so very irregularly.[3, 6, 7] The lower limb inserts more or less at the B ring, also irregularly.[3, 6, 7] Fibers of the phrenoesophageal membrane pass between the muscle bundles and become continuous with the elastic trabeculae that pass through the wall of the esophagus to the submucosa.[7] Swallowing causes the esophagus to rise, so there is tension on the phrenoesophageal membrane (see Fig 16–4,B); on deep inspiration, the hiatus descends, so that there is again tension on the phrenoesophageal membrane (see Fig 16–3,C).[3] In either case the membrane could pull out part of the wall, creating a pseudoulcer.

The radiologic findings in our patient are compatible with type 1 pseudoulcer (see Fig 16–1).

There is a definite proved anatomical or pathological explanation for the radiological appearance of type 2 pseudoulcer. One possible explanation is the entrapment of barium between the sling fiber notch and the diaphragmatic hiatus in a patient with a sliding hiatal hernia. As the esophagus distends with further swallowing, the typical appearance of the sling fiber notch becomes evident, so that the cause of the pseudoulcer becomes clear. The sling fiber notch was not visible in our patient, thus excluding this diagnosis.

Type 2 pseudoulcer occurs when a herniated pouch of stomach overlaps the distal esophagus, producing the appearance of an ulcer.[5] However, if the patient is rotated to a different position the overlap is separated and the cause of the pseudoulcer becomes apparent. No such overlap was present in our patient.

Epiphrenic diverticulum can simulate a type 1 pseudoulcer or a penetrating ulcer (Fig 16–7). The important consideration in this case is that the diverticulum will be most obvious when the esophagus is partially collapsed, whereas a type 1 pseudoulcer is best seen on a well-distended distal esophagus. The lesion in our patient was best seen when the distal esophagus was well distended, suggesting that it was not a diverticulum.

Pseudodiverticulosis[10] can simulate type 1 pseudoulcer or true ulcer (Fig 16–8). The glands in the esophagus lie either superficial or deep relative to the muscularis mucosae.[6] Superficial glands occur only at the pharyngoesophageal and gastroe-

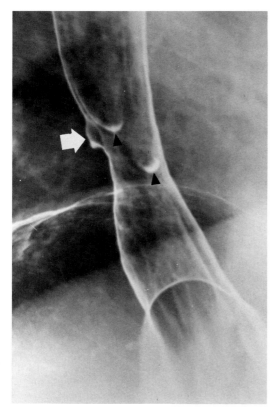

also a miscellaneous group of conditions causing esophagitis and ulcers.[11]

Reflux esophagitis usually can be distinguished from esophagitis due to infection by the patient's history, physical examination, and esophagogram.[11] For example, patients with reflux esophagitis complain of heartburn, whereas those with infectious esophagitis usually complain of pain on swallowing.[11]

Types of esophagitis due to infection that can cause ulcers include candidiasis, herpes, tuberculosis, histoplasmosis, and other fungal infections.[11] In such cases it is important to examine the patient's mouth and the back of the throat for ulcers or other evidence of candidiasis or herpes. In addition, patients with infectious esophagitis frequently are debilitated and usually are immunocompromised, which makes them susceptible to infection.[11] Our patient did not complain of heartburn or pain on swallowing; his pain was located primarily over the anterior aspect of the chest. He was not debilitated or immunocompromised, and his mouth and throat appeared normal.

The radiographic distribution of the lesions on

FIG 16–7.
Barium-air contrast esophagogram demonstrating two small epiphrenic diverticula *(arrowheads)* and an esophageal ulcer *(arrow).*

sophageal junctions.[6] A pseudodiverticulum is an enlarged inflamed deep esophageal gland,[10] which can be differentiated from type 1 pseudoulcer in that it is commonly multiple, usually smaller, and best seen when the esophagus is completely collapsed. A pseudodiverticulum is commonly associated with candidiasis or reflux esophagitis. The esophageal protrusion in our patient was much larger than a pseudodiverticulum and was best seen when the esophagus was well distended, making this diagnosis extremely unlikely.

A similar protrusion can be due to an ulcer in a patient with esophagitis (Fig 16–9). Several conditions can produce esophagitis resulting in ulcers in the distal esophagus and yielding an appearance similar to that seen in our patient.[11] Esophagitis usually is caused by gastroesophageal reflux (peptic esophagitis), but esophagitis secondary to infection, which also can cause ulcers, may exist, and there is

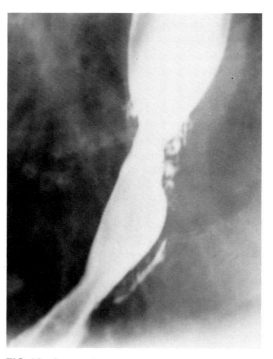

FIG 16–8.
Intramural pseudodiverticulosis. Note multiple small barium-filled protrusions.

CHAPTER 17

Pharyngeal Diverticula

Bronwyn Jones, M.B., B.S.
Martin W. Donner, M.D.

Case Presentation

Two patients had difficulty swallowing. In both, barium esophagograms were obtained (Fig 17–1,A and B). Describe the findings in these two patients. What are the most likely diagnoses? What might the initial symptoms be? How should the lesions be treated?

DISCUSSION

In Figure 17–1,A the most likely diagnosis is Zenker's diverticulum (also known as pharyngoesophageal diverticulum). This kind of diverticulum was first described in 1769 by Ludlow[1] as a "preternatural dilatation" of the pharynx. Currently, Zenker's diverticulum is thought to be a type of pulsion (and false) diverticulum in which there is protrusion of mucosa and submucosa through the posterior muscle layers of the pharynx, commonly through an anatomically weak area on the posterior wall. The most common site is between the oblique and horizontal fibers of the cricopharyngeal muscle; this triangular area is known as Killian's triangle or dehiscence. In fact, this is only one of several possible sites of weakness and potential herniation in this area.[2] Another less common site is through Laimer's triangle, bordered cranially by the cricopharyngeal muscle and caudally by the circular and longitudinal fibers of the cervical esophagus. Zenker's diverticulum is always found on the posterior wall of the pharynx. As it enlarges it tends to flop to one side, more commonly to the left (approximately, 50% are slightly to the left of midline, 30% in the midline, and 20% to the right of midline).

In 20,000 routine examinations, 22 patients had Zenker's diverticulum,[3] whereas 1.8% of patients with dysphagia[4] and 4% of those with esophageal disease had Zenker's diverticulum.[5] The entity is about three times more common in men than in women.[6]

Three developmental stages of Zenker's diverticulum have been described[3]:

Stage 1: A small protrusion.
Stage 2: A larger diverticulum; the lumina of the pharynx and the cervical esophagus still lie in a straight line.
Stage 3: The lumen of the large diverticulum lies in line with the hypopharynx.

Some authorities claim that stage 1 diverticula are not true diverticula but should be known as "inconstant or unstable diverticula" because they rarely enlarge and are commonly asymptomatic.[7] Early diverticula may not be visible during swallowing but may remain filled after swallowing. Ekberg and Nylander[8] differentiate between a true diverticulum and a pseudodiverticulum caused by cricopharyngeal prominence, with trapping of contrast between the peristaltic wave of the pharynx and the cricopharyngeal muscle.

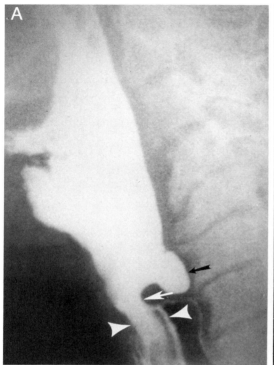 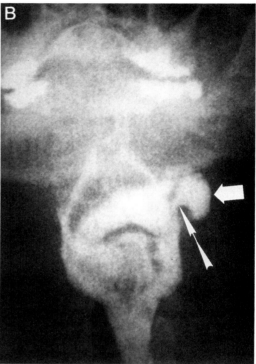

FIG 17–1.

A, lateral freeze frame from a cinepharyngogram shows a small Zenker's diverticulum posteriorly *(black arrow)* with the cricopharyngeal muscle prominent below the diverticulum *(white arrow)* and a jet of contrast inferiorly due to luminal compromise *(arrow-heads).* **B,** frontal stop frame from a cinepharyngogram demonstrates a lateral pharyngeal pouch on the left *(arrow)*. Note that it originates from the left piriform sinus and that it has a narrow neck *(arrow-heads).*

The pathogenesis of Zenker's diverticulum remains unclear, although dyscoordination between pharyngeal contraction and cricopharyngeal relaxation may be a contributing factor. Some manometric and cineradiographic studies have demonstrated premature sphincter closure in some patients with Zenker's diverticulum; many of the studies in the literature, however, were performed in patients with fully developed diverticula, at which point pharyngeal contraction and cricopharyngeal relaxation do not appear to be out of synchronization. Further studies are necessary, including those of the early stages of development, to clarify the contributing factors.

Gastroesophageal reflux may play a role in the development of Zenker's diverticulum.[9] Indeed, many patients with Zenker's diverticulum have radiographic findings suggestive of gastroesophageal reflux, such as segmental spasm with neutral barium, acid-induced spasm (acid-sensitive esopha-gus), hiatal hernia, and Schatzki's ring, sometimes with free gastroesophageal reflux during the radiographic examination.[10, 11]

The diverticulum bulges inferiorly as it enlarges, and the neck is narrow and higher than the diverticulum itself; hence the diverticulum often fills preferentially to the cervical esophagus. After a swallow or as the next swallow begins and the pharynx begins to rise, the diverticulum will often empty back into the pharynx, with the potential for overflow aspiration. Stasis is a prominent finding (often resulting in halitosis as an initial symptom). The diverticulum tends to collect ingested particulate matter (e.g., peas and corn kernels), and the patient may regurgitate undigested particles several hours after their ingestion. An air-fluid level may be identified within the diverticulum on soft-tissue radiographs of the neck.

Treatment depends on symptoms and on the size of the diverticulum. Many patients learn to empty the diverticulum by applying gentle manual pressure to the neck. Others adjust their dietary intake to exclude foods that easily lodge in the diverticulum. However, surgery may be necessary for symptomatic diverticula, especially when progressive enlargement occurs. Surgical treatment varies from simple diverticulopexy (tucking the diverticulum up so that it drains by gravity), to excision alone, to excision with cricopharyngeal myotomy. Recurrence is common, especially if cricopharyngeal myotomy is not performed with the original surgery.

Other diverticula or pouches may be demonstrated in the pharynx or pharyngoesophageal area. Although much less common than the posterior Zenker's diverticulum, lateral diverticula have also been described at the pharyngoesophageal junction.[12] These are thought to form at the level of a lateral slit near the outer and lateral border of the cricoid cartilage at the insertion of the cricopharyngeal muscle; this corresponds to the passage of the inferior laryngeal nerve. Diverticula with narrow and wide necks have been described at this level. Diverticula with wide openings may represent merely pouches or bulges due to a weak wall; those with narrow necks appear to be true diverticula (Fig 17–2).

Figure 17–1,B shows a unilateral lateral pharyngeal pouch, "ear," or diverticulum. Bachman et al.[13, 14] distinguish between tonsillar and piriform fossa ears, which they consider a common normal variant, and actual acquired diverticula, which arise from the piriform sinus ear when the bulging mucosa actually breaks through the poorly supporting fascia of the thyrohyoid membrane. Radiographically these appear to originate from the piriform sinus ear. Using this ter-

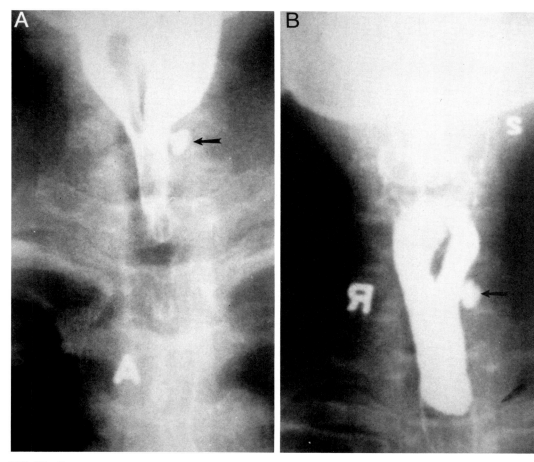

FIG 17–2.
A and **B,** two films from a cinepharyngogram show a diverticulum with a narrow neck *(arrows)* extending from the left lateral border of the pharyngoesophageal junction.

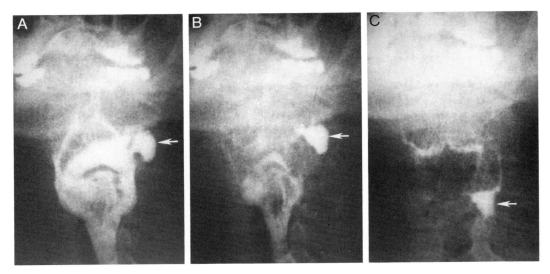

FIG 17–3.
(Same patient as in Fig 17–1,B) Three consecutive stop-frame prints from a cinepharyngogram. **A,** the pouch *(arrow)* is filled during actual bolus passage through the piriform sinus area. **B,** the pouch remains filled after swallowing. **C,** subsequently the pouch empties into the left piriform sinus, raising the potential for overflow aspiration of retained bolus.

minology, our patient (see Fig 17–1,B) may have a true diverticulum. The term "pouch" is preferable.

Opinions vary with regard to whether pouches represent a normal variant and whether they can be symptomatic. Incidence of pouches increases with age and in patients with pharyngeal paresis or muscular or neuromuscular disease affecting the pharynx. An association also has been proposed between the development of pouches and esophageal disease such as gastroesophageal reflux.[15] Pouches that empty with swallowing may be less significant than those that retain barium (and by inference other ingested liquids) after swallowing (Fig 17–3). These empty into the valleculae or piriform sinuses after the main bolus has passed, resulting in retention with the potential for overflow aspiration or even choking episodes.

Congenital diverticula also occur in the pharynx as a result of persistent branchial cleft tracts.[13, 14] The most common is that derived from the second cleft, which opens into the tonsillar fossa or vallecula. The third and fourth cleft tract remnants open into the piriform fossa.[14]

REFERENCES

1. Ludlow A: A case of obstructed deglutition, from a preternatural dilation of, and bag formed in the pharynx, in *Medical Observations and Inquiries,* vol 3. London, Society of Physicians, 1769, p 85.
2. Perrott JW: Anatomical aspects of hypopharyngeal diverticula. *Aust NZ J Surg* 1962; 31:307–317.
3. Wheeler D: Diverticula of the foregut. *Radiology* 1947; 49:476–481.
4. MacMillan AS: Statistical study of diseases of the esophagus. *Surg Gynecol Obstet* 1935; 60:394–402.
5. Hardy JD, Conn JH: Diseases of the esophagus. An analysis of 308 consecutive cases. *Ann Surg* 1962; 155:971–990.
6. Harrington SW: The surgical treatment of pulsion diverticula of the thoracic esophagus. *Ann Surg* 1949; 192:606–618.
7. VanOverbeek JJM: The hypopharyngeal diverticulum. Endoscopic treatment and manometry. Assen, The Netherlands, VanGorcum BV, 1977.
8. Ekberg D, Nylander G: Dysfunction of the cricopharyngeal muscle. *Radiology* 1982; 143:481–486.
9. Knuff TE, Benjamin SB, Castell DO: Pharyngeal (Zenker's) diverticulum: A reappraisal. *Gastroenterology* 1982; 82:734–736.
10. Smiley TB, Caves PK, Porter DC: Relationship between posterior pharyngeal pouch and hiatus hernia. *Thorax* 1970; 25:725–731.
11. Delahunty JE, Margulies SI, Alonso UA, et al:

The relationship of reflux esophagitis to pharyngeal pouch (Zenker's diverticulum). *Laryngoscope* 1971; 81:570–577.

12. Ekberg O, Nylander G: Lateral diverticula from the pharyngoesophageal junction area. *Radiology* 1983; 146:117–122.

13. Bachman AL, Seaman WB, Macken KL: Lateral pharyngeal diverticula. *Radiology* 1968; 91:774–782.

14. Bachman AL: Benign non-neoplastic conditions of the larynx and pharynx. *Radiol Clin North Am* 1978; 16:273–290.

15. Jones BJ, Ravich WJ, Donner MW, et al: Pharyngoesophageal interrelationships: Observations and working concepts. *Gastrointest Radiol* 1985; 10:225–233.

CHAPTER 18

Ingested Foreign Bodies: Radiological Diagnosis and Management

Gary G. Ghahremani, M.D.

Case Presentation

A clinical history of sore throat and swallowing discomfort associated with a recent choking episode in two patients prompted radiological examination for possible foreign body ingestion (Figs 18–1 and 18–2). Can you recognize the precise nature of the demonstrated findings? What are the differential diagnosis and recommended course of action?

DISCUSSION

Radiologic diagnosis of an ingested foreign body is relatively simple if the item is a dense metallic object, such as a coin, often swallowed accidentally by children. In many instances, however, accurate clinical information regarding the incident and the physical properties of the ingested particle are not available. Furthermore, the detection of radiolucent or faintly opaque items on plain radiographs poses a formidable challenge because a variety of normally occurring calcifications are potential sources of confusion and diagnostic error. This is illustrated in both of the cases presented.

The apparent round density visible on the chest radiograph in the child (see Fig 18–1) could represent a semiopaque foreign body lodged in the proximal esophagus, for example, a large button seen en face with its thick rim casting a ringlike shadow. On careful evaluation of the original chest films, however, an experienced radiologist would identify it as the normal ossification center of the manubrium.

This anatomic structure, as well as other associated sternal calcifications, is sometimes quite prominent in the pediatric age group.[1] These are best seen on oblique views of the chest and should not be mistaken for foreign bodies (Fig 18–3).

The cluster of calcifications visible in the pharyngoesophageal region in the adult patient (see Fig 18–2) may present a similar diagnostic problem. Because most of it projects over the posterior aspect of the air-containing laryngotracheal junction, it is recognizable as the calcified cricoid cartilage. The smaller density located horizontally behind it might be considered an extraneous piece of bone stuck in the throat but actually represents an ossified part of the cricoid lamina. Knowledge of cartilaginous components of the larynx and various patterns of their calcification is crucial in differentiating these normal structures from an ingested bone or other object trapped in the same area[2-4] (Fig 18–4).

Most foreign bodies are swallowed accidentally, and numerous blunt objects less than 1 to 2

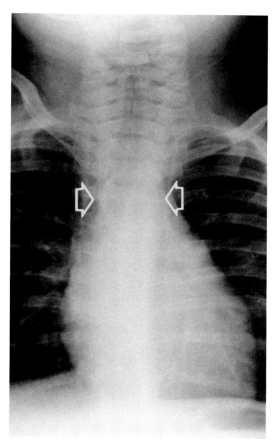

FIG 18–1.
Chest film in a 1-year-old girl demonstrates a circular, 2 cm density located in the midline at the level of aortic arch *(arrows)*.

ways provided but should be suspected whenever children or adults experience acute dysphagia and suprasternal discomfort following a choking or gagging episode. Respiratory difficulty and wheezing also may develop if a large bolus of meat or other bulky object is lodged in the pharyngoesophageal region, causing extrinsic compression of the trachea.[2, 8–10] More commonly, however, such symptoms are associated with food or foreign body impaction in the larynx and airways. They can lead to an often fatal "cafe coronary," whereby the choking person becomes mute because of laryngospasm and unable to exchange air despite vigorous respiratory efforts. The Heimlich maneuver (abdominal thrust) should be applied promptly to expel the obstructing object by forced increase in intrathoracic pressures.

Sometimes patients are unaware of foreign

cm in diameter may pass uneventfully through the alimentary tract.[5] Therefore this discussion is limited to symptomatic cases in which the pharynx or esophagus is the principal site of impaction. Such complications are not infrequent among children, the mentally retarded, and senile patients, who tend to place inedible items in their mouths and swallow them inadvertently. Similar incidents occur in certain occupations, notably among carpenters and dressmakers, who have the habit of holding nails or needles with their lips. Other contributing factors include careless preparation of food that may contain fragments of bone, gluttonous eating of improperly masticated meat, and artificial dentures that cover the sensitive area of the hard palate in edentulous patients.[6, 7]

A history of foreign body ingestion is not al-

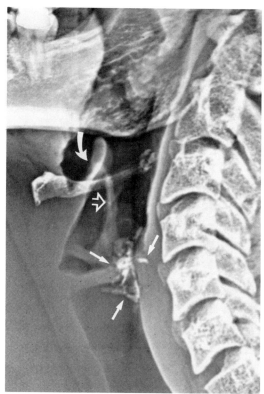

FIG 18–2.
Xeroradiography of the lateral neck in a 42-year-old man shows a cluster of irregular calcifications in the region of the hypopharynx and laryngotracheal junction *(arrows)*. Note that the epiglottis *(curved arrow)* and aryepiglottic folds *(open arrow)* are clearly outlined by air during phonation.

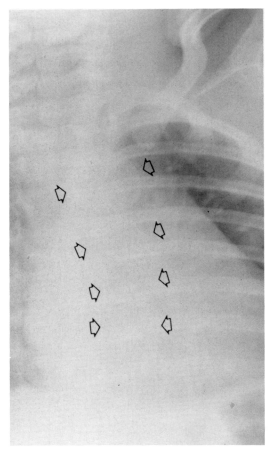

FIG 18–3.
Chest radiograph of a 15-month-old boy in the left posterior oblique projection reveals multiple round densities related to sternal ossification centers *(arrows)*. These should not be mistaken for foreign bodies.

cervical esophagus usually produce pain and discomfort in the adjacent region. Therefore the most useful initial study is a radiograph or xeroradiograph of the lateral neck,[2, 3] centered just below the angle of the mandible and covering an area between the base of the skull and the thoracic inlet. The exposure is made with the patient in an upright or sitting position with the neck well extended while the shoulders are held low and posteriorly. It is of utmost importance that the patient be instructed to say a prolonged "Eeee. . ." during filming. This phonation maneuver distends the pharyngoesophageal region with air, enhancing the visibility of soft tissue structures that serve as important anatomic landmarks. The same technique should be used to obtain an anteroposterior view of the neck, although it is less informative than the lateral projection. If the

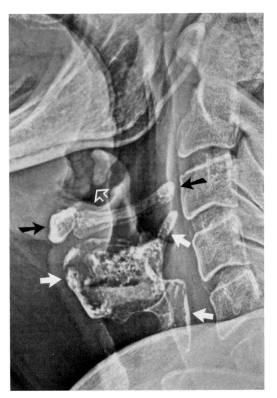

FIG 18–4.
Xeroradiograph of the lateral neck in an elderly patient shows extensive ossification of the thyroid and cricoid cartilages *(white arrows)* and the body and greater horns of the hyoid bone *(black arrows)*. The lingual tonsils are visible within the air-distended valleculae *(open arrow)*. (Courtesy Claire Smith, MD, Rush Medical College, Chicago.)

body ingestion but seek medical attention because of progressive retrosternal pain and dysphagia. These symptoms may reflect blockage of a preexisting lower esophageal stricture or tight Schatzki's ring by food particles, tablets, or other materials (Fig 18–5).

Radiologists play a crucial role in the evaluation and management of ingested foreign bodies. The principal goals of radiologic examinations are detection of the impacted object and documentation of its nature, location, and associated complications. A tailored approach is recommended based on the available clinical history and symptoms.

Foreign bodies lodged in the hypopharynx or

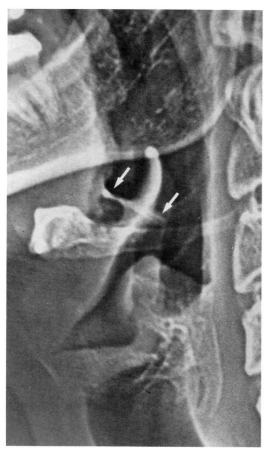

FIG 18–5.
Demonstration of a fish bone lodged in the vallecula *(arrows)*, with coexistent ossification of various laryngeal cartilages, in a middle-aged woman.

suspected foreign body is not visible, the radiologist may assume that it has moved distally into the alimentary tract. Accordingly, radiographs of the chest and abdomen should be obtained. When these plain films also fail to show an opaque item or extraluminal air due to perforation, a search for a possible radiolucent object should be pursued in the symptomatic patient.[7–10] In such cases careful fluoroscopic evaluation of the upper gastrointestinal tract with orally administered contrast media is a safe and simple alternative to endoscopy.

Small but dangerously sharp foreign bodies such as fish bones commonly are entrapped in the pharynx and are often retained in the piriform sinuses, valleculae, or palatine or lingual tonsils. It is of critical importance to evaluate each of these areas

on radiographs or xerograms of the neck. Particular attention should be given to the cartilaginous parts of the larynx. They calcify or ossify with advanced age and become a major source of diagnostic error in differentiation from foreign bodies[2–4] (see Fig 18–5).

As a general rule, ingested bony fragments appear as linear or slightly curved densities with well-defined margins as a result of edge enhancement or xeroradiography.[2] Sometimes the sharp tip of an entrapped needle or piece of bone may be seen piercing the pharyngeal wall while the rest of it projects into the air-containing lumen. Most glass particles also are sufficiently opaque to be readily visible,[11] but pieces of radiolucent plastic or wood can pose diagnostic difficulties.[12] In such cases radiographs may provide evidence for the induced mucosal

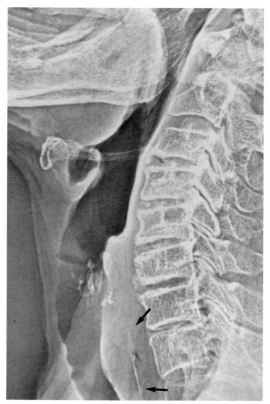

FIG 18–6.
Xeroradiograph of the lateral neck shows perforation of the cervical esophagus by a chicken bone *(arrows)*. The surrounding soft tissue abscess contains some gas and causes compression of the posterior tracheal wall. (Courtesy Claire Smith, MD, Rush Medical College, Chicago.)

constrictor muscles but stop in the cervical esophagus, where the muscular activity is much weaker (Fig 18–7). If the object is sufficiently opaque, its presence can be discerned on lateral neck radiographs; otherwise an esophagogram is necessary for accurate diagnosis. The examination also may disclose an underlying abnormality such as cervical esophageal web. A simple technique for detection of bone spicules or other pointed nonopaque objects in the pharyngoesophageal region is to have the patient swallow a barium-soaked cotton pledget, which will tend to become entangled in the foreign body (Fig 18–8). The radiographs obtained after oral administration of barium also can be helpful in demonstrating objects that become impregnated

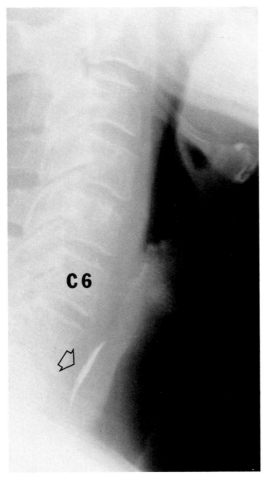

FIG 18–7.
Lateral neck film shows a fragment of oyster shell in the cervical esophagus *(arrow)*. It is lodged in the typical location just below the cricopharyngeal muscle at the C6 level.

trauma, manifesting as localized soft tissue emphysema, retropharyngeal edema, hematoma, or abscess (Fig 18–6). The posterior walls of the pharynx and cervical esophagus normally are parallel to the anterior edge of the cervical spine. Because their thickness is usually less than 70% of the diameter of the C4 vertebral body, a pathologic process should be suspected if there is either a localized lump or diffuse widening of the retropharyngeal soft tissues.[2, 3]

An area predisposed to foreign body impaction is the cervical esophagus just below the cricopharyngeal muscle at the C6 level. Many swallowed objects are forced distally by the strong pharyngeal

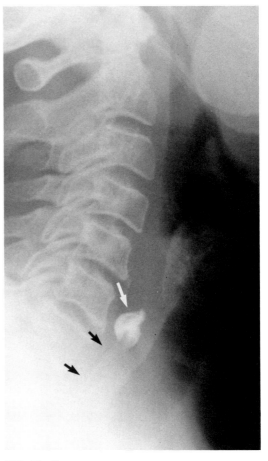

FIG 18–8.
This patient had ingested a faintly opaque chicken bone *(black arrows)*, which was made apparent by the entangled piece of cotton soaked in barium *(white arrow)*.

with or retain contrast material on their surface (Fig 18–9).

The adult tubular thoracic esophagus is approximately 25 to 30 cm long and 2 to 2.5 cm in diameter. Nevertheless, it is subject to food or foreign body impaction at several levels, including the area of indentation by the aortic arch or the left bronchus, the gastroesophageal junction, and proximal to any pre-existing narrowing due to peptic stricture, Schatzki'sring, or benign or malignant neoplasm.[6–8] Chest radiographs may reveal the presence of a radiopaque object in the esophagus. The correct localization is simplified because flat objects, such as a coin, orient themselves in the coronal plane if in the esophagus (Fig 18–10); in contrast, those located in the larynx or trachea lie in the sagittal plane. The presence of a nonopaque foreign body is suggested by indirect signs of obstruction: air-fluid level in the distended esophageal lumen and lack of gas in the gastric fundus. Esophagography can confirm the site and nature of impacted material as well as the cause of associated luminal narrowing. Clinical or radio-

graphic findings indicative of perforation warrant initial esophagography with iodinated water-soluble agents. If there is no apparent extraluminal leakage, however, additional films should be obtained during administration of barium. This approach allows more accurate identification of small perforations, which are sometimes difficult to visualize with aqueous contrast medium.[13]

Radiologic studies will not demonstrate a foreign body if it has passed through the gastrointestinal tract. Nevertheless, it could have caused enough mucosal trauma and local irritation of the pharynx or esophagus to account for persistent dysphagia. If such symptoms do not disappear within a 24-hour period of clinical observation, endoscopy should be performed to search for a retained foreign body.

REMOVAL OF FOREIGN OBJECTS

The management of objects lodged in the pharynx or esophagus depends on their physical character-

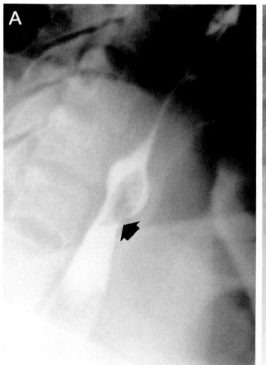 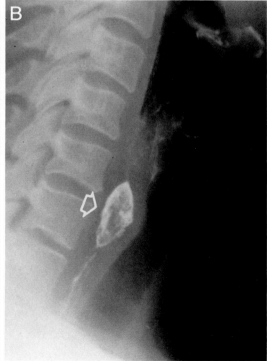

FIG 18–9.

A, spot film exposed during ingestion of barium reveals a radiolucent object above a cervical esophageal web *(arrow).* **B,** subsequent film shows retention of barium on the surface of this foreign body *(arrow),* an almond that was retrieved by endoscopy.

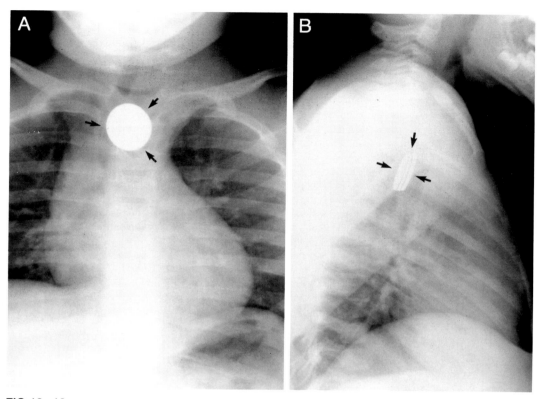

FIG 18–10.
Chest films in frontal **(A)** and lateral **(B)** projections disclose a stack of three coins impacted in the proximal esophagus *(arrows)*. Note that such flat discoid objects are retained in the coronal plane with the esophagus, whereas they are oriented sagittally when aspirated into the trachea.

istics and associated complications. Prompt surgical-intervention is warranted when there is evidence for perforation of the wall or impaction secondary to an underlying obstruction process.[5-7] Endoscopic removal under direct vision is recommended for sharp-edged and irregularly shaped foreign bodies.[10, 14] However, several radiologic techniques are available for the retrieval of blunt objects and disimpaction of food particles from the esophagus.

A conservative approach might be justified in dealing with intraesophageal foreign bodies that have a smooth surface and a diameter of less than 1.5 to 2.0 cm. These may pass spontaneously through the alimentary tract, and digestible materials will be dissolved once they reach the stomach.[5-7] Their passage beyond the narrowed segment of the esophagus can be facilitated by oral administration of effervescent agents used in double-contrast radiography.[15] The released carbon dioxide gas distends the esophagus and increases the intraluminal pressure, pro-moting disimpaction and distal movement of the entrapped material (Fig 18–11).

Several pharmacologic agents have proved useful by relieving spasm of the lower esophageal sphincter. For this purpose anticholinergic drugs such as probantheline bromide may be injected intravenously at a dose of 25 mg.[16] Similarly, glucagon in doses of 0.5 to 1.0 mg intravenously can be used to relieve esophageal food impaction.[17]

The use of proteolytic enzymes such as papain to induce artificial digestion of impacted food is not recommended. This process may take several hours and can cause serious mucosal injury or even perforation of the esophageal wall.[18, 19] Endoscopic removal of a large meat bolus may cause problems because the retraction of multiple fragments requires repeated insertion of the instrument, with increasing risk for perforation.[14, 20]

The extraction of coins and other blunt objects from the esophagus can be achieved easily under fluoroscopic guidance. A safe and simple approach is to insert a Foley catheter through the mouth and advance the tip of it beyond the intraluminal foreign body.[21, 22] The inflatable balloon of the catheter is then filled with water-soluble contrast material; with the patient in the prone oblique position, the Foley catheter is generally withdrawn so that its opacified balloon pulls along the retained foreign body (Fig 18–12). When the object reaches the oropharynx, it can be expelled by the patient or removed manually to avoid possible aspiration. Utmost care must be exercised in patients with esophagitis or stricture to prevent overdistention of the Foley balloon and perforation.

A similar technique is the removal of ferromagnetic objects with a feeding tube that has a cylindrical magnet attached to its distal end.[23] This procedure is particularly useful for the retrieval from the esophagus and stomach[24] of small disk batteries that contain toxic and corrosive agents such as potassium hydroxide and mercury. These batteries may leak or disintegrate within the gastrointestinal tract, causing caustic injury and possible mercury poisoning.[25] Therefore prompt retrieval of ingested alkaline batteries is recommended, although their small size may suggest spontaneous passage through the alimentary tract.

The radiologist should also be acquainted with the technique of esophageal foreign body extraction using a Dormia-type wire basket.[26] This procedure can be done safely under fluoroscopy and is particularly useful for the retrieval of blunt spherical objects and food boluses lodged in the esophagus.

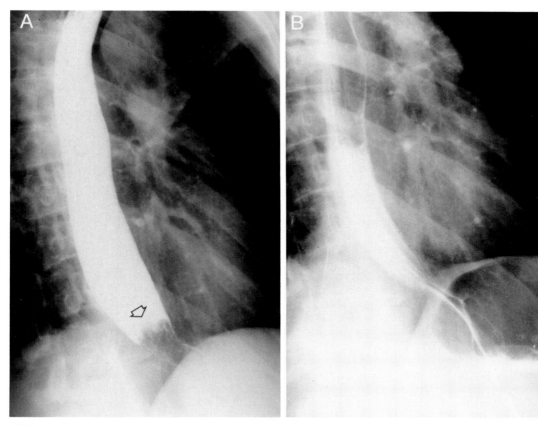

FIG 18–11.

A, barium examination of the esophagus demonstrates an impacted meat bolus *(arrow)* causing complete obstruction of the lumen, with absent gas in the gastric fundus. **B,** repeat study after intravenous glucagon (0.5 mg) and oral administration of an effervescent agent shows disimpaction of food. The gastroesophageal region and gas-filled fundus now appear normal.

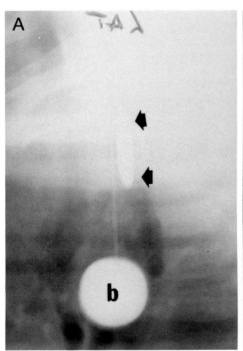 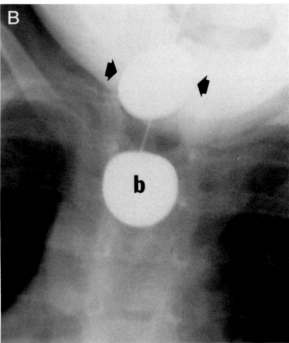

FIG 18–12.
Radiologic technique for the extraction of blunt esophageal foreign bodies. **A,** with the patient in the right lateral position, a Foley catheter is advanced beyond the ingested coin *(arrows),* and its balloon *(b)* is opacified with water-soluble contrast material. **B,** with patient in the prone oblique position, the Foley catheter is gently withdrawn under fluoroscopic control, bringing along the coin *(arrows)* into the oropharynx and mouth.

PATIENT MANAGEMENT

Because foreign body impaction may signify the presence of organic or functional esophageal disorder, the removal of an impacted object is best followed by contrast esophagography (Fig 18–13). This simple examination permits assessment of the motor function and patency of the pharynx and esophagus and detection of any injuries caused by the foreign body or instrumentation during its retrieval.[20, 27]

In this context, a wide spectrum of clinical findings may be associated with mucosal trauma induced by an ingested object. Sharp metallic items such as a needle can produce a silent perforation because of their small size and the relatively low bacterial content of the upper gastrointestinal tract.[28] On the other hand, serious complications may result due to an intramural abscess, generalized sepsis, and massive hemorrhage.[6, 7, 14]

The passage of foreign bodies beyond the pharynx and esophagus carries a more favorable prognosis because 95% to 98% are excreted uneventfully;[5, 29] the remaining 2% to 5% are retained within the alimentary tract but only occasionally cause perforation at the sites of narrowing or angulation (e.g., the pylorus, duodenal flexures, and ileocecal valve).[28]

In contrast to densely opaque objects, the radiographic detectability of toxic or radiolucent material is limited. This is particularly important in pediatric cases involving accidental ingestion of plastic or wooden toys, medications, and adulterated food. In one series, foreign bodies were documented radiographically in only 62% of 125 children.[30] Several manufacturers in the United States have initiated the process of opacifying plastic toys with barium sulfate.[31] Similar problems are encountered after certain types of foreign body ingestion in adults. For example, large numbers of cocaine-filled packets sometimes are swallowed by drug dealers during international smuggling operations. These

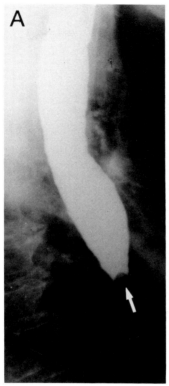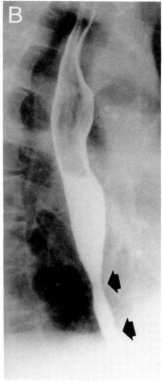

FIG 18–13.
A, complete obstruction of the distal esophagus by an ingested cherry seed *(arrow).* **B,** repeat study after administration of glucagon and effervescent material shows disimpaction of the foreign body but also a long peptic stricture *(arrows),* which was subsequently dilated under fluoroscopy using the inflatable balloon catheter technique.

nonopaque rubber balloons may produce intestinal blockage or systemic intoxication if their contents are released within the gastrointestinal tract.[32] Several authors have described the radiologic features that permit correct preoperative diagnosis of these conditions.[32–34] There are also a few reports concerning ingestion of pull-tabs from beverage cans.[35] Such pieces of thin aluminum are almost radiolucent and easily overlooked on the en face projection. When exposed in profile or on edge, however, their presence can be more readily appreciated on chest or abdominal radiographs.

REFERENCES

1. Ogden JA, Conlogue GJ, Bronson ML, et al: Radiology of postnatal skeletal development. II. The manubrium and sternum. *Skeletal Radiol* 1979; 4:189–195.
2. Smith C, Ramsey RG: Xeroradiography of the lateral neck. *Radiographics* 1982; 2:306–328.
3. Muroff LR, Seaman WB: Normal anatomy of the larynx and pharynx, and differential diagnosis of foreign bodies. *Semin Roentgenol* 1974; 9:267–280.
4. Chamberlain WE, Young BR: Ossification (so-called "calcification") of normal laryngeal cartilages mistaken for foreign body. *AJR* 1935; 33:441–450.
5. Pellerin D, Fortier-Beaulieu M, Gueguen J: The fate of swallowed foreign bodies. Experience with 1,250 instances of subdiaphragmatic foreign bodies in children. *Prog Pediatr Radiol* 1969; 2:286–302.
6. Chaikhouni A, Kratz JM, Crawford FA: Foreign bodies of the esophagus. *Am Surg* 1985; 51:173–179.
7. Selianov V, Sheldon GF, Cello JP, et al: Management of foreign body ingestion. *Ann Surg* 1984; 199:187–191.

8. Handler SD, Beaugard ME, Canalis RF, et al: Unsuspected esophageal foreign bodies in adults with upper airway obstruction. *Chest* 1981; 80:234–236.

9. Humphry A, Holland WG: Unsuspected esophageal foreign bodies. *J Can Assoc Radiol* 1981; 32:17–20.

10. O'Neill JA Jr, Holcomb GW Jr, Neblett WW: Management of tracheobronchial and esophageal foreign bodies in childhood. *J Pediatr Surg* 1983; 18:475–479.

11. Felman AH, Fisher MS: The radiographic detection of glass in soft tissue. *Radiology* 1969; 92:1529–1531.

12. Newman DE: The radiolucent esophageal foreign body: An often forgotten cause of respiratory symptoms. *J Pediatr* 1978; 92:60–63.

13. Foley MJ, Ghahremani GG, Rogers LF: Reappraisal of contrast media used to detect upper gastrointestinal perforations: Comparison of ionic water-soluble media with barium sulfate. *Radiology* 1982; 144:231–237.

14. Ricote GC, Torre LR, Perez De Ayala V, et al: Fiberendoscopic removal of foreign bodies of the upper gastrointestinal tract. *Surg Gynecol Obstet* 1985; 160:499–504.

15. Rice BT, Spiegel PK, Dombrowski PJ: Acute esophageal food impaction treated by gas-forming agents. *Radiology* 1983; 146:299–301.

16. Ghahremani GG, Heck LL, Williams JR: A pharmacologic aid in the radiographic diagnosis of obstructive esophageal lesions. *Radiology* 1972; 103:289–293.

17. Trenkner SW, Maglinte DDT, Lehman GA, et al: Esophageal food impaction: Treatment with glucagon. *Radiology* 1983; 149:401–403.

18. Goldner F, Danley D: Enzymatic digestion of esophageal meat impaction: A study of Adolph's meat tenderizer. *Dig Dis Sci* 1985; 30:456–459.

19. Holsinger JW Jr, Fuson RL, Sealy WC: Esophageal perforation following meat impaction and papain ingestion. *JAMA* 1968; 204:734–735.

20. Meyers MA, Ghahremani GG: Complications of fiberoptic endoscopy. I. Esophagoscopy and gastroscopy. *Radiology* 1975; 115:293–300.

21. Nixon GW: Foley catheter method of esophageal foreign body removal: Extension of applications. *AJR* 1979; 132:441–442.

22. Campbell JB, Quattromani FL, Foley LC: Foley catheter removal of blunt esophageal foreign bodies. Experience with 100 consecutive children. *Pediatr Radiol* 1983; 13:116–119.

23. Himadi GM, Fischer GJ: Magnetic removal of foreign bodies from the upper gastrointestinal tract. *Radiology* 1977; 123:226–227.

24. Jaffe RB, Corneli HM: Fluoroscopic removal of ingested alkaline batteries. *Radiology* 1984; 150:585–586.

25. Votteler TP, Nash JC, Rutledge JC: The hazard of ingested alkaline batteries in children. *JAMA* 1983; 249:2504–2506.

26. Shaffer HA Jr, Alford BA, DeLange EE, et al: Basket extraction of esophageal foreign bodies. *AJR* 1986; 147:1010–1013.

27. Bladergroen MR, Lowe JE, Postlethwait RW: Diagnosis and recommended management of esophageal perforation and rupture. *Ann Thorac Surg* 1986; 42:235–239.

28. Hashmonai M, Kaufman T, Schramek A: Silent perforations of the stomach and duodenum by needles. *Arch Surg* 1978; 113:1406–1409.

29. Joseph AE, Crampton AR, Agha FP, et al: Impacted foreign bodies in the duodenum. *Am J Gastroenterol* 1987; 82:1074–1077.

30. Bender L, Anderson WA: Pediatric gastrointestinal foreign body ingestions. *Ann Emerg Med* 1984; 13:112–117.

31. Glassbrenner K: Giving visibility to accidentally swallowed toy. *JAMA* 1984; 252:323–324.

32. Trent MS, Kim U: Cocaine packet ingestion. Surgical or medical management? *Arch Surg* 1987; 122:1179–1181.

33. McCarron MM, Wood JD: The cocaine "body packer" syndrome: Diagnosis and treatment. *JAMA* 1983; 250:1417–1420.

34. Beerman R, Nunez D Jr, Wetli CV: Radiographic evaluation of the cocaine smuggler. *Gastrointest Radiol* 1986; 11:351–354.

35. Rogers LF, Igini JP: Beverage can pull-tabs. Inadvertent ingestion or aspiration. *JAMA* 1975; 233:345–348.

CHAPTER 19

Ingestion of Caustic Material

Howard J. Ansel, M.D.

Case Presentation

This 20-year-old man came to the hospital emergency room with severe burns of the mouth following ingestion of a drain cleaner in a suicide attempt. An esophagogram obtained shortly after admission (Fig 19–1) demonstrates some spasm of the upper esophagus but normal distensibility without ulceration distally. Air bubbles are present within the esophagus. What is the likely outcome of this event? What complications might arise?

DISCUSSION

The ingestion of caustic materials, whether acid or alkaline, may cause considerable damage to the upper gastrointestinal tract. The damage results from the direct contact of the offending agent with the mucosa of the involved organ. Traditionally it has been taught that the ingestion of an alkaline material causes esophageal lesions but spares the stomach. When alkaline materials are ingested, severe esophageal spasm results in prolonged contact of the agent with the esophageal mucosa. Material that reaches the stomach may be partially neutralized by the gastric acid. On the other hand, it has been taught that swallowed acid often spares the esophagus but summates with the acid in the stomach, to cause severe gastric injury. However, studies with air contrast techniques showed that acid also may severely affect the esophagus.[1]

Immediately and during the first several days after ingestion of caustic material intense inflammatory reaction occurs. Pharyngeal burns may lead to aspiration and airway compromise. Radiographically, severe spasm may be seen. Manifestations of abnormal motility, either severe rigidity with an atonic esophagus or marked tertiary contractions, may be present. Pathologically, protein coagulation, epithelial destruction, inflammatory changes, and vascular thrombosis with liquification of the submucosa and occasionally the muscularis occur.[2]

Over the next 2 to 5 days the dead tissue sloughs, extensive ulceration occasionally leading to perforation occurs, and healing by granulation begins. Fibroblasts appear by day 5, and begin laying down collagen by days 8 to 12. Free or contained perforations of the viscus may occur soon after ingestion or during the ulcerative and early repair phases of the injury, when the organ wall is weakest. Contained perforations adjacent to the trachea and aorta may lead to mediastinitis, tracheoesophageal fistulas, or esophageal aortic fistulas. Severe pneumonitis, pulmonary abscess, or exsanguinating hemorrhage is the result.

During the next several weeks healing by granulation and fibrosis continues. In the esophagus this leads to stricture formation and shortening. Shorten-

are seen. In addition, the stomach may be dilated and the antrum and pylorus rigid. In a smaller percentage of patients perforation may ensue or gastric emphysema, an ominous sign, may be seen. If the material enters the duodenum the duodenal bulb may become atonic and dilate. Marked edema of the mucosa and ulceration frequently are present. The distal duodenum also may be damaged.[5]

As the stomach heals and fibrosis occurs, the distal stomach is most frequently affected. The lesser curvature contracts and the antrum narrows. Achlorhydria is common. The radiographic picture is reminiscent of infiltrating carcinoma of the stomach, tuberculosis, syphilis, or granulomatous disease (Fig 19–3). This narrowing may be so severe that total gastric outlet obstruction results[6] (Fig 19–4,A and B). In some cases pneumatosis intestinalis also occurs. When the duodenum is affected it

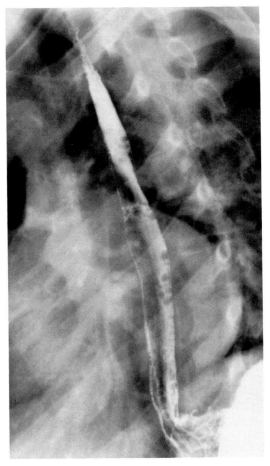

FIG 19–1.
A single esophagogram film demonstrates distensibility of the esophagus with no evidence for mucosal ulceration or spasm. The filling defects in the film are air bubbles. At fluoroscopy the esophagus was atonic; no peristaltic activity was demonstrated.

ing of the esophagus pulls the gastroesophageal junction into the chest, resulting in hiatal hernia, frequently associated with gastroesophageal reflux (Fig 19–2). A much delayed complication of caustic esophageal injury is development of carcinoma.[3]

The newer concentrated liquid alkaline cleaners may produce more severe damage. Full-thickness mural necrosis and gangrene might appear within hours of ingestion, causing mediastinitis perforation and peritonitis.[4]

When caustic material enters the stomach it courses along the lesser curvature of the antrum. Atony, rigidity, ulceration, and thickening of folds

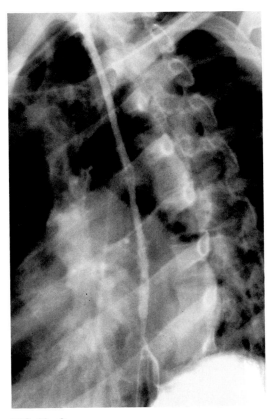

FIG 19–2.
Radiograph of our patient 1 month after suicide attempt demonstrates a severe stricture of the esophagus with shortening and presence of a hiatal hernia. Reflux was demonstrated.

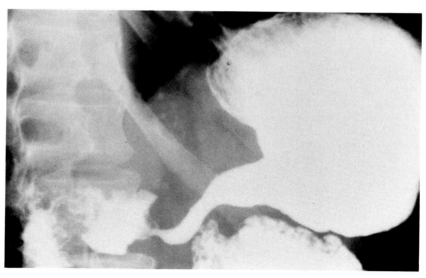

FIG 19–3.
This patient's stomach at the time of ingestion appeared normal. Approximately 1 month later, marked narrowing of the distal body and antrum of the stomach suggests infiltrating carcinoma.

may remain atonic. If the agent reaches the small bowel, ulceration with gastrointestinal bleeding may occur.

In the case presented, severe esophageal stricture with hiatal hernia and severe scarring of the gastric antrum with gastric outlet obstruction was the result of caustic ingestion. In such cases it is important to remember to evaluate the entire upper gastrointestinal tract to evaluate the extent of damage adequately.

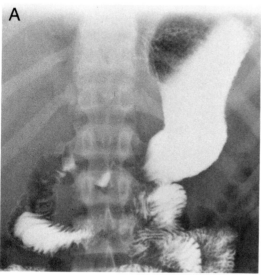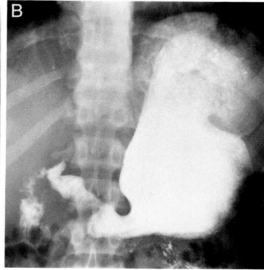

FIG 19–4.
A, our patient's stomach at the time of ingestion demonstrates mucosal irregularities and ulceration along the body and antrum. **B,** radiograph obtained 1 month after ingestion; the stomach is grossly deformed, with contraction of the antrum and duodenum, and there is evidence of outlet obstruction.

REFERENCES

1. Muhletaler CA, Gerlock AJ, DeSoto L, et al: Acid corrosive esophagitis: Radiographic findings. *Am J Roentgenol Radium Ther* 1980; 134:1137–1140.
2. Johnson EE: A study of corrosive esophagitis. *Laryngoscope* 1963; 73:1651–1696.
3. Franken EA: Caustic damage of the gastrointestinal tract: Roentgen features. *Am J Roentgenol Radium Ther* 1973; 118:77–85.
4. Martel W: Radiologic features of esophagogastritis secondary to extremely caustic agents. *Radiology* 1972; 103:31–36.
5. Muhletaler CA, Gerlock AJ, DeSoto L, et al: Gastroduodenal lesions of ingested acids: Radiographic findings. *Am J Roentgenol Radium Ther* 1980; 135:1247–1252.
6. Karon AB: The delayed gastric syndrome with pyloric stenosis and achlorhydria following the ingestion of acid—A definite clinical entity. *Am J Dig Dis* 1962; 7:1041–1046.

CHAPTER 20

Abnormal Esophageal Peristalsis

E. T. Stewart, M.D.

Wylie J. Dodds, M.D.

Case Presentation

A 24-year-old man was referred by his internist for examination because of progressive dysphagia that had worsened over the past several years. The morphologic appearance of the esophagus is recorded on an overhead film (Fig 20–1). Based on this study, without having had a chance to observe the fluoroscopic appearance of the esophageal motility, what should be included in the differential diagnosis?

DISCUSSION

Detailed discussion of the differential diagnosis is preceded by a review of the anatomy and physiology of the esophagus and by consideration of proper technique for examining the esophagus to evaluate motility disorders and morphologic abnormalities.

Normal Anatomy and Physiology

Swallowing is a complex process.[1-4] The act of deglutition involves interaction of neuromuscular events primarily controlled by cranial nerves. The oral and pharyngeal phases of swallowing are not considered here but should not be ignored in the day-to-day observations of swallowing and esophageal motor disorders. The esophagus is a tubular structure that, by definition, begins at the cricopharyngeal muscle, also known as the upper esophageal sphincter (UES), and ends at the esophagogastric junction, which lies just below the lower esophageal sphincter (LES). The esophagus is lined by stratified squamous epithelium. The transition between squamous epithelium and columnar epithelium, which lines the remainder of the gut, occurs at the squamocolumnar junction, better known to the endoscopist as the gastroesophageal junction or Z line. Two features are unique to the esophagus. One concerns the intrinsic muscles. As with the other viscera, there are two muscle layers, an inner circular and an outer longitudinal layer. Unique to the esophagus, these muscles are striated in the upper part of the esophagus and smooth in the distal part. There is a transition zone in the mid-portion of the esophagus so that the lower two thirds is primarily smooth muscle. Neutral control of peristalsis is mediated primarily by motor fibers in the vagus nerve. The UES is a distinct muscle, composed mostly of the striated cricopharyngeal muscle. The LES is a zone of smooth muscle but is not a distinct muscle group. The second feature unique to the esophagus, as opposed to the other viscera, is the lack of a serosal covering. This has implications when consid-

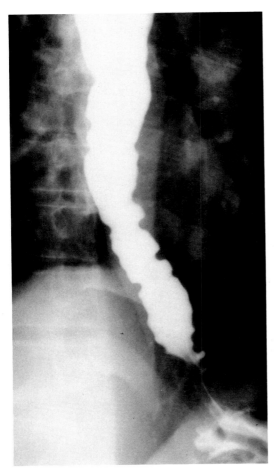

FIG 20–1.
Single film from a barium swallow.

ering spread of primary neoplasms of the esophagus.

Esophageal motility refers to the peristaltic events that occur during the transport of a bolus from the mouth to the stomach (Fig 20–2). Normally, in the resting state the UES and LES are actively contracted. The remainder of the musculature is at rest. During swallowing and transport of the bolus the UES and LES relax and a stripping wave, consisting of contracting circular muscle, travels the length of the esophagus in an aboral direction, stripping the bolus into the stomach. This action is the peristaltic sequence. The speed of the peristaltic wave in the pharynx is rapid, between 10 and 25 cm/sec; in the esophagus the velocity slows to between 2 and 4 cm/sec.

By convention, the mechanical events that oc-

cur in the body of the esophagus include primary peristalsis, secondary peristalsis, and tertiary, nonpropulsive contractions. Primary peristalsis is the peristaltic sequence initiated by the act of swallowing. Secondary peristalsis is identical to primary peristalsis in every way but mode of initiation. Secondary peristaltic activity is initiated simply by the presence of a bolus within the lumen of the esophagus, such as regurgitated air or food. Secondary peristalsis can be initiated at any level in the esophagus simply by the presence of a bolus at that point. Once initiated, a secondary peristaltic sequence is identical to a primary wave as it clears the esophagus. Secondary peristalsis can be used to examine the esophagus in the patient who cannot or will not swallow. This is done by inserting a nasoesophageal tube and injecting an appropriate bolus, usually 5 to 10 ml. Tertiary or nonpropulsive contractions are not peristaltic events but are simply lumen-obliterating or non-lumen-obliterating segmental nonpropulsive contractions. Tertiary contractions are a frequent phenomenon and may be superimposed on otherwise normal appearing primary or secondary peristaltic activity. Tertiary nonpropulsive contractions often accompany severe motility abnormalities; however, they are seen frequently in normal individuals as well. Nonperistaltic or tertiary contractions are limited to the smooth muscle portion of the esophagus.

Radiologic Examination

A comprehensive examination of the esophagus should provide information concerning morphologic features and motility as well as such phenomena as gastroesophageal reflux. The examination can be tailored to answer the clinician's specific questions about the presence or absence of obstruction, stricture, tumor, or inflammatory disease. In most cases the technique should provide answers to either avoid additional examination or direct the patient for more specific evaluation, such as direct visualization with or without biopsy or manometry.

Fluoroscopic examination of esophageal motor disturbances is highly accurate. The qualitative assessment of abnormal fluoroscopic mechanical events is specific. The only advantage of manometry over fluoroscopic observations is the quantitative information added by pressure recordings. Because the radiographic examination is highly sensitive for detection of motility disorders, it should be the primary screening method. Careful observation and recording of fluoroscopic events are therefore essential. Esophageal motility cannot be adequately examined with the patient erect, because of the influence of gravity. For proper assessment of motility the esophagus must be made to work to clear itself. Therefore the patient should be recumbent, either prone or supine; the prone oblique position is used most commonly for initial observations of esophageal motility. Although bolus size can be varied, a suitable bolus for examining motility is between 5 and 10 ml barium. Repetitive swallowing will inhibit peristaltic events; therefore the patient should be instructed that only a single swallow is necessary while peristalsis is being observed. The essential

portion of the peristaltic sequence is the lumen-obliterating contraction immediately proximal to the contrast bolus; the stripping wave is observed as it traverses the length of the esophagus (Fig 20–3). Several swallows may be necessary to evaluate peristalsis adequately, because of subtle mechanical alterations that are insignificant but might at first glance appear unusual. For example, it is not unusual for a small amount of barium to escape from the primary peristaltic sequence in the mid-portion of the esophagus. This can be a normal event due to the somewhat lower pressures in the esophagus near the region of the aortic arch. Also, occasional

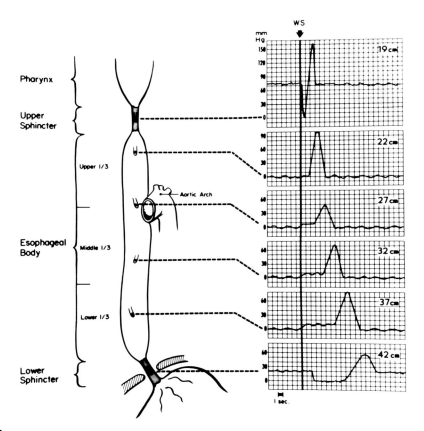

FIG 20–2.
Manometric recording of normal peristalsis. The thoracic esophagus is bounded by two sphincter muscles, the upper esophageal sphincter (UES) and the lower esophageal sphincter (LES). This schematic represents the pressure events that might be measured during normal peristalsis. The UES and LES are contracted between swallowing sequences. Following a "wet swallow" *(WS),* the UES and LES relax. The aboral progress of the stripping wave can be measured manometrically as the tail of the bolus passes the recording catheter. Notice how the two sphincters contribute to the peristaltic sequence following relaxation. After the bolus passes, the UES and LES return to their resting tonic contraction. (From Dodds WJ: Radiology. V. Esophagus and esophagogastric region, in Margulis AR, Burhenne HJ (eds): *Alimentary Tract Radiology,* ed 3, vol 1. St Louis, CV Mosby Co, 1983, pp 529–603. Used by permission.)

A. Normal Peristalsis - No Proximal Escape of the Barium Bolus

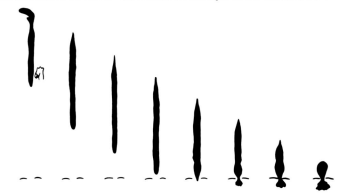

B. Normal Peristalsis - Some Escape of Barium in Proximal Esophagus

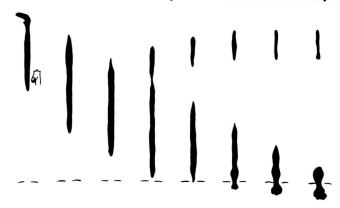

FIG 20–3.
Schematic of normal peristalsis. **A,** primary peristalsis initiated by swallowing. The lumen-obliterating aboral contraction wave progresses the length of the esophagus uninterrupted, resulting in complete emptying. As the wave reaches the distal esophagus, slowing occurs. These events are primarily manifestations of circular muscle contractions. Although the longitudinal muscles are also contracting, their shortening effects are not seen unless some marker, such as a diverticulum or ring, is present that dramatizes the longitudinal motion. **B,** some escape of barium from the primary peristaltic wave in the upper esophagus is a frequent finding and is due to lower pressure in this region, which can be normal. This phenomenon should not be confused with abnormal peristalsis. (From Dodds WJ: Radiology. V. Esophagus and esophagogastric region, in Margulis AR, Burhenne HJ (eds): *Alimentary Tract Radiology,* ed 3, vol 1. St Louis, CV Mosby Co, 1983, pp 529–603. Used by permission.)

breaking of the primary wave occurs in normal subjects. Tertiary contractions can be seen superimposed on otherwise normal appearing peristaltic activity and generally represent an incidental finding. Most significant motility disorders are not random but are reproducible and can be demonstrated with diligence and repeated swallows.

The morphologic assessment of esophageal mucosa and anatomy is best accomplished by a combination of single- and double-contrast techniques, with the patient in erect and recumbent positions, and should include documentation of strictures, webs, rings, and hiatal hernia. Spontaneous gastroesophageal reflux and reflux induced by stress maneuvers are important observations. Use of a marshmallow or, in some cases, a barium-impregnated tablet of known dimensions is of value in demonstrating the significance of narrowed areas of the esophagus, suggesting either benign or malignant stricture. Subtle strictures are easily overlooked, but their significance is readily apparent when the patient is challenged with a solid bolus, such as a marshmallow. Attention to the UES and

LES should allow an adequate assessment of whether the sphincters open normally.

Abnormal Esophageal Motility

Abnormalities demonstrated in esophageal motility are limited. Peristaltic abnormalities are (1) diminished incidence of peristalsis induced by swallowing, (2) inadequate peristaltic waves or breaking of the waves, and (3) absence of peristaltic activity, or aperistalsis. Tertiary or nonpropulsive contractions are frequently superimposed on normal peristalsis or abnormal peristaltic events.

Table 20–1 divides esophageal motility disorders into primary and secondary groups. Primary esophageal motility disorders are motility disturbances that have no associated underlying systemic disease and appear to represent isolated phenomena in the esophagus. Secondary motility disorders are associated with an underlying disease in which the manifestations of esophageal involvement are only part of the disease spectrum.

Discussion

The clinical history is of paramount importance in the assessment of motor disturbances involving the esophagus. The patient presented has symptoms that have progressed slowly over several years. The patient is young and has no history of an underlying disease process. Even this meager history suggests a chronic, possibly primary process. We are asked to assess a single radiograph and make some comment about a motility disorder without access to the dynamic events observed fluoroscopically. Figure 20–1 shows a mildly dilated esophagus. The most striking findings are the numerous segmental non-lumen-obliterating tertiary contractions. The LES segment is not readily identified anatomically, but the general area is somewhat narrowed. Because the esophagus seems to be entirely full of barium, this narrowing of the LES could be due to the fact that the patient is drinking rapidly or to retained barium within a mildly dilated esophagus in which there is no adequate peristaltic activity or possibly a distal obstruction.

Possible causes include diffuse esophageal spasm, achalasia, or stricture with proximal obstruction. Is this related to underlying disease such as diabetes or myasthenia gravis? Could the findings be associated with a chemical ingestion, caustic burn, or scleroderma?

Although scleroderma is a chronic disease, this appearance would be unusual. Patients with sclero-

TABLE 20–1.
Classification of Esophageal Motility Disorders*

Primary
  Achalasia
  Diffuse esophageal spasm
  Intestinal pseudo-obstruction
  Presbyesophagus
  Congenital tracheoesophageal fistula
  Chalasia
Secondary
  Connective tissue
  Chemical or physical
    Reflux (peptic) esophagitis
    Caustic esophagitis
    Vagotomy
    Radiation
  Infection
    Fungal moniliasis
    Bacterial: tuberculosis, diphtheria, etc.
    Parasitic: Chagas' disease
    Viral: herpes simplex
  Metabolic
    Diabetes
    Alcoholism
    Amyloidosis
    Serum pH and electrolyte disturbances
  Endocrine disease
    Myxedema
    Thyrotoxicosis
  Neurologic disease
    Parkinsonism
    Huntington's chorea
    Wilson's disease
    Cerebrovascular disease
    Multiple sclerosis
    Amyotrophic lateral sclerosis
    CNS neoplasm
    Bulbar poliomyelitis
    Pseudobulbar palsy
    Friedreich's or hereditary spastic ataxia
    Familial dysautonomia (Riley-Day syndrome)
    Stiff man's syndrome
    Ganglioneuromatosis
  Muscular disease
    Myotonic dystrophy
    Muscular dystrophy
    Oculopharyngeal dystrophy
    Myasthenia gravis (neuromotor end plate)
  Vascular
    Varices?
    Ischemia?
  Neoplasm
    Invasion
    Systemic effects
  Pharmacologic
    Atropine, propantheline, curare, etc.

*From Dodds WJ: Radiology. V. Esophagus and esophagogastric region, in Margulis AR, Burhenne HJ (eds): *Alimentary Tract Radiology*, ed 3, vol 1. St Louis, CV Mosby Co, 1983, pp 529–603. Used by permission.

derma initially may manifest tertiary activity as an early motor abnormality; however, the striking segmental contractions in this case would be unusual. The principle abnormality in scleroderma is atrophy of the smooth muscle, which is found in the distal half to two thirds of the esophagus.[6, 7] The atrophy leads to breaking of the primary wave in the distal esophagus. In as much as the LES is also involved, there may be incompetence of the LES segment and free gastroesophageal reflux. A demonstrable hiatal hernia also is common in these patients. Scleroderma is an unlikely explanation for the findings in our patient; the features of scleroderma are demonstrated in Figure 20–4. It should be remembered that it is not unusual for patients with scleroderma with severe reflux esophagitis to develop a peptic stricture, most commonly seen in the distal esophagus. This can result in an appearance that may mimic achalasia. Other manifestations of scleroderma, such as pulmonary disease or musculoskeletal changes, can help with the diagnosis.

Ingestion of a caustic substance results in the immediate appearance of a severe chemical burn and coagulation necrosis of the mucosa. This precedes the rapid appearance of superficial ulceration and sloughing of the esophageal mucosa.[8] Within weeks, severe fibrosis may result in marked stricturing of the esophagus. Accompanying the acute burn is a nonspecific motility disturbance, characterized mainly by absence of normal peristaltic activity and breaking of the primary peristaltic wave in the involved segments. The absence of ulceration and atony in this case are not indicative of acute caustic injury. Further, this patient's history is not consistent with this diagnosis because his symptoms are chronic.

One of the most common metabolic disorders encountered in clinical practice is diabetes. Abnormalities frequently seen in the esophagus of diabetic patients are mild motor disturbances that, almost without exception, are unassociated with clinical symptoms.[9, 10] Breaking of the primary peristaltic wave, inadequate clearance with escape from the primary wave, and tertiary contractions are among the most common motility alterations. Occasionally there may be mild dilation of the esophagus. The very striking segmental contractions and dilatation seen in this case are much more marked than normally encountered in patients with diabetes. For these reasons, diabetes is excluded from consideration.

Myasthenia gravis, a neuromuscular disease characterized by weak skeletal muscle contraction, would be expected to present primarily as a pharyn-

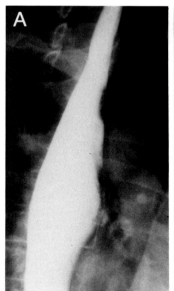
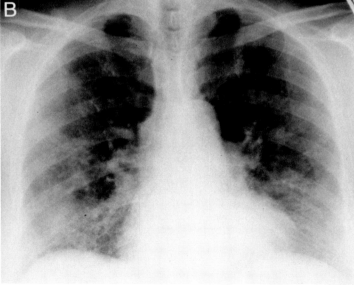

FIG 20–4.
Scleroderma. **A,** features of scleroderma include absent peristalsis in the distal esophagus, mild dilation, and reflux, which was present in this patient. **B,** usually the chest film is abnormal, with parenchymal changes consistent with the diagnosis of scleroderma. Other clinical features of systemic sclerosis, such as Raynaud's phenomenon, also herald the correct diagnosis.

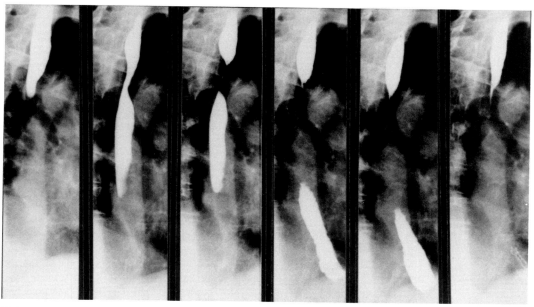

FIG 20–5.
Myasthenia gravis. Fatigue and inadequate contraction in the striated muscle have allowed considerable barium to escape the primary peristaltic sequence. The remaining thoracic esophagus clears itself adequately. These motility changes are rapidly reversed by the injection of a cholinesterase inhibitor. (From Dodds WJ: Radiology. V. Esophagus and esophagogastric region, in Margulis AR, Burhenne HJ (eds): *Alimentary Tract Radiology,* ed 3, vol 1. St Louis, CV Mosby Co, 1983, pp 529–603. Used by permission.)

geal or upper esophageal motor abnormality.[11] Symptoms in myasthenia frequently manifest after the patient is asked to swallow repetitively, because the muscles tire with use. Escape from the primary wave in the proximal third of the esophagus after passage of the primary peristaltic sequence is the usual appearance (Fig 20–5). There is nothing in Figure 20–1 to suggest that this patient has myasthenia. In fact, his motor disturbance appears to involve the entire esophagus. Therefore myasthenia is unlikely.

Obstruction alters the appearance of the esophagus, depending on whether it is acute or chronic and on the level of obstruction. Obstructing lesions can be benign, such as a peptic stricture, or malignant due to primary or secondary tumor. The patient almost always has dysphagia. As obstruction becomes more severe, the esophagus begins to dilate proximal to the obstruction and peristalsis becomes ineffective. Motility may vary. Early in obstruction the esophagus tries vigorously to empty itself and may appear to contract actively, with weakening of the peristaltic sequence due to the obstruction. With time peristalsis becomes less active and the decompensated esophagus dilates. In cases of high-grade long-standing distal obstruction, the esophagus may appear dilated and atonic. It is this situation that may resemble achalasia[12] (Fig 20–6). The appearance of the esophagus in our patient does not demonstrate a definite distal obstruction, and we can exclude this diagnosis with reasonable confidence even with a single film. In addition, most patients with malignant obstruction with dysphagia have had symptoms for less than 6 months.

The two most likely causes of the findings in Figure 20–1 are diffuse esophageal spasm (DES) or achalasia.

Diffuse esophageal spasm is considered a primary motor disorder of the esophagus and is characterized by clinical symptoms of dysphagia with segmental lumen-obliterating contractions on radiologic examination.[13] The wall of the esophagus often is thickened as a result of hypertrophy of the smooth muscle. Patients with DES are generally middle-aged and the dysphagia is somewhat unusual in that it is accompanied by significant chest pain or odynophagia. When these patients are studied manometrically, the lumen-obliterating contractions may be of high amplitude. Although the LES segment generally relaxes normally, in some patients it re-

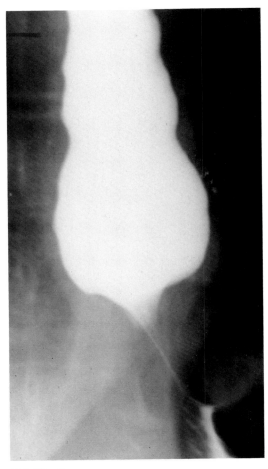

FIG 20–6.
Pseudoachalasia due to infiltrating carcinoma. Tumor infiltrating submucosally in the distal esophagus is producing a 2 to 3 cm narrowing at the esophago-gastric junction. Note dilation of the body of the esophagus. Peristalsis is ineffective in clearing the esophagus. Some tertiary activity is seen in the distal esophagus. This patient with adenocarcinoma of the stomach has findings mimicking achalasia. Unlike achalasia, symptoms have been present for only a short time, usually less than 6 months.

laxes incompletely. The lumen-obliterating contractions are generally reproducible, and when they are severe they compartmentalize the esophagus (Fig 20–7,A and B). Dysphagia and odynophagia are due to the forceful nonpropulsive contractions on a bolus as it passes.

Achalasia, the correct diagnosis in this case, is also a primary motor abnormality. Achalasia is interesting in that it has a spectrum at its presentation.

The early literature demonstrating the radiographic appearance of achalasia typically showed a markedly dilated aperistaltic esophagus with a "bird beak" appearance caused by failure of the LES segment to relax (Fig 20–8,A). In many patients, however, achalasia, is now discovered before massive dilation of the esophagus occurs. The early manifestations of the disease often include impaired relaxation of the LES, vigorous nonpropulsive contractions primarily in the distal half of the esophagus, and only mild dilation. This "vigorous achalasia," as seen in Figure 20–1, may be misinterpreted as esophageal spasm. In fact, some evidence suggests that DES and achalasia are closely related diseases.[14] Achalasia generally is considered to be caused by denervation of the esophagus. There is either impairment or loss of ganglion cells in Auerbach's plexus. In some cases there may be wallerian degeneration and a decreased number of cells in the medullary dorsal motor nucleus. Because the esophagus was denervated, methacholine chloride (Mecholyl Chloride) was used as an early test to confirm the diagnosis of achalasia. Subcutaneous administration of methacholine produces prompt and vigorous contraction in the denervated esophagus, most marked in the distal third to half of the esophagus. Since the advent of esophageal manometry and direct measurements of LES pressure, the methacholine test is less commonly used. The failure of the LES segment to relax is easily documented at the time of manometry. The radiologic counterpart of direct manometric measurements of the LES is the use of amyl nitrite. Amyl nitrite is a smooth muscle relaxant; after its inhalation the LES segment relaxes, allowing confirmation of the suspicion of achalasia (Fig 20–8,B).

The management of achalasia varies. Currently, pneumatic dilation is the preferred initial procedure in the majority of patients. Pneumatic dilation is best performed as a joint procedure by a gastroenterologist and a radiologist. Usually, pneumatic dilation with balloon pressures between 8 and 12 pounds per square inch achieves adequate sphincter dilation (Fig 20–8,C). During dilation of the LES in patients with achalasia there is mucosal disruption, evidenced by superficial hemorrhage. In approximately 3% of these patients esophageal perforation can be expected as a complication of the procedure and appears to be unavoidable. Examination with water contrast immediately following pneumatic dilation is the preferred method to identify such esophageal perforation.[15] Immediate iden-

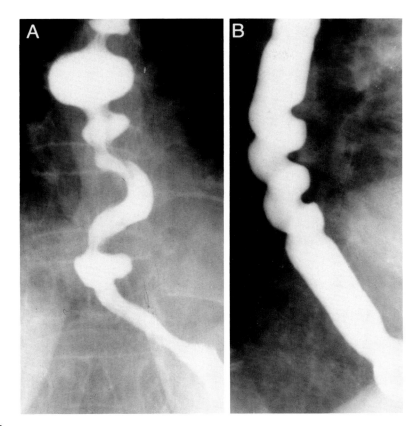

FIG 20−7.
Diffuse esophageal spasm (DES). **A,** Lumen-obliterating contractions of DES. This phenomenon is seen on repeated swallows, and generally the segmental contractions occur at the same location and have a "shish kebab" appearance. **B,** segmental contractions in the mid-esophagus. The "curling" appearance, as seen here, occasionally is seen in patients with DES.

tification of perforation results in the lowest morbidity.

A myotomy through the region of the sphincter (Heller myotomy) generally is done in patients who do not respond well to pneumatic dilation or in whom complications arise. After the LES is ablated by Heller myotomy the patient is at risk for gastroesophageal reflux. Impaired peristaltic activity in patients with achalasia may then predispose these patients to reflux esophagitis. Therefore an antireflux procedure may be performed at the same time as myotomy.

Although patients with achalasia are at increased risk for subsequent development of esophageal carcinoma, there are no established guidelines for surveillance of this patient population. However, during any radiologic study it is important to evaluate the mucosal surface throughout the esophagus

and to document the motility disturbance. For the same reasons, it is important that the endoscopist visualize the entire esophagus in patients with achalasia and not concentrate attention on the LES segment.

Many cases of disturbed esophageal motility elude classification. Minor and subtle transient motility disturbances are not uncommon in otherwise normal patients. These phenomenon may be related to anxiety, drugs, or the examination technique. On the other hand, significant motility disturbances usually are reproducible, dramatic, and commonly associated with significant clinical symptoms. The radiographic examination should be the primary screening method when a motility disturbance is suspected. An understanding of the normal peristaltic events and the method for examining the esophagus is essential. Extrapolating a motility disorder

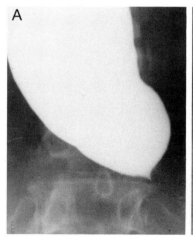 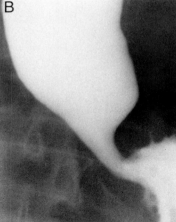 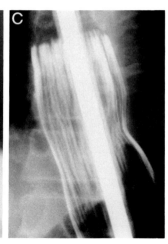

FIG 20–8.
Achalasia. **A,** the classic "bird beak" deformity at the tonic lower esophageal sphincter (LES) is displayed. The proximal aperistaltic esophagus is markedly dilated. **B,** film taken 60 seconds after the inhalation of amyl nitrite (with the patient standing) dramatically demonstrates relaxation of the LES. This maneuver allows a confident diagnosis of achalasia. Other conditions, such as an obstructing tumor or benign peptic stricture, will not change under the influence of amyl nitrite, which is a smooth muscle relaxant. **C,** pneumatic dilation of the LES segment is the preferred initial treatment for achalasia. Indentation of the bag identifies the location of the LES during the procedure.

after viewing a single static film of the esophagus can be extremely difficult, because dynamic observations of esophageal motility seen at the time of fluoroscopy are an essential part of the examination. Although it is unfair to ask the reader to commit to a diagnosis on the basis of a single film, it does allow a basis for discussion of the possibilities.

REFERENCES

1. Ingelfinger FJ: Esophageal motility. *Physiol Rev* 1958; 38:533.
2. Dodds WJ: Radiology. V. Esophagus and esophagogastric region, in Margulis AR, Burhenne HJ (eds): *Alimentary Tract Radiology,* ed 3, vol 1. St Louis, CV Mosby Co, 1983, pp 529–603.
3. Stewart ET: Radiographic evaluation of the esophagus and its motor disorders. *Med Clin North Am* 1981:1173–1194.
4. Dodds WJ: Cannon Lecture. Current concepts of esophageal motor function: Clinical implications for radiology. *AJR* 1977; 128:549.
5. Hogan WJ, Dodds WJ, Stewart ET: Comparison of roentgenology and intraluminal manometry for evaluating oesophageal peristalsis (abstract). *Rendic Gastroenterol* 1973; 5:28.
6. Creamer B, Andersen HA, Code CF: Esoph-
ageal motility in patients with scleroderma and related diseases. *Gastroenterologia* 1956; 86:763.
7. Treacy WL, et al: Scleroderma of the esophagus: A correlation of histologic and physiologic findings. *Ann Intern Med* 1963; 59:351.
8. Martel W: Radiologic features of esophagogastritis secondary to extremely caustic agents. *Radiology* 1972; 103:31.
9. Hollis JB, Castell DO, Braddom RL: Esophageal motor function in diabetes mellitus and its relation to peripheral neuropathy. *Gastroenterology* 1977; 73:1098.
10. Vix V: Esophageal motility in diabetes mellitus. *Radiology* 1969; 92:363.
11. Fischer RA, et al: Esophageal motility in neuromuscular disorders. *Ann Intern Med* 1965; 63:229.
12. Lawson TL, Dodds WJ: Infiltrating carcinoma simulating achalasia. *Gastrointest Radiol* 1976; 1:245.
13. Creamer B, Donoghue FE, Code CF: Pattern of esophageal motility in diffuse spasm. *Gastroenterology* 1958; 34:782.
14. Kramer P, Harris LD, Donaldson RM Jr: Transition from symptomatic diffuse spasm to cardiospasm. *Gut* 1967; 8:115.
15. Stewart ET, et al: Desirability of roentgen examination immediately after pneumatic dilatation for achalasia. *Radiology* 1979; 130:589.

PART 3

Stomach-Duodenum

CHAPTER 21

Gastric Outlet Obstruction

Howard J. Ansel, M.D.

Case Presentation

This 70-year-old man had a several-month history of abdominal pain that had become progressively worse. During the previous week he had noted increasing pain with progressive vomiting; he was vomiting after every meal, and the vomitus contained nondigested food. An upper gastrointestinal examination was performed (Fig 21–1,A and B). What is the cause of the vomiting? What conditions must be considered in the differential diagnosis for the cause of this condition?

DISCUSSION

The vomiting of nondigested food, the presence of food within the stomach 8 to 12 hours after meals, and positive saline load test findings suggest the presence of a gastric outlet obstruction. Of the numerous causes of gastric outlet obstruction the two most common are peptic disease and carcinoma. Peptic ulcer disease, whether of the duodenal bulb, pyloric channel, or distal antrum, accounts for nearly two thirds of cases of gastric outlet obstruction. Patients usually have evidence of chronic ulcer disease, with the obstruction caused by a combination of edema and scarring (Fig 21–2). Some patients respond to medical management of the obstruction, but more than 90% require surgical intervention within 1 year.[1]

Because of the considerable amount of retained material within the stomach, endoscopy frequently is markedly hampered. The upper gastrointestinal examination probably is the study of choice in the evaluation of these patients. Entubation and aspiration of the stomach contents permits a better examination. Every effort should be made to visualize the pylorus and duodenum with contrast material; the presence of scarring and deformity in the duodenal bulb and postbulbar area is highly suggestive of duodenal ulcer disease as a cause for the obstruction.[2, 3]

Nearly one third of cases of gastric outlet obstruction are due to gastric adenocarcinoma (Fig 21–3). These lesions usually involve the gastric antrum. An infiltrating tumor or tumor mass results in marked narrowing of the lumen and obstruction. The presence of retained material may hinder the differentiation between benign peptic ulceration with edema and infiltrating adenocarcinoma. Other primary gastric malignancies, such as lymphoma, and prolapsing benign tumors may obstruct. Carcinoma of the duodenum is rare but may be signalled by outlet obstruction. Extension of tumor from adjacent structures such as the pancreas is an additional cause.[4–7]

Inflammatory conditions, especially granulomatous processes, may involve the antrum. Although infrequent, Crohn's disease, gastric syphilis

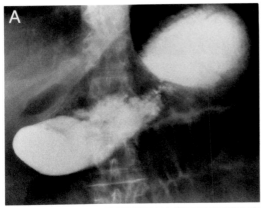

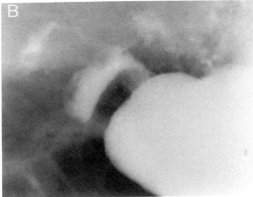

FIG 21–2.
Considerable retention of food particles mixed with barium is evident present in the stomach of this patient with peptic disease. Because of the retained material, the cause for the obstruction could not be seen radiographically.

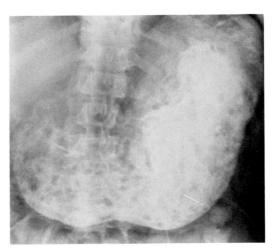

FIG 21–1.
A, barium and secretions remain in the stomach 30 minutes after ingestion of contrast material. **B,** coned down view of a deformed duodenal bulb shows no contrast passing beyond into the more distal duodenum.

sarcoidosis, and tuberculosis should be considered when antral narrowing is encountered. Adhesions from previous gallbladder surgery, irradiation, and amyloidosis have a similar radiographic appearance on rare occasions.[8, 9]

Acute inflammatory conditions, such as pancreatitis and pseudocyst, may involve the gastric wall with edema, spasm, and subsequent outlet obstruction. The clinical findings are helpful in identifying such a case.

Antral diaphragms, enteric duplications, and heterotopic pancreatic tissue are other rare causes for outlet obstruction.[10, 11]

The ingestion of caustic materials (Fig 21–4), especially acids, causes severe damage to the stomach. Ulceration and necrosis and subsequent spasm and scarring result in marked narrowing of the an-

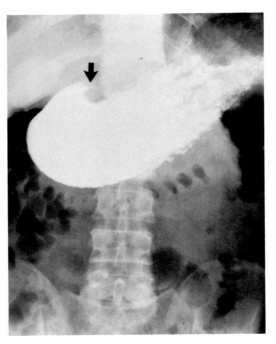

FIG 21–3.
Contrast fails to empty from the stomach. The distal antrum is tightly narrowed, with a suggestion of shouldering effect from a mass *(arrow).* An infiltrating adenocarcinoma was found at surgery.

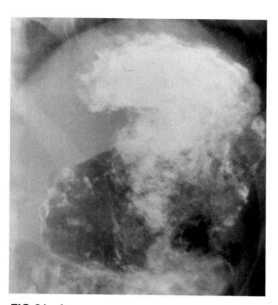

FIG 21–4.
One month after ingestion of a caustic agent in a suicide attempt, this patient arrived in the emergency room with symptoms of outlet obstruction. The stomach is distended and filled with secretions. Almost no contrast left the stomach. Surgical drainage was required.

trum that often resembles infiltrating carcinoma radiographically. Clinically, outlet obstruction frequently is present at this stage.[12, 13]

In infants, hypertrophic pyloric stenosis is the most common form of outlet obstruction. These infants, who usually are boys about 1 month old, have projectile vomiting and a palpable "olive" in the epigastrium. In adults hypertrophic pyloric stenosis may be associated with gastric ulcer. Whether the ulcer causes the stenosis or the stenosis causes the ulcer is unknown. Because the lesion may be indistinguishable from that in children, some believe it represents a milder version of pediatric pyloric stenosis that has remained asymptomatic since infancy. Radiographically these patients have a long (often several centimeters) narrowed pyloric canal; they usually do not have high-grade gastric outlet obstruction, as is seen in some of the previously mentioned conditions.[5, 14]

The prolapse of gastric lesions through the pyloris and into the duodenal bulb may cause intermittent obstructive symptoms. Gastric polyps and on occasion gastric mucosa have been described as the source of prolapse.[7]

Gastric outlet obstruction frequently is diag-

nosed clinically. Radiographically, we consider lesions confined to the antrum, duodenal bulb, and pylorus. Clinically, however, lesions in the distal duodenum may present a similar picture. Depending on the site of the lesion and its relationship to the duodenal papilla, there may or may not be bile in the patient's vomitus. Among the more distal lesions to consider as obstructive are postbulbar duodenal ulcers, carcinoma of the pancreas, annular pancreas, duodenal webs, intraduodenal hematomas, and pseudocysts. Metastatic disease, superior mesenteric artery syndrome, Crohn's disease, and tuberculosis also should be considered.[15–19]

The radiologist has two main tasks in evaluating gastric distention. The first is to demonstrate whether the cause is obstructive or nonobstructive (Fig 21–5). If an obstruction is present, the radiologist must try to demonstrate its nature. Because the most common cause for outlet obstruction is peptic ulcer disease, demonstration of deformity of the duodenal bulb or an ulcer may result in a greatly different therapeutic approach than the demonstration of an annular lesion in the antrum. Although patients with peptic ulcer disease frequently require surgery, a significant number can be brought

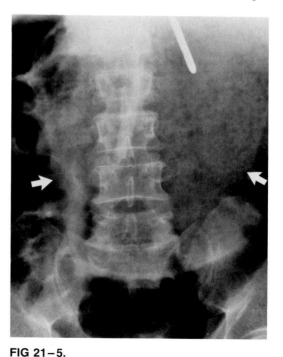

FIG 21–5.
Acute gastric dilation in a patient with diabetes. The stomach is considerably distended and filled with fluid *(arrows)*. No obstructing lesion was found.

through the acute phase of outlet obstruction without emergency surgery.[20]

In the case presented, duodenal deformity and a perforating duodenal ulcer are demonstrated. The patient underwent surgery and subsequently recovered.

REFERENCES

1. Weiland D, Dunn D, Humphrey E, et al: Gastric outlet obstruction in peptic ulcer disease: An indication for surgery. *Am J Surg* 1982; 143:90–93.
2. Eisenberg RL, Margulis AR, Moss AA: Giant duodenal ulcers. *Gastrointest Radiol* 1978; 2:347–353.
3. Kressel HY: Peptic disease of the stomach and duodenum, in Margulis AR, Burhenne HJ (eds): *Alimentary Tract Radiology*, ed 3. St Louis, CV Mosby Co, 1983, pp 789–790.
4. Balthazar EJ, Rosenberg H, Davidian MM: Scirrhous carcinoma of the pyloric channel and distal antrum. *AJR* 1980; 134:669–673.
5. Ellis H: Pyloric stenosis, in Nyhus L, Wastel C (eds): *Surgery of the Stomach and Duodenum,* ed 4. Boston, Little Brown & Co, 1986, pp 475–489.
6. Blatt CJ, Burnstein RG, Lopez F: Uncommon roentgenologic manifestations of pancreatic carcinoma. *Am J Roentgenol Radium Ther* 1971; 113:119–124.
7. Short WF, Young BR: Roentgen demonstration of prolapse of benign polypoid gastric tumors into the duodenum including a dumbell-shaped leiomyoma. *Am J Roentgenol Radium Ther* 1968; 103:317–320.
8. Nelson SW: Some interesting and unusual manifestations of Crohn's disease ("regional enteritis") of the stomach, duodenum, and small intestine. *Am J Roentgenol Radium Ther* 1969; 107:86–101.
9. Thompson W, Cockrill H, Rice RP: Regional enteritis of the duodenum. *Am J Roentgenol Radium Ther* 1974; 123:252–261.
10. Clements JL Jr, Jinkins JR, Torres WE, et al: Antral mucosal diaphragms in adults. *AJR* 1979; 113:1105–1111.
11. Mandell GA: Association of antral diaphragm and hypertrophic pyloric stenosis. *AJR* 1978; 131:203.
12. Muhletaler CA, Gerlock AJ, DeSoto L, Halter SA: Gastroduodenal lesions of ingested acids: Radiographic findings. *AJR* 1980; 135:1247–1252.
13. Karon AB: The delayed gastric syndrome with pyloric stenosis and achlorhydria following the ingestion of acid—A definite clinical entity. *Am J Dig Dis* 1962; 7:1041–1046.
14. Mindelzun RE, McCort JJ: Acute abdomen, in Margulis AR, Burhenne HJ (eds): *Alimentary Tract Radiology,* ed 3. St Louis, CV Mosby Co, 1983, pp 422–431.
15. Stassa G, Klugensmith WC: Primary tumors of the duodenal bulb. *Am J Roentgenol Radium Ther* 1969; 107:105–110.
16. Bosse G, Nelly JA: Roentgenologic findings in primary malignant tumors of the duodenum. *Am J Roentgenol Radium Ther* 1969; 107:111–118.
17. Wallace RG, Howard WB: Acute superior mesenteric artery syndrome in the severely burned patient. *Radiology* 1970; 94:307–310.
18. Lockwood IH, Smith AB, Shook LD: Lesions in and about the second portion of the duodenum. *Am J Roentgenol Radium Ther* 1954; 71:573–580.
19. Basemann EF, Auerbach SH, Wolfe WW: The importance of roentgenologic diagnosis of aberrant pancreatic tissue in the gastrointestinal tract. *Am J Roentgenol Radium Ther* 1967; 107:71–76.
20. Joffe N: Some unusual roentgenologic findings associated with marked gastric dilatation. *Am J Roentgenol Radium Ther* 1973; 119:291–299.

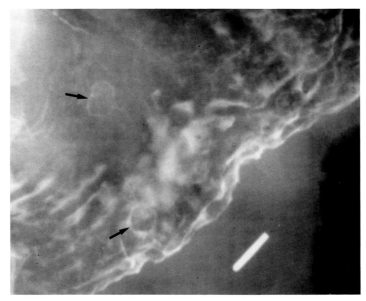

FIG 22–5.
Mid-body of the stomach in a patient with Gardner's syndrome who already has had a colectomy. The small polyps *(arrows)* are hyperplastic, although there is also an increased incidence of adenomatous polyps in these patients.

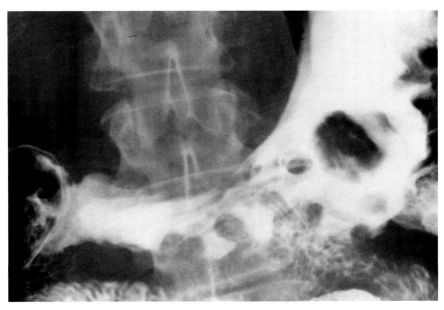

FIG 22–6.
Several large mural and intraluminal masses secondary to neurofibromas in a patient with neurofibromatosis.

and present as polypoid lesions. Spindle cell tumors (leiomyomas) are the most common, but lipomas, hemangiomas, and neurogenic tumors occur as well. Typically these tumors are solitary, but in some conditions, such as neurofibromatosis, they can be multiple (Fig 22–6). These lesions can be relatively large and may have surface ulceration, with a radiographic appearance similar to Figure 22–1.

There are several other benign causes of multiple polyps of the stomach, although most are rare. One that may be encountered in daily practice is severe gastritis. In severe erosive disease small mounds of edematous mucosa are seen, and the punctate central barium collections may not be identifiable. Also, patients with severe gastritis have enlarged rugal folds, which may assume a polypoid appearance. The enlarged rugal folds of Menetrier's disease also can mimic polypoid filling defects. Another inflammatory process that causes polypoid excrescences is candidiasis in immunocompromised patients. Other rare causes include gastric varices, amyloid, granulomatous processes such as tuberculosis, sarcoid, and even Crohn's disease. Patients with eosinophilic gastroenteritis may have multiple polyps throughout the gastrointestinal tract, including the stomach; these are benign mucosal polyps with heavy eosinophilic infiltration (Fig 22–7).

Polypoid lesions of the stomach due to a malignant neoplastic process are less common. Malignant neoplasms presenting as polyps tend to be larger and more irregular than benign polyps, although there is enough overlap that this criterion can be misleading. The most common gastric malignancy, adenocarcinoma, seldom occurs as a well-defined polyp, and usually appears as a large bulky mass or infiltrates the bowel wall. In a review of early gastric carcinoma, one study showed that an isolated polyp was one of the least common presentations for adenocarcinoma.[18] However, adenomas and less frequently hyperplastic polyps are associated with carcinomatous degeneration in adjacent mucosa. Thus any unusual or irregular polyp occurring against a background of benign-appearing polyps should be considered with suspicion and warrants biopsy (see Fig 22–2).

Lymphoma of the gastrointestinal tract is a great imitator of a variety of benign and malignant processes. In the stomach its appearance ranges from irregular rugal folds to large masses. Although rarely seen, lymphoma may occur as multiple polyps in the gastrointestinal tract, including the stomach.

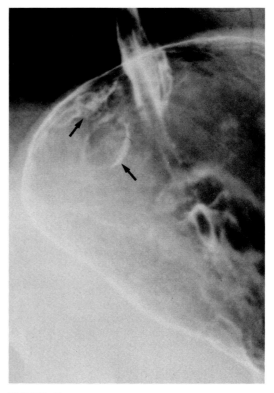

FIG 22–7.
Two small fundal polyps *(arrows)* in a patient with eosinophilic gastroenteritis. These polyps were heavily infiltrated with eosinophils.

Perhaps the most common malignant process to appear in the stomach as multiple polyps is hematogenous metastases. The major neoplasms to metastasize to the stomach are melanoma and breast and lung carcinoma.[19] Although these are among the most common neoplasms encountered, the total number of patients with these diseases who have gastric metastases is low. Melanoma is perhaps one of the most common to produce hematogenous metastases to the gastrointestinal tract, including the stomach. Typically, these are well-circumscribed lesions of variable size, sometimes with central ulceration or umbilication, giving the so-called bull's-eye appearance. When they occur they are almost always diffuse and will be seen not only in the stomach but in the small bowel and in other organs. Breast and lung carcinomas also metastasize to the stomach, although discrete polypoid lesions are the less common presentation. Classically breast carcinoma produces more of a linitis plastica appearance.[19] A tumor that is becoming identified more frequently is Kaposi's sarcoma. Although once considered rare, it is now seen in patients with acquired immune deficiency syndrome.[20] This tumor is well known for its metastases to the gastrointestinal tract (Fig 22–8) and occasionally develops central ulceration, producing a bull's-eye lesion. The patient presented could have one of these processes.

Although there are numerous causes of polypoid lesions in the stomach, a skilled radiologist often can narrow the diagnostic possibilities considerably and aid the clinician in evaluating these patients. When confronted with findings such as in the case presented, there are several logical steps. First the entire gastrointestinal tract must be evaluated, particularly the small bowel. If lesions are evident in the small bowel, the likelihood increases that the polyps are of great clinical significance, usually due to a neoplastic process. The major categories that cause both stomach and small bowel polyps are hematogenous metastases or a polyposis syndrome. Benign causes are relatively rare. Size and location of polyps also can be strong criteria. When all polyps encountered are smaller than 1 cm, they usually are due to a benign process and generally are hyperplastic.[13] Polyps larger than 1 cm (especially greater than 2 cm) should be viewed with suspicion and warrant biopsy and perhaps removal.[12, 13] Location is a weak criterion for evaluating polyps and should not be a determining factor. As a general rule, adenomatous polyps are in the distal stomach and hyperplastic polyps proximal.[10–13] Surface features also are less important but sometimes may be helpful, as in the case of central ulceration, which is seen in leiomyomas and metastatic disease such as melanoma and Kaposi's sarcoma.

Clinical information can be helpful but should not be relied on to include or exclude significant disease. Most patients with disease of the upper gastrointestinal tract have nonspecific symptoms such as pain, nausea, and emesis; even asymptomatic individuals may harbor significant disease. Age and gender are nonspecific; gastric polyps may be one instance in which young patients have more significant disease than older patients.

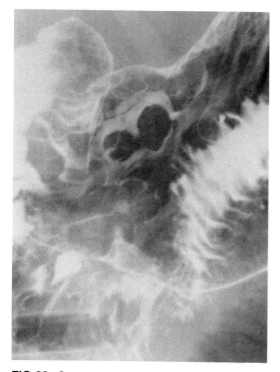

FIG 22–8.
Multiple polyps of various sizes in the distal stomach in a 28-year-old man with metastatic Kaposi's sarcoma from acquired immune deficiency disease (AIDS).

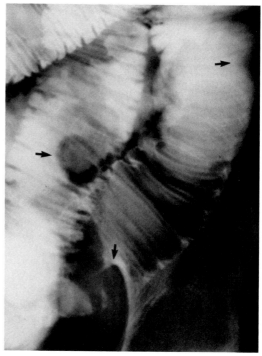

FIG 22–9.
(Same patient as in Fig 22–1) Small bowel enteroclysis demonstrates several small polyps *(arrows)* from metastatic melanoma.

In patients with gastric polyps, even when all criteria have been evaluated, the wisest course of action may be further examination by endoscopy and biopsy. The procedure is simple, with low morbidity, and substantial diagnostic errors can be avoided.

CONCLUSION

In the case presented, vague abdominal complaints were correctly diagnosed by the radiologist from just the upper gastrointestinal examination as due to metastatic melanoma to the gastrointestinal tract. Diagnosis was based on the presence of several broad-based lesions, one of which had central ulceration (see Fig 22–1,A and B). Further questioning of the patient revealed that he had had a mole removed from his back several years previously without further follow-up. Small bowel enteroclysis (Fig 22–9) revealed several other lesions in the small bowel. The patient responded poorly to therapy and died within a year.

REFERENCES

1. Yarnis H, Marshak RH, Friedman AI: Gastric polyps. *JAMA* 1952; 148:1088–1094.
2. Gordon R, Laufer I, Kressel HY: Gastric polyps found on routine double-contrast examination of the stomach. *Radiology* 1980; 134:27–30.
3. Feczko PJ, Halpert RD, Ackerman LV: Gastric polyps: Radiological evaluation and clinical significance. *Radiology* 1985; 155:581–584.
4. Montesi A, De Nigris E, Pesaresi A, et al: Diagnostic accuracy of double-contrast examination in the detection of gastric polyps. *Radiol Med (Torino)* 1981; 67:509–513.
5. Kamiya T, Morishita T, Asakura H, et al: Histoclinical longstanding follow-up study of hyperplastic polyps of the stomach. *Am J Gastroenterol* 1981; 75:275–281.
6. Monaco AP, Roth SI, Castleman B, et al: Adenomatous polyps of the stomach. A clinical and pathological study of 153 cases. *Cancer* 1962; 15:456–467.
7. Ming S-C, Goldman H: Gastric polyps. A histogenetic classification and its relation to carcinoma. *Cancer* 1965; 18:721–726.
8. Tomasulo J: Gastric polyps. Histologic types and their relationship to gastric carcinoma. *Cancer* 1971; 27:1346–1355.
9. Op den Orth JO, Dekker W: Gastric adenomas. *Radiology* 1981; 141:289–293.
10. Snover DC: Benign epithelial polyps of the stomach. *Pathol Annu* 1985; 20:303–329.
11. Ming S-C: The adenoma-carcinoma sequence in the stomach and colon. II. Malignant potential of gastric polyps. *Gastrointest Radiol* 1976; 1:121–125.
12. Neimark S, Rogers AI: Gastric polyps: A review. *Am J Gastroenterol* 1982; 77:585–587.
13. Morrissey JF: Small polypoid lesions of the stomach. *Gastrointest Endosc* 1982; 28:266–267.
14. Smith HJ, Lee EL: Large hyperplastic polyps of the stomach. *Gastrointest Radiol* 1983; 8:19–21.
15. Lee RG, Burt RW: The histopathology of fundic gland polyps of the stomach. *Am J Clin Pathol* 1986; 86:498–503.
16. Sarre RG, Frost AG, Jagelman DG, et al: Gastric and duodenal polyps in familial adenomatous polyposis: A prospective study of the nature and prevalence of upper gastrointestinal polyps. *Gut* 1987; 28:206–314.
17. Jarvinen HJ, Sipponen P: Gastroduodenal polyps in familial adenomatous and juvenile polyposis. *Endoscopy* 1986; 18:230–234.
18. Gold RP, Green PHR, O'Toole KM, et al: Early gastric cancer: Radiographic experience. *Radiology* 1984; 152:283–290.
19. Menuck LS, Amberg JR: Metastatic disease involving the stomach. *Am J Dig Dis* 1975; 20:903–913.
20. Frager DH, Frager JD, Brandt LJ, et al: Gastrointestinal complications of AIDS: Radiologic features. *Radiology* 1986; 158:597–602.

CHAPTER 23

Epigastric Pain – Gastritis

R. Kristina Gedgaudas-McClees, M.D.

Case Presentation

A 30-year-old woman with rheumatoid arthritis had severe epigastric pain that improved after antacid therapy. An upper gastrointestinal examination revealed an abnormality in the gastric antrum (Fig 23–1). What is the diagnosis?

DISCUSSION

The upper gastrointestinal examination illustrates classic shallow longitudinal ulcers in the gastric antrum, which have formed as the result of coalescence of multiple aphthoid erosions. This patient has aspirin-induced erosive gastritis.

In contrast to true gastric ulceration, acute erosive gastritis is confined to the mucosa, without involvement of the muscularis layer. In acute gastritis, histologic study of biopsy tissue reveals that the cells of the surface epithelium have lost their normal columnar shape and have assumed a cuboidal form. Infiltration occurs, with polymorphonuclear leukocytes grouping within the glandular layer of the mucosa. The gastric mucosa is lined with small linear or round superficial petechiae and central erosions, the latter measuring 2 to 3 mm in diameter. In contrast to a true gastric ulcer, erosions never extend into the muscularis layer of the mucosa. Complete healing occurs without scarring, and after the lesions have healed the prognosis is excellent. Clinically acute gastritis is seen in up to 10% of the general population.[1]

The condition pathologists and gastroenterologists designate as gastritis has a spectrum of presentations and is associated with diseases of greater clinical importance, such as gastric carcinoma and gastric ulcer.

Gastritis is a multifactorial disease with many causes, including genetic and environmental factors. The occurrence of gastritis among first-degree relatives in spite of varied environmental conditions suggests a familial pattern.[2] Pernicious anemia and gastric atrophy are common in some families due to an inborn inherent tendency.[3-5] Environmental factors predisposing to the presence of acute erosive gastritis include diet, the use and abuse of alcohol, drugs (aspirin, tetracycline, phenylbutazone, morphine, chemotherapeutic agents), tobacco, infections *(Staphylococcus aureus, Escherichia coli, Clostridium, Candida,* herpesvirus, cytomegalovirus), acids, and alkalis.[1, 6, 7]

It is presumed that drugs lead to gastritis by irritating the gastric mucosa and reducing resistance to other irritants. The acidity of the stomach also plays a role in the toxicity of certain drugs on the mucosa. Aspirin, for example, requires an acid pH to effect damage; patients with achlorhydria are less susceptible to gastritis than is the general population.[8]

Some patients with acute gastritis may have no symptoms; others may have upper abdominal distress. Upper gastrointestinal hemorrhage, occult or massive, is the most common presentation. Radiographically, acute erosive gastritis secondary to any cause may have a variety of appearances. Findings on upper gastrointestinal examination may be nor-

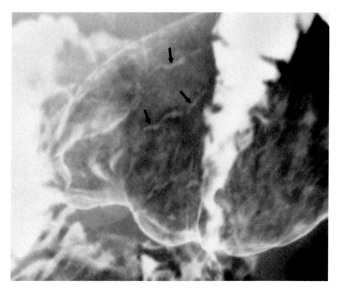

FIG 23–1.
Aspirin-induced erosive gastritis. Shallow, longitudinal collections of barium *(arrows)* are surrounded by edema. These represent coalescence of numerous aphthoid erosions.

mal in the milder cases. Criteria in both double-contrast and conventional techniques include (1) poor distensibility, seen as flattening and incomplete distention along the lesser, greater, or both curvatures of the antrum; (2) crenulations along the antrum, generally along the lesser curvature; (3) thickened folds; (4) spasm; or (5) aphthoid erosions characterized by pinpoint central collections of barium surrounded by a smooth halo of edema[9] (Fig 23–2). Any or a combination of the first four criteria is sug-

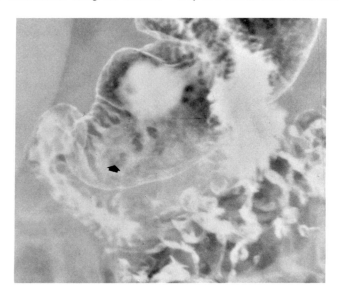

FIG 23–2.
This patient has several features of acute erosive gastritis. Aphthoid erosions are present *(arrow)*. Also, the lesser curvature is not distended as on the greater curvature side of the antrum. A finely crenulated or serrated border is present, due to intense local inflammation.

gestive of the diagnosis. The presence of erosions is pathognomonic, as seen in the case described. Their natural history is to heal completely (sometimes within several days) or to progress, with coalescence and the formation of deeper, frank ulcerations.

Chronic gastritis is a separate condition, probably occurring as the result of continuous, longstanding irritation to the mucosa. Studies have suggested the role of parietal cell antibodies of the immunoglobulin G and A varieties, especially in patients with genetic predisposition to gastritis.[2, 10] Parietal cell antibodies are common in older patients, in nearly all patients with pernicious anemia, and in more than half of patients with other forms of gastritis.[11] As chronic superficial gastritis develops, acid and pepsin secretions decrease. Because subsequent degeneration of gastric mucosa occurs in stages, true gastric atrophy develops in a small percentage of patients.[12] Radiographic findings of chronic gastritis vary. Superficial gastritis is essentially an endoscopic diagnosis, whereas atrophic gastritis is manifested radiographically by the absence of folds in localized or generalized areas of the stomach.

The term hypertrophic gastritis is a misnomer because there is no inflammation.[13, 14] Hyperplasia of the surface epithelium creates marked thickening of the folds. Menetrier's disease is a classic example of hypertrophic gastritis. Patients have marked protein loss from the stomach. Biopsy findings include giant hypertrophy of the mucosa, without edema. Cystic glandular enlargement is present. The disease is often confined to the fundus and the body of the stomach. Radiographically, all forms of hypertrophic gastritis can be difficult to distinguish from other acute forms of gastritis and from diffuse infiltrative forms of non-Hodgkin's lymphoma. The gastric folds, which appear markedly thickened radiographically, are soft and pliable and can be effaced on double-contrast examination. The antrum usually is spared (Fig 23–3).

Another distinctive form of hypertrophic gastritis is Zollinger-Ellison syndrome. Patients with this disease have non-beta, islet cell, gastrin-secreting tumors of the pancreas. Histologically, gastric hyperplasia in conjunction with an increase in parietal cells eventually leads to aggressive peptic ulceration.[1] The presence of intractable gastric ulcer or multiple ulcers within the stomach or proximal small bowel suggests the disease. Severe edema may be present, and hypersecretion is common. However, the radiologist should be aware that all

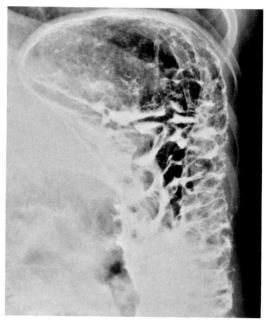

FIG 23–3.
Menetrier's disease. Giant rugal folds are present along the fundus and body of the stomach. The antrum was spared. Differentiating this from other forms of gastritis is impossible. Non-Hodgkin's lymphoma can have this appearance, although it tends to cause more nodular thickening of the rugae.

three manifestations need not be present. Gastrin immunoassays confirm the diagnosis. Selective angiography and computed tomographic angiography are useful in localizing the tumors, 50% of which are malignant, and in identifying metastatic disease.

Granulomatous gastritides[9, 15] include Crohn's disease, sarcoidosis, syphilis, tuberculosis, histoplasmosis, and actinomycosis. Of these, Crohn's disease is the most common. Initially the radiographic findings are identical to those of other forms of acute gastritis with aphthoid erosions. The mucosa can be edematous, with nodular fold thickening. As the disease progresses, resultant scarring causes narrowing and rigidity, particularly in the antrum. Severe cases may be indistinguishable from linitis plastica (Fig 23–4).

Eosinophilic gastritis is characterized by infiltration of eosinophils into the stomach either focally, creating a polypoid "eosinophilic granuloma," or diffusely with "eosinophilic gastritis."[16, 17] The cause may be a gastrointestinal response to an allergen; patients generally have histories or family histories of allergies (60%). A peripheral eosinophilia

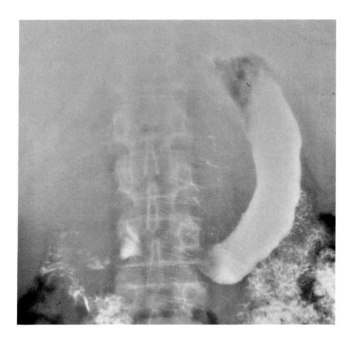

FIG 23–4.
Chronic gastric sarcoidosis. Findings resemble those of linitis plastica in loss of a normal rugal pattern, contracted shape and narrowed lumen, and general loss of peristalsis. The diagnosis was made by open surgical biopsy. Adenocarcinoma eventually developed in the antrum, presumably due to the presence of chronic gastritis and its metaplastic effects on the gastric mucosa.

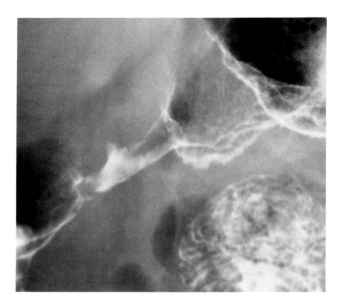

FIG 23–5.
Corrosive gastritis. This patient swallowed a drain cleaner and suffered severe mucosal sloughing of the entire stomach. This examination was performed only 1 month later, revealing the intense scarring and narrowing that ensued.

is present in most patients. The disease also can involve the small bowel with malabsorption symptoms. Radiographically the gastric folds are thickened, with discrete polypoid lesions arising from the submucosa. The chronic form reveals scarring within the affected areas of the stomach, indistinguishable from the other chronic forms of gastritis.

Corrosive agents such as acids and alkalis can have devastating effects on the stomach.[18, 19] Corrosive alkalis damage the esophagus more than the stomach, because of the potentially neutralizing effects of gastric acids, whereas strong acids injure the gastric mucosa. Initially there is marked edema, with mucosal sloughing and ulcer formation. Within weeks severe scarring shrinks the stomach, often causing outlet obstruction (Fig 23–5).

Radiation-induced gastritis occurs when the stomach is exposed to levels of radiation exceeding 3,500 rads.[9] Mucosal edema and superficial ulceration can be observed. Radiographic abnormalities develop within an average of 6 months after radiation but can be seen within 1 or 2 months after intensive therapy. After the acute inflammatory response scarring occurs, as with other forms of acute gastric injury.

Phlegmonous gastritis is an often fatal infection of the stomach, resulting in gastric necrosis and generalized sepsis. Bacteria implicated in this disorder include alpha hemolytic streptococci, *S. aureus*, *E. coli*, *Clostridium*, *Proteus*, and pneumococci. When gas-forming organisms are present a form of phlegmonous gastritis, termed emphysematous gastritis, can be readily identified radiographically.[9] On plain films, linear or small mottled collections of gas can be identified in the wall of the stomach (Fig 23–6). Their intramural location can be verified by the use of oral contrast material. Computed tomography is also an excellent method for identifying or confirming the diagnosis. Other causes of intramural gastric pneumatosis include infarction, trauma (including endoscopy), and erosive gastritis.

Patients who have undergone subtotal gastrectomy with gastroduodenostomy or gastroenterostomy frequently have reflux of bile and pancreatic secretions into the gastric remnant. This can have toxic consequences on the stomach, creating hemorrhage and mucosal disease. There are data to support the theory that chronic bile reflux gastritis lasting more than 10 years can increase the likelihood of gastric carcinoma. Many of the chronic gastritides have been implicated in subsequent development of carcinoma, although the incidence generally is believed to be low.

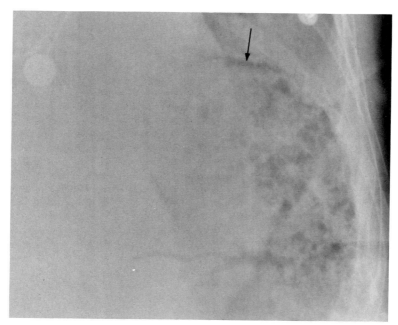

FIG 23–6.
Emphysematous gastritis. Linear gas collections line the wall of the stomach *(arrow)* in this patient who recently had undergone endoscopy. He recovered, with no symptoms.

REFERENCES

1. Spiro HM (ed): *Clinical Gastroenterology.* New York, Macmillan Publishing Co, 1970, pp 155–180.
2. Siurala M, Varis K: Gastritis, in Sircus W, Smith AN (eds): *Scientific Foundations of Gastroenterology.* Philadelphia, WB Saunders Co, 1980, pp 357–369.
3. Taylor KB: Immune aspects of pernicious anemia and atrophic gastritis. *Clin Haematol* 1976; 5:497.
4. Siurala M, Lehtola J, Ihamaki T: Atrophic gastritis and its sequelae. Results of 19–23 years: Follow-up examinations. *Scand J Gastroenterol* 1977; 9:441.
5. Glass GBJ, Pitchumoni CS: Atrophic gastritis. *Hum Pathol* 1975; 6:219.
6. Croft DN, Wood PH: Gastric mucosa and susceptibility to occult gastrointestinal bleeding caused by aspirin. *Br Med J* 1967; 1:137–141.
7. Davenport HW: Salicylate damage to the gastric mucosal barrier. *N Engl J Med* 1967; 276:1307–1312.
8. Winawer S, Bejar J, Zamcheck N: Recurrent massive hemorrhage in patients with achlorhydria and atrophic gastritis. *Arch Intern Med* 1967; 120:327.
9. Gedgaudas-McClees RK, McClees EC: The stomach, in Gedgaudas-McClees RK (ed): *Gastrointestinal Imaging.* New York, Churchill-Livingstone, 1987, pp 41–47.
10. Vilardell E: Chronic gastritis, in Bockus HL (ed): *Gastroenterology,* Philadelphia, WB Saunders Co, pp 150–155.
11. Kravetz R, Van Noorden A, Spiro H: Parietal cell antibodies in patients with duodenal ulcer and gastric cancer. *Lancet* 1967; 1:235–237.
12. Siurala M, Varorinen Y: Follow-up studies of patients with superficial gastritis and patients with a normal gastric mucosa. *Acta Med Scand* 1963; 173:45–52.
13. Butz WC: Giant hypertrophic gastritis. *Gastroenterology* 1960; 39:183–190.
14. Chocas WV, Connor DH, Innes RC: Giant hypertrophy of the gastric mucosa, hypoproteinemia and edema (Menetrier's disease). *Am J Med* 1959; 27:125–131.
15. Johnson OA, Hoskins DW, Todd J, et al: Crohn's disease of the stomach. *Gastroenterology* 1966; 50:571–577.
16. Edelmann MJ, March TC: Eosinophilic gastroenteritis. *Am J Roentgenol* 1964; 91:773–778.
17. Morson BC: Intestinal metaplasia of gastric mucosa. *Gastroenterologia* 1956; 85:181–190.
18. Marks IN, Bank S, Werbeloff L, et al: The natural history of corrosive gastritis. Report of five cases. *Am J Dig Dis* 1963; 8:509–524.
19. Poteshman NL: Corrosive gastritis due to hydrochloric acid ingestion. *Am J Roentgenol* 1968; 99:182–185.

Enlarged Gastric Folds

Janis Gissel Letourneau, M.D.

Case Presentation

A 79-year-old female Russian immigrant was seen in the medicine clinic for treatment of hypertension. The interviewing physician obtained a history of a 10-pound weight loss and mild epigastric discomfort. An abdominal computed tomographic (CT) scan showed thickening of the gastric wall (Fig 24−1,A and B). The presence of thickened and disorganized gastric folds was confirmed on an upper gastrointestinal series (Fig 24−1,C). What diagnostic considerations should be made in this patient, and how should they be approached?

DISCUSSION

Diffuse thickening of the gastric folds is not an uncommon radiographic finding. It can be seen in association with disorganization and nodularity of the folds, increased gastric secretions, and diminished gastric pliability. The presence or absence of these secondary findings helps to limit the differential diagnosis of this nonspecific finding.

Thickening of the gastric wall, specifically thickening of the gastric rugal folds, can be detected by a variety of radiographic techniques. The most common of these is a standard single- or double-contrast upper gastrointestinal series. A single-contrast study permits ready identification of thickened gastric folds, because the rugal pattern is not obliterated by gaseous distention of the stomach. Use of a biphasic technique permits imaging of the nondistended stomach, overcoming a potential limitation of the double-contrast examination. The width of normal gastric folds is 5 mm in the regions of the body and antrum[1]; slightly wider folds may be seen in the normal fundus. The pattern of the folds as well as their width must be assessed. Gastric folds in the body and antrum parallel the long axis of the

stomach. As the folds approach the gastroesophageal junction the pattern becomes more complex and can be difficult to assess.

Computed tomography also can be used to assess gastric wall thickness. With this technique it is difficult to differentiate fold thickening (involving the epithelium, lamina propria, muscularis mucosa, and a portion of the submucosa) from more diffuse gastric wall thickening. Occasionally individual folds are outlined by intraluminal contrast medium and can be measured. The upper limit for normal gastric wall thickness in a distended stomach is 1 cm by CT.[2−4] Ultrasonography can detect wall thickening in various segments of the gastrointestinal tract. This method is used most frequently in the characterization of focal gastrointestinal lesions.[4] Its value in assessing a diffuse process, such as gastric fold thickening, is limited.

Thickened gastric folds are seen in a variety of conditions (Table 24−1) and as a normal variant. In cases such as the one presented the differential diagnosis can be narrowed by means of historical considerations and by secondary radiologic findings. Diffuse gastric fold thickening can be seen with a variety of forms of gastritis, including alcoholic,

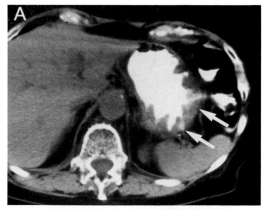

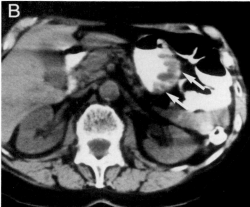

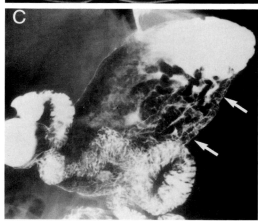

FIG 24–1.
A, computed tomographic scan of the upper abdomen after opacification of the gastrointestinal system reveals thickening of the posterior wall of the gastric body *(arrows)*. **B,** a slightly lower section reveals extension of this process into the distal gastric body *(arrows)*. **C,** thickened and disorganized folds in the gastric body *(arrows)* are confirmed by double-contrast upper gastrointestinal radiographic series.

TABLE 24–1.
Causes of Gastric Fold Thickening

Normal variant
Gastritis
  Alcoholic
  Corrosive
  Infectious
  Post-irradiation
Infiltrative processes
  Crohn's disease
  Eosinophilic gastritis
  Sarcoidosis
  Amyloidosis
Peptic ulcer disease
  Zollinger-Ellison syndrome
  Menetrier's disease
Malignancy
  Adenocarcinoma
  Lymphoma
  Leukemia
  (Pseudolymphoma)
Varices
Pancreatic disease
  Pancreatitis
  Pancreatic carcinoma

corrosive, and infectious (e.g., tuberculous or syphilitic) gastritis.[1, 5, 6] Infiltrative processes can cause thickening of the gastric folds, and may be associated with mucosal inflammation. The most common of these entities are Crohn's disease and eosinophilic gastritis. Other infiltrative processes that cause fold thickening are sarcoidosis and amyloidosis.[7]

Peptic ulcer disease can be associated with diffuse gastric fold thickening.[1] This is particularly well demonstrated in Zollinger-Ellison syndrome, in which a gastrin-secreting tumor causes severe gastritis and gastric duodenal ulceration. Zollinger-Ellison syndrome is characterized by diffuse gastric fold thickening, postbulbar ulcers, and gastric hypersecretion (Fig 24–2).

Menetrier's disease, one of the protein-losing enteropathies, also known as giant hypertrophic gastritis, is associated with thickened gastric folds.[8] It typically involves the gastric fundus and body but can involve the antrum as well (Fig 24–3). In this disease, the cause of which is unknown, thickened, distorted folds are seen in the setting of impaired peristalsis.

Several malignant processes can produce thickened gastric folds. Thickened, distorted, and sometimes nodular gastric folds are one radiographic form of gastric lymphoma.[9, 10] Pliability and disten

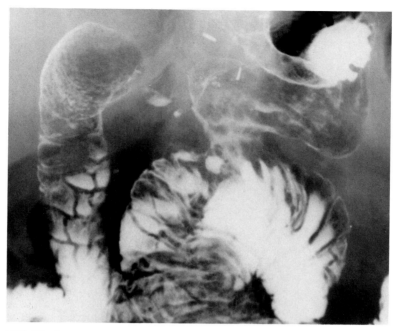

FIG 25–1.
Case presentation.

scopically. Judicious use of the correct contrast material and proper patient positioning relative to the type of surgery assure that the surgical site is well visualized and reliably examined, rather than flooded and obscured by too much of the wrong type of contrast material.

Choice of Contrast Material and Examination Method

Barium remains the agent of choice in postoperative examination, when anastomotic leakage, staple-line dehiscence, or bowel perforation, all of which are better investigated with a water-soluble contrast agent, are not suspected. The choice of single- or double-contrast technique may be more difficult, because there is debate as to whether there is any significant difference in diagnostic yield.[2] Single-contrast examination is the method of choice for detecting a fistula, evaluating the rate and direction of flow, and examining a patient who is immobile and unable to cooperate for a study requiring rapid changes in patient position.[3] Palpation, pressure, and mucosal relief films allow visualization of the perianastomotic area. However, compression films may be difficult to obtain postoperatively because of the smaller gastric size and interference from the

overlying ribs. Films should be obtained with the patient in the upright and recumbent positions. All portions of the stomach and small bowel should be filled.

Double-contrast techniques afford a good view of the mucosa and of the anastomosis, with the stomach and duodenum well distended. The gastric remnant can be examined easily without the need for vigorous palpation. The anastomosis remains well visualized with fine mucosal detail despite filling of the distal bowel loops with contrast material.[4-6]

Examination

Whichever method is chosen, examination of any postoperative patient should begin with a plain film of the abdomen that includes the site of surgery. The pattern of surgical clips or staples may provide useful information about the operative procedure, particularly in patients who have had surgery for control of obesity.[7] In gastric restrictive operations, more than in any other type of gastric procedure, staple patterns are definite and recognizable (Table 25–2) and allow precise identification of the type of surgery. Also, plain films show any unsuspected densities or retained contrast material, which

TABLE 25–1.

Complications After Gastric Surgery That Can Produce Recurrent Abdominal Pain

Esophagitis
  Gastroesophageal reflux
  Bile reflux
  Nasogastric tube use
Gastric atony after vagotomy
  Bezoar formation
Gastritis and gastric remnant ulceration
  Bile reflux
  Ulcerogenic substance use
Neoplasm
  Recurrent tumor
  Primary or gastric remnant cancer
Anastomotic leak (usually an early postoperative problem)
  Fistula
  Abscess
Bowel obstruction
  Narrow anastomotic or channel diameter
    Edema
    Hemorrhage
    Marginal ulcer
    Stricture after ulcer healing
    Mucosal prolapse and intussusception
  Afferent loop obstruction
  Paralytic ileus with gastric atony
  Bezoar formation
  Distal obstruction
Gastrojejunocolic fistula
Jejunitis

may add to confusion during the study, and abdominal films show abnormal gas patterns, which may indicate unsuspected bowel obstruction.

Because each patient is unique and surgical modifications are varied, the upper gastrointestinal examination often requires creative radiology. Protocols for position changes and film sequences are not standardized easily, but traditional principles of fluoroscopic evaluation apply.[3–6] For a double-contrast examination the study begins with the patient sitting on the side of the fluoroscopy table. Glucagon (0.5 mg) is given intravenously to induce bowel hypotonia. Although this is optional, it helps retard the loss of contrast material into the small bowel and displays the anastomotic stoma.[2, 5, 6] The patient places the contents of one packet of effervescent granules in the back of the mouth and washes it down with 10 to 20 ml high-density barium sulfate preparation. The patient then lies prone and the head of the table is lowered. An additional 100 ml barium sulfate is administered via a straw while the

esophageal motility is monitored. The patient rotates through a full circle in both directions to coat the mucosa, and films are taken with the patient in various positions. Patients must be positioned promptly, because egress of gastric contents is rapid in individuals who have had gastric drainage procedures. Anything that delays filming is detrimental to the examination. As long as the patient is head-down, barium will remain mostly in the stomach, but the gas may disperse distally through the anastomosis. When films of the stomach have been obtained, the head of the table may be elevated and the patient rotated to negotiate the barium and gas through the anastomosis and into the distal bowel loops. Single-contrast views with compression of the anastomotic area complete the study. If the barium sulfate suspension and gas have passed distally before satisfactory films are obtained, additional amounts of both materials should be given without hesitation.

Modified Examination Methods in Obese Patients[7, 8]

Traditional fluoroscopic methods may fail in morbidly obese patients, especially in the first postoperative week. The patient's large body precludes rapid position changes, and some views may be impossible to obtain in patients who can barely squeeze between the x-ray tube and the fluoroscopy table. Fluoroscopic tracking of the contrast material may be nearly impossible, because the contrast material is often barely discernible in the morbidly obese patient. Fluoroscopic methods must be modified or the study will frustrate the examiner and yield erroneous results. For obese patients, accurate examination necessitates prompt filming of the first swallow of contrast material, without prolonged attempts at fluoroscopic study. The patients must be turned into the best position possible to demonstrate the staple lines, depending on the type of operation (see Table 25–2)[8]; otherwise the surgical site is obscured (Fig 25–2).

If a double-contrast study is performed, half a packet of effervescent granules is used because of the small gastric pouch size. Because egress of contrast material through the narrow channel is slow, continued administration of contrast material should be judicious to prevent overdistention of the proximal pouch and vomiting. With steady administration of contrast material the distal stomach and duodenum can be satisfactorily examined in a patient who has had a gastroplasty. If the patient has had a

TABLE 25–2.
Staple-line Geometry Predicts Optimal Examination Position*

Staple Geometry	Probable Surgery	Optimal Initial Position
Vertical	Gastroplasty, lesser curvature channel	Right posterior oblique
Horizontal	Gastroplasty, greater curvature channel	Left posterior oblique
Mixed or confusing	Gastric bypass	Left posterior oblique
	Revision operation	Left posterior oblique
	Unknown anatomy	Right posterior oblique
	Vertical gastroplasty	

*Modified from Smith C, Gardiner R, Kubicka RA, et al: Gastric restrictive surgery for obesity: Early radiologic evaluation. *Radiology* 1984; 153:321–327.

gastric bypass with anastomosis to the small bowel, the anastomotic site and small bowel loops are localized and examined as in any other postoperative patient.

Review of Surgical Anatomy and Terminology

Terminology describing postoperative anatomy may need clarification, especially eponyms that are used in different parts of the world.[1, 9] Billroth I operation refers to any antrectomy with gastroduodenostomy. The anastomosis may be end-to-end (Fig 25–3) or a variant. Billroth II operation is any gastric resection with gastrojejunostomy. The two most common configurations are the Roux-en-Y and loop types. In the Roux-en-Y (Fig 25–4), the jejunum is divided, the proximal end or side of the distal segment of jejunum is attached to the stomach, and the

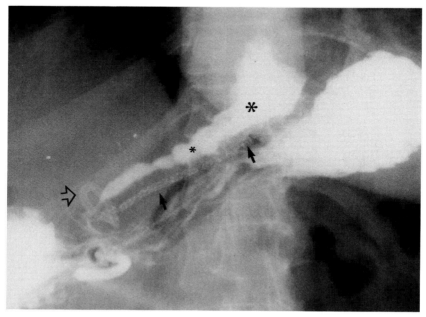

FIG 25–2.
Normal vertical banded gastroplasty. The triangular small capacity proximal pouch *(asterisks)* projects away from the staple lines *(arrows)* in the right posterior oblique view, allowing for accurate evaluation. An opaque ring *(open arrow)* surrounds the intentionally narrow channel. A gastrostomy tube in the distal stomach is filled with contrast material.

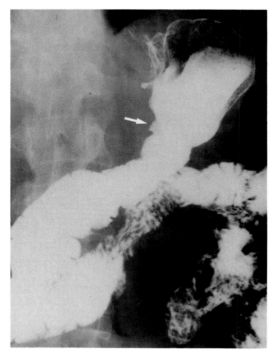

FIG 25–3.
Anastomotic ulceration following antrectomy with end-to-end gastroduodenostomy (Billroth I). There is a small ulcer crater *(arrow)* on the lesser curvature at the anastomosis. Deformity at the gastroesophageal junction is technical.

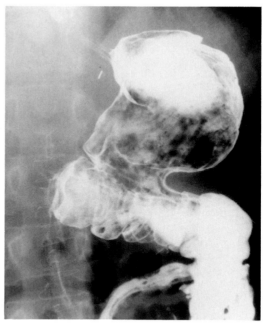

FIG 25–4.
Normal Billroth II with Roux-en-Y gastrojejunostomy. The proximal jejunal segment is not included on this radiography.

distal end of the proximal jejunal segment is anastomosed to the side of the distal jejunal segment. In the loop type (Fig 25–5), the small bowel is brought up intact and anastomosed to the stomach, with formation of an afferent (proximal) loop that carries contents toward the stomach and an efferent (distal) loop that empties beyond and away from the stomach.

The anastomosis may be further identified as either anterior or posterior and as either left-to-right or right-to-left. With an anterior gastrojejunostomy the jejunum is brought up to the stomach in a position anterior to the transverse colon, or antecolic. Posterior anastomoses usually are retrocolic; that is, the jejunum and stomach are brought together posterior to the transverse colon through a surgically created foramen in the transverse mesocolon. In a left-to-right gastrojejunostomy (see Fig 25–5) the afferent (proximal) loop is located on the left side of the stomach, or on the greater curve, when there has been gastric resection and the efferent (distal) loop is located on the right side, or lesser curve side of

the stomach. A right-to-left gastrojejunostomy (Fig 25–6) describes the reverse: the afferent loop is attached to the right side of the stomach, or to the lesser curve, after gastric resection and the efferent loop is located on the left, or the greater curve side. Choice of jejunal orientation relates to the surgeon's preference and the patient's body habitus. Formerly the terms antiperistaltic (against peristalsis) and isoperistaltic (with peristalsis) were used to describe the relationship of the peristalsis of the stomach and the small bowel. These terms are confusing and may be misleading when describing the mechanics of gastric and small bowel motility.[10]

For gastric restrictive operations a different set of terms specifies the anatomy. Unlike small bowel bypass procedures, which cause weight loss by controlled malabsorption, gastric restrictive operations control weight by limiting gastric capacity and restricting gastric egress. Small bowel bypass procedures are no longer performed because of life-threatening complications, and in patients with an ileojejunal bypass still intact the bypass should be reversed and normal small bowel anatomy restored.[11] In gastroplasty procedures rows of staples are placed either vertically or horizontally partway

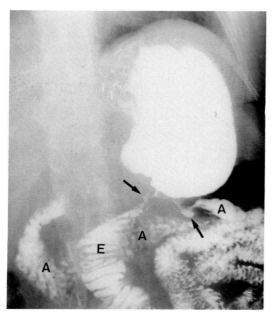

FIG 25–5.
Recurrent ulceration after vagotomy, antrectomy, and a left-to-right gastrojejunostomy (Billroth II). The afferent (proximal) loop *(A)* is attached to the left, or greater curve, side of the stomach; the efferent (distal) loop *(E)* is along the right side of the stomach. There is partial gastric outlet obstruction caused by the edema that surrounds two ulcer craters *(arrows)*.

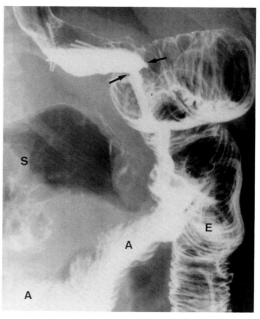

FIG 25–6.
Normal gastric bypass with right-to-left loop gastrojejunostomy. The anastomosis *(arrows)* is intentionally narrow to restrict overeating. The afferent (proximal) loop *(A)* is filled, with gas and barium faintly outlining the distal stomach *(S)*, which has been stapled and transected from the proximal stomach. The efferent (distal) loop *(E)* is well distended because of hypotonia induced by glucagon.

across the stomach to form a small-volume food-receiving segment, or proximal pouch (Fig 25–2), that empties into the distal stomach by way of a channel 1 cm in diameter. The channel is supported by an opaque ring or nonopaque band. In gastric bypass operations (Fig 25–6) the small proximal pouch is anastomosed to the jejunum by either a standard loop or Roux-en-Y gastrojejunostomy. Unlike anastomoses in bypass procedures done because of ulcer disease or tumor, the diameter of the anastomosis in a gastric bypass is intentionally limited to 1 cm or less. The distal stomach is functionally separate from the proximal pouch but may not be transected.[7, 8]

Review of Surgical Case Presentation and Analysis

In the case presented (Figs 25–1 and 25–7), double-contrast views were obtained by standard methods. The history indicates a truncal vagotomy, evidenced by surgical clips (see Fig 25–7) near the

gastroesophageal junction. There has not been any gastric resection, but the gastric antrum is scarred, contracted, and nondistensible. Variable degrees of antral contraction can be seen in patients with a long-standing gastroenterostomy that was performed because of benign disease. It is not clear how soon after gastroenterostomy such contraction may be expected to develop, and the causes for the deformity remain elusive.[6, 12] The appearance of the antrum mimics infiltrating tumor, which should be, and was, excluded by endoscopy.

There is a 5 cm diameter side-to-side loop-type left-to-right gastrojejunostomy, with contrast material outlining small bowel loops. During fluoroscopy, when the patient was in the lateral position, the anastomosis was seen on the anterior wall of the stomach.

Although the anastomosis is patent, there is evidence for gastritis with mucosal edema, which is characterized by fold thickening. Closer inspection reveals a well-defined barium-filled crater (see Fig

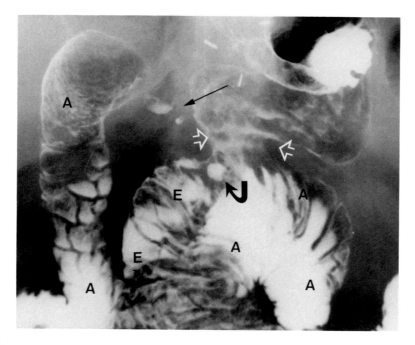

FIG 25-7.
Stomal ulceration after vagotomy with left-to-right gastrojejunostomy. The anastomosis *(open arrows)* is widely patent, but there are thickened folds near edema, with an ulcer crater *(curved arrow)* in the ef- ferent (distal) loop *(E)* of jejunum. The afferent (proximal) loop *(A)*, including the duodenum, is normal. The gastric antrum *(long arrow)* is atrophic and contracted, but was otherwise normal on endoscopy.

25-7), representing an ulcer in the distal loop of the jejunum distal to the anastomosis. At endoscopy this ulcer proved to be a site of active bleeding.

Recurrent Ulceration and Sequelae

Although recurrent ulcers are termed marginal or stomal, they have a predilection for the small bowel. They are seen more frequently in the efferent loop, usually within 2 cm of the anastomosis (see Fig 25-5).[3, 6, 9, 10] Recurrent ulcers following Billroth I partial gastrectomy are usually near or at the anastomosis (see Fig 25-3).[13] Ulceration in the gastric remnant is rare.[13] Of all recurrent ulcers, about 95% occur after surgery because of duodenal ulcer; only 2% to 4% occur after surgery because of gastric ulcer.[14] They generally result from inadequate therapy, that is, incomplete vagotomy or insufficient resection of the parietal cell mass during subtotal gastrectomy.[14] However, other causes of recurrent ulceration, such as Zollinger-Ellison syndrome with a gastrin-secreting tumor, hypercalcemia, smoking, and ulcerogenic drug abuse, should not be forgotten.[14] The incidence of recurrent ulcer- ation varies with the type of antiulcer surgery performed, but an acceptable recurrent ulcer rate is about 3% for any type of operation done because of duodenal ulcer.[14] In general, operations that effect a greater reduction in gastric secretion, such as vagotomy and hemigastrectomy, have a lower incidence of ulcer recurrence than those that reduce gastric secretion to a lesser extent, such as antral exclusion or gastroenterostomy alone.[15] However, these operations are more likely to have untoward side effects, including undesirable postprandial symptoms, bilious vomiting, diarrhea, and weight loss, with increased postoperative mortality and morbidity.[16] Surgical trends change, but with the advent of medical agents including histamine H_2-receptor antagonists, recurrent ulceration may be less of an unacceptable complication than the other problems associated with ulcer-curing operations requiring extensive gastric resection.[14, 16] Ulcer disease following gastric restrictive surgery is unusual; most patients do not have an underlying cause for ulceration and the stomach is not resected, so the normal physiologic mechanisms of gastric acid secretion are not disturbed. When ulcerations do occur, they are usu-

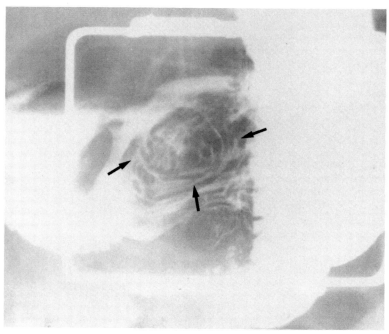

FIG 25–8.
Retrograde intussusception. A compression film shows a striated filling defect with small bowel folds *(arrows)* identified in the gastric lumen near the site of gastrojejunostomy.

ally in the stomach, associated with some degree of stasis above a narrowed channel.[8]

Radiologic detection of marginal ulceration varies widely.[2, 4, 5, 17, 18] If the radiologic diagnosis of ulceration is questionable or if the patient's symptoms persist in the face of normal findings on upper gastrointestinal study, endoscopy can be a valuable supplement. At present endoscopy may be superior to radiography in the detection of small stomal ulcers.[3, 4, 18]

Complications of recurrent ulcer include hemorrhage, bowel perforation, abscess formation, and gastrojejunocolic fistula.[3, 9, 10, 14] Hemorrhage occurs in as many as 60% of patients.[14] Although bleeding usually is chronic, acute massive hemorrhage requiring emergency surgery can occur. Perforation follows marginal ulceration in about 10% of patients.[14] Symptoms in these patients are similar to those seen in nonsurgical patients with ulcer perforation.

Occasionally an anterior abdominal wall abscess occurs after antecolic gastrojejunostomy; if the anastomosis is retrocolic, a gastrojejunocolic fistula may occur. The incidence of gastrojejunocolic fistula ranges from 5% to 23%.[14] Diarrhea, weight loss with emaciation, electrolyte imbalance, and abdominal distention may be present, but patients may not have abdominal findings. The most reliable diagnostic procedure for a fistula is a barium enema.[3]

Other Complications After Gastric Surgery

Outlet obstruction from perianastomotic edema, hemorrhage, scarring, or stricture from prior ulceration can develop.[3, 6, 9, 10, 13, 14] With attention to detail during the upper gastrointestinal study, the radiologist can obtain a reliable film of the proximal bowel loop and exclude obstruction of the afferent loop. However, endoscopy may be required to evaluate for stomal patency. If this is not technically feasible, computed tomography or ultrasonographic studies can show abnormal fluid-filled bowel.

Other obstructing anastomotic lesions include antegrade or retrograde intussusception.[6, 10, 19] Symptoms usually suggest an intermittent obstruction, with colicky bouts of vomiting and abdominal pain; however, intussusception may be asymptomatic. A striated filling defect (Fig 25–8) with small bowel folds, usually the efferent limb, is outlined in the gastric lumen.[9]

Neoplasm at the anastomosis can occur secondarily as a recurrent process after resection performed because of gastric cancer or as a primary process in a patient whose original surgery was done because of benign disease.[3, 6, 9, 10, 13] Surgical deformity makes evaluation for tumor at the anastomosis difficult except in gross cases. Gastric remnant cancer after surgery because of benign disease may be as high as 10%.[20] On average, the carcinoma develops in about 23 years, but monitoring for cancer should start at 7 to 10 years.[6] The tumor usually develops in the gastric remnant near the stoma, with polypoid mucosal changes occurring near the gastroenterostomy.[20] The cause for tumor development is not fully known, but it may relate to the presence of atrophic gastritis.[13, 20] Radiographic findings include localized nodularity (Fig 25–9) or diffuse infiltrating tumor causing constriction of the gastric remnant.

Narrowing of the channel in patients with gastroplasty or gastric bypass surgery (Fig 25–10) can occur, causing outlet obstruction. Some patients tolerate channel narrowing better than others and may endure uncomfortable symptoms as long as they continue to lose weight.[8] Gastroesophageal reflux and its sequelae usually cause them to seek follow-up care.

Retained food or debris is well known to occur proximal to an obstructing lesion, but gastric bezoars also can be seen as a complication of vagot-

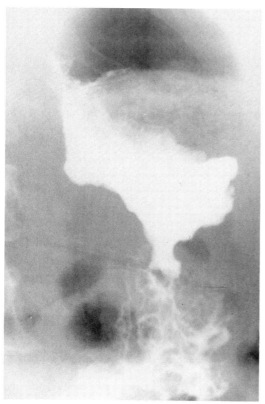

FIG 25–9.
Recurrent carcinoma. The inferior border of the gastric remnant is nodular and nondistensible in this patient who had undergone subtotal gastric resection with a loop-type gastrojejunostomy because of gastric cancer. Outlet obstruction is evident with gas-debris level.

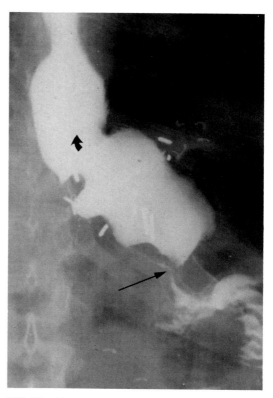

FIG 25–10.
Roux-en-Y gastric bypass with channel stenosis, pouch dilation, and gastroesophageal reflux. The channel *(long arrow)* is severely narrowed, with minimal contrast material filling the small bowel and dilation of the proximal pouch. Despite symptoms of gastroesophageal reflux *(curved arrow)* and subsequent esophagitis, the patient was reluctant to seek follow-up care because postoperative weight loss was rapid and sustained.

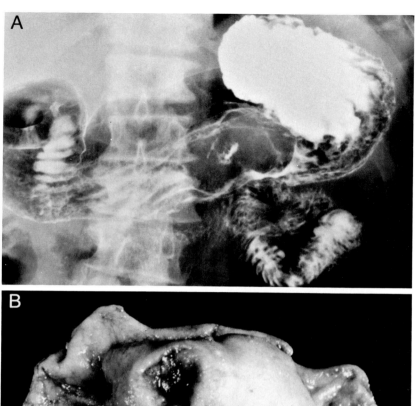

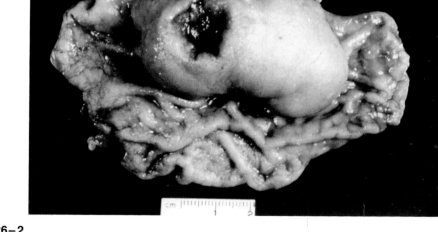

FIG 26–2.
A, large ulcerated submucosal mass is seen within the body of the stomach. This appearance is compatible with a variety of submucosal gastric tumors, including carcinoid, which ulcerates in approximately 40% of cases. **B,** gross surgical specimen confirms the radiologic findings. Pathologic examination revealed a carcinoid.

dominant cells in eosinophilic granuloma are fibroblasts and inflammatory cells; thus the alternate designation for this condition, inflammatory fibroid polyp.[10] These lesions are well circumscribed and completely benign. They have no relationship to eosinophilic granuloma of bone and are distinct from eosinophilic gastroenteritis.[11] Peripheral eosinophilia does not occur, and there is no association with allergies.[10] Therapy for eosinophilic granuloma usually is simple resection.

Lipoma

Gastric lipomas (Fig 26–5) occur most commonly in the antrum and account for 5% of gastrointestinal lipomas, the colon being the favored lo-

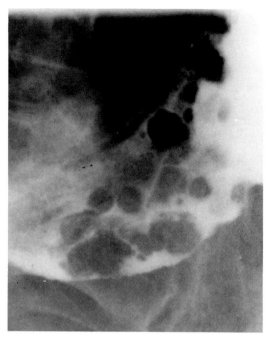

FIG 26–3.
Multiple submucosal filling defects are visualized within the body of the stomach. This is an unusual example of multiple islands of ectopic pancreas.

cation. Ninety percent of gastric lipomas are of submucosal origin, the rest are subserosal; approximately 10% are multiple.[12] Initial symptoms include massive hemorrhage and abdominal pain.[13] Upper gastrointestinal series demonstrates a smooth well-defined mass that can change in configuration, especially with external compression. In addition the radiolucent fatty quality of the tumor can be seen if soft tissue technique is used. The diagnosis can be better made by CT, in which attenuation of the mass is of fat density (i.e., from 80 to −120 Hounsfield units).[14] Pathologically the mass should be homogeneous without septa. Liposarcomas of the stomach have not been reported. Because gastric lipoma is a benign tumor, it should be treated conservatively; symptomatic lesions can be biopsied and resected.

Vascular Tumors

Hemangioma is the most common submucosal vascular lesion in the stomach, accounting for approximately 2% of all benign tumors. This lesion can be specifically diagnosed on upper gastrointestinal series when phleboliths are present[15] (Fig

26–6). These benign tumors usually are round and lobulated. Histologically there is no infiltration of the surrounding tissues. Most patients with hemangioma have hemorrhage, which may be slow and chronic. Sarcomatous transformation is rare, and simple resection is the treatment of choice.[16]

Hemangiopericytoma and lymphangioma are two other vascular tumors that occur in the submucosal layer of the stomach. The hemangiopericytoma originates from muscular elements surrounding capillary walls, specifically from the pericytes of Zimmermann. Most of these tumors occur in the subcutaneous tissues of the lower extremities and the retroperitoneum; rarely, however, they occur in the gastrointestinal tract, most commonly in the stomach. These are bulky, slow-growing tumors that bleed. They do have malignant potential but also have a better prognosis than hemangiopericytoma in other parts of the body.[17] Lymphangiomas are benign tumors that rarely occur in the stomach;

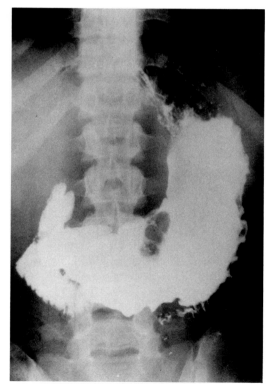

FIG 26–4.
A polypoid mass is visualized along the lesser curvature of the stomach. Examination of biopsy tissue revealed the lesion to be eosinophilic granuloma (also called inflammatory fibroid polyp).

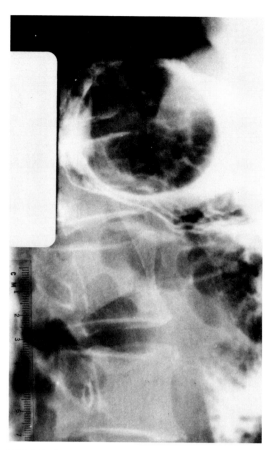

FIG 26–5.
A large, well-defined round gastric mass, which changed in configuration on fluoroscopy, was surgically proved to be a lipoma.

they are found most commonly in the neck, axilla, and trunk. These tumors (also known as lymphatic cysts, mesenteric cysts, cystic hygromas, and cavernous lymphangiomas) are composed of dilated endothelial-lined spaces surrounded by connective tissue and smooth muscle. The most common symptoms of gastric lymphangioma are caused by an enlarging mass, although these tumors can be asymptomatic. No malignant degeneration has been reported.[18]

Neural Tumors

The two major types of benign gastric neural tumors are neurofibroma and schwannoma.[19] Approximately half of all gastric neurofibromas are associated with neurofibromatosis. The stomach is second only to the jejunum as the location of gas-

trointestinal neurofibromas in neurofibromatosis.[20] Schwannomas usually are not associated with neurofibromatosis. Chronic bleeding and anemia are the most common symptoms in both groups. Neurogenic tumors (Fig 26–7) usually have a broad-based attachment to the stomach wall or can be pedunculated.[19] If the tumor is pedunculated, it can prolapse through the pylorus and cause obstruction. Deep punched-out ulcerations are often present. Malignant degeneration of benign neural tumors has been reported.[20] Neurogenic sarcomas are locally invasive early and metastasize late. Because neural tumors are known to recur locally, treatment is usually wide surgical resection.[19]

CONCLUSION

Many different types of benign and malignant submucosal neoplasms arise within the stomach

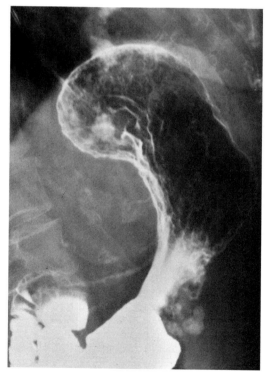

FIG 26–6.
Filling defect along the greater curvature of the stomach contains round calcific densities (some with central lucencies) typical of phleboliths. Note that the epicenter of the mass is within the wall of the stomach. These findings are highly suggestive of hemangioma.

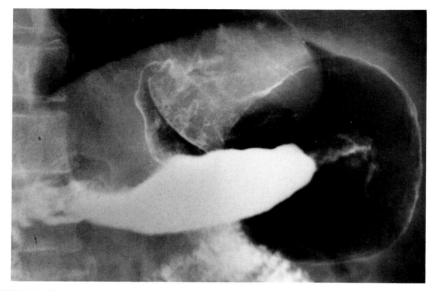

FIG 26–7.
A large mass in the fundus of the stomach is causing considerable irregularity of the adjacent wall. This lesion was resected and found to be a neurofibroma.

wall. When occasional phleboliths or an accessory-barium-filled pancreatic duct are seen, the diagnosis can be made on an upper gastrointestinal series. Similarly, if a tumor is thought to be a lipoma, a CT scan can be obtained to give the definitive diagnosis. Because most gastric submucosal tumors are similar in appearance, however, usually only a differential diagnosis can be offered and pathologic analysis is required.

Excellent radiologic technique fostering identification of these masses is of prime importance. Whereas certain characteristics of a gastric lesion are suggestive of a benign submucosal tumor, the radiologist must always be aware that these tumors can sometimes be mimicked by their malignant counterparts (e.g., leiomyoma versus leiomyosarcoma) and occasionally by malignant mucosal neoplasms, including carcinoma and lymphoma. Each lesion should be carefully examined for malignant characteristics, such as infiltration of the gastric wall or presence of metastases.

Through systematic analysis, a differential, and occasionally a specific, diagnosis of a submucosal gastric tumor can be suggested and proper management provided.

Acknowledgments

The authors thank Mrs. Kathleen Jensen for expert editorial and transcription assistance, and the Department of Radiologic Pathology at the Armed Forces Institute of Pathology and their contributors for our figures.

REFERENCES

1. Delikaris P, Golematis B, Missitzis J, et al: Smooth muscle neoplasms of the stomach. *South Med J* 1983; 76:440–442.
2. Scatarige JC, Fishman EK, Jones B, et al: Gastric leiomyosarcoma: CT observations. *J Comput Assist Tomogr* 1985; 9:320–327.
3. O'Riordan D, Levine MS, Yeager BA: Complete healing of ulceration within a gastric leiomyoma. *Gastric Radiol* 1985; 10:47–49.
4. Nauert TC, Zornoza J, Ordonez N: Gastric leiomyosarcomas. *AJR* 1982; 139:291–297.
5. Balthazar EJ, Megibow A, Bryk D, et al: Gastric carcinoid tumors: Radiographic features in eight cases. *AJR* 1982; 139:1123–1127.
6. Goldfarb JP, Gross F, Maxfield R, et al: Gastric carcinoid: Two unusual presentations. *Am J Gastroenterol* 1983; 78:332–334.
7. Marshak RH, Lindner AE, Maklansky D: *Radiology of the Stomach.* Philadelphia, WB Saunders Co, 1983, pp 205–215.
8. Thoeni RF, Gedgaudas RK: Ectopic pancreas: Usual and unusual features. *Gastrointest Radiol* 1980; 5:37–42.
9. Kilman WJ, Berk RN: The spectrum of radiological features of aberrant pancreatic rests

involving the stomach. *Radiology* 1977; 123:291–296.

10. Shimer GR, Helwig EB: Inflammatory fibroid polyps of the intestines. *Am J Clin Pathol* 1984; 81:708–714.

11. Ishikura H, Sato F, Naka A, et al: Inflammatory fibroid polyp of the stomach. *Acta Pathol Jpn* 1986; 36:327–335.

12. Agha FP, Dent TL, Fiddian-Green RG, et al: Bleeding lipomas of the upper gastrointestinal tract. *Am Surg* 1985; 51:279–285.

13. Maderal F, Hunter F, Fuselier G, et al: Gastric lipomas—An update of clinical presentation, diagnosis and treatment. *Am J Gastroenterol* 1984; 79:964–967.

14. Imoto T, Nobe T, Koga M, et al: Computed tomography of gastric lipomas. *Gastrointest Radiol* 1983; 8:129–131.

15. Flannery MG, Caster MP: Hemangioma of the stomach with a roentgenologic diagnostic point. *Am J Roentgenol* 1957; 77:38–39.

16. Simms SM: Gastric hemangioma associated with phleboliths. *Gastrointest Radiol* 1985; 10:51–53.

17. Cueto J, Gilbert EF, Currie RA: Hemangiopericytoma of the stomach. *Am J Surg* 1966; 112:943–946.

18. Drago JR, DeMuth WE: Lymphangioma of the stomach in a child. *Am J Surg* 1976; 131:605–606.

19. Canney RL: Neurogenic tumors of the stomach. *Br J Surg* 1948; 36:139–147.

20. Petersen JM, Ferguson DR: Gastrointestinal neurofibromatosis. *J Clin Gastroenterol* 1984; 6:529–534.

CHAPTER 27

Gastric Fundal Masses

Hal D. Safrit, M.D.
Reed P. Rice, M.D.

Case Presentation

A 50-year-old woman had intermittent dysphagia and increasing epigastric pain for 4 months. An upper gastrointestinal examination performed 5 years previously was remarkable only for a sliding hiatal hernia. The present study reveals a lobulated fundal mass (Fig 27–1). What is the differential diagnosis? What additional maneuvers may be helpful?

DISCUSSION

The gastric fundus, defined as the region of the stomach proximal to the esophogastric junction, presents a challenge to the combined technical and interpretive skills of the radiologist. The difficulty in accurate delineation of disease involving the fundus has been addressed repeatedly since the first application of contrast studies to the upper gastrointestinal tract. Early authorities clearly understood this problem and emphasized the importance of close scrutiny on conventional single-contrast examinations. More recently authors have advocated double-contrast techniques to improve fundal distention, mucosal coating, and visualization. However, even with a satisfactory examination the correct interpretation of radiographic findings can be hindered significantly by the many normal variants, benign tumors, and other conditions that may mimic fundal malignancies.[1–3]

In the fundal region the overlying rib cage limits effective compression, the essential component of a single-contrast examination. Not surprisingly, recent literature has indicated that the double-contrast examination permits a more consistent demonstration of the normal and abnormal fundus.[4, 5] It is not our purpose to debate the relative merits of these techniques; however, no examination of the stomach is complete unless there is sufficient fundal distention and visualization of mucosal detail. Many radiologists routinely perform a biphasic examination by following a double-contrast upper gastrointestinal study with thin barium and palpation. When an initial single-contrast examination does not adequately evaluate the fundus the reverse sequence may be used. We have found that after poor visualization of the fundal region by a single-contrast examination a supplementary double-contrast study with the administration of effervescent crystals and heavy-density barium can result in excellent fundal distention and mucosal coating (Fig 27–2).

Assuming a satisfactory examination, the radiologist not only must detect the presence of an abnormality but also determine its significance. An extensive differential diagnosis of fundal deformities is listed in Table 27–1. Malignant tumors are the most important fundal lesions and may have a variety of radiographic appearances. Several of their salient features are reviewed in order to arrive at an appropriate differential diagnosis. In the United States the most common radiographic presentation

11. Klinefelter EW: Invagination of the esophagus in hiatal hernia. *Radiology* 1956; 67:562–568.
12. Rice RP, Thompson WM, Kelvin FM, et al: Gastric varices without esophageal varices. *JAMA* 1977; 237:1976–1979.
13. Muhletaler C, Gerlock AJ, Goncharenko V, et al: Gastric varices secondary to splenic vein occlusion: Radiographic diagnosis and clinical significance. *Radiology* 1979; 132:593–598.
14. Evans JA, Delany F: Gastric varices. *Radiology* 1953; 60:46–51.
15. Balthazar EJ, Megibow A, Naidach D, et al: Computed tomographic recognition of gastric varices. *AJR* 1984; 142:1121–1125.
16. Skucas J, Mangla JC, Adams JT, et al: An evaluation of the Nissen fundoplication. *Radiology* 1976; 118:539–543.
17. Feigin DS, James AE, Stitik FP, et al: The radiological appearance of hiatal hernia repairs. *Radiology* 1974; 110:71–77.
18. Balthazar EJ: Miscellaneous disorders of the stomach, in Taveras JM, Ferrucci JT (eds): *Radiology: Diagnosis, Imaging, Intervention,* vol 4. *Gastrointestinal Radiology.* Philadelphia, JB Lippincott Co, 1987, pp 1–14.
19. Wright FW, Matthews JM: Hemophilic pseudotumor of the stomach. *Radiology* 1971; 98:547–550.
20. Eisenberg R: Intrinsic/extrinsic masses of the fundus, in *Gastrointestinal Radiology: A Pattern Approach.* Philadelphia, JB Lippincott Co, 1983, pp 296–308.

CHAPTER 28

Gastric Ulceration in the Cancer Patient

David Frager, M.D.
Thomas C. Beneventano, M.D.

Case Presentation

A 72-year-old woman with metastatic carcinoma of the breast had epigastric pain and melena. An upper gastrointestinal roentgenographic series performed to determine the source of the bleeding (Fig 28–1) demonstrated two gastric ulcers. Endoscopy and biopsy were performed to exclude metastatic involvement. What is the likelihood that these gastric ulcerations are malignant? Does the upper gastrointestinal roentgenographic series help resolve this question?

DISCUSSION

Carcinoma of the breast is one of the leading causes of gastric metastases and is found in 6% to 18% of such patients at autopsy.[1, 2] Carcinoma of the lung (gastric metastases in 10% to 26% of patients) is the other major malignant lesion with a predilection for gastric involvement.[1, 2] Thus in the case presented an ulcerating gastric metastasis is a major clinical consideration.

Metastatic disease to the stomach from carcinoma of the breast typically is of the constricting infiltrating form, which mimics linitis plastica of primary gastric adenocarcinoma (Fig 28–2). In approximately 50% to 89% of patients with gastric metastases due to carcinoma of the breast the metastasis has the appearance of linitis plastica.[3, 4] This form of submucosal metastatic infiltration from breast cancer occasionally produces mucosal ulceration and bleeding.

The polypoid form of submucosal metastasis can be single or multiple. In some instances this form ulcerates and produces a "bull's-eye" or "target" appearance (Fig 28–3). Ulcerating submucosal masses that are large, intraluminal, necrotic, and have an irregular appearance can mimic a primary ulcerating gastric carcinoma (Fig 28–4). Submucosal masses with a large extraluminal component (exoenteric) can undergo necrosis and form large aneurysmal cavities or ulcers. This kind of ulcerating lesion usually is secondary to a sarcoma, lymphoma, or melanoma involving the bowel (Figs 28–3 to 28–5).

Serosal gastric metastases usually are due to direct extension from contiguous tumors of the transverse colon or pancreas; in cases of diffuse peritoneal carcinomatosis with "omental cake" they may be due to carcinoma of the ovary or colon. Peritoneal carcinomatosis secondary to carcinoma of the lung or breast is uncommon. In these rare cases and in cases of omental cake secondary to ovarian carcinoma the appearance of the stomach may be similar. Infrequently serosal lesions extend through the mucosa and produce ulceration, such as in carcinoma of the pancreas.

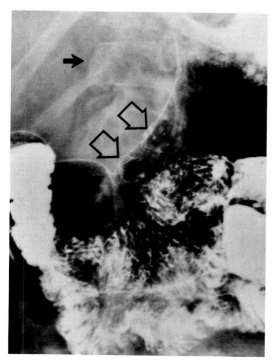

FIG 28–1.
Anteroposterior view of the stomach demonstrates two gastric ulcers *(open arrows)* and vertebral metastasis *(arrow).*

No characteristic appearance has been associated with gastric metastases due to carcinoma of the lung (see Fig 28–4), which can vary from bull's-eye lesions to linitis plastica. Metastatic melanoma, however, characteristically assumes a bull's-eye configuration or rarely the appearance of aneurysmal ulceration.

The upper gastrointestinal roentgenographic series in our case reveals two gastric ulcers on the lesser curvature in the region of the angulus (see Fig 28–1). No mass is associated with these ulcers. At least one ulcer is extraluminal and regular in shape. These findings are characteristic of a benign gastric ulcer. The disturbing facts in this case are the known clinical history of metastatic breast carcinoma and the multiplicity of the ulcers. The number of gastric ulcers, however, does not predict whether they are benign or malignant.[5, 6] In several reviews of benign peptic gastric ulcers the percentage of multiple (two or more) gastric ulcers ranged from about 3% to 30%[7, 8]; most recent reviews put the number of multiple gastric ulcers between 10% and 24%.[5, 9, 10] The corollary holds true that 18% of pa-

tients with multiple gastric ulcers have an underlying malignant lesion,[6] often lymphoma. In our experience, patients who are severely debilitated from underlying benign or malignant disease tend to have multiple benign ulcers (Fig 28–6). These ulcers often fail to show evidence of an associated inflammatory (edema) or healing (radiating folds) response. Multiple benign gastric ulcers also have been associated with ingestion of aspirin or related compounds.

A clinical history of underlying breast carcinoma does not necessarily indicate that a gastric lesion is malignant. Several endoscopic studies of patients with cancer with hematemesis or significant melena showed that the cause of bleeding is usually benign.[11–13] In Lightdale et al.'s[11] series from Memorial Sloan-Kettering Cancer Center, among 81 patients with malignant disease and upper gastrointestinal tract hemorrhage, 47% had severe gastritis, 11% had duodenal ulcers, and 11% had gastric ulcers as the leading cause of hemorrhage. Causes of severe gastritis were severe stress due to sepsis, shock, renal, or hepatic insufficiency; the postoperative state; and exogenous agents including nonsteroidal anti-inflammatory drugs, corticosteroids, ethanol, chemotherapeutic agents (e.g., 5-fluorouracil, cyclophosphamide, methotrexate, bleomycin), and radiotherapy. Although systemic chemotherapy usually does not produce frank gastric or duodenal ulcers, large ulcers have been produced by direct hepatic artery infusion of chemotherapeutic agents.[14] These results were supported by a study from the M.D. Anderson Hospital and Tumor Institute,[12] where only 27% of bleeding gastroduodenal lesions in patients with known cancer were malignant. The metastatic tumor most likely to bleed was due to systemic lymphoma with gastric involvement.[11]

Thus in the case presented, the radiographic finding of multiple benign gastric ulcers is helpful in patient treatment. The treatment and prognosis for benign peptic ulcer disease and metastatic disease differ. The need for endoscopic biopsy under these circumstances is controversial. However, when the policy of an institution is to perform a biopsy in all gastric ulcers, this patient would undergo endoscopy. Alternatively, if the clinician is willing to rely on the radiographic diagnosis of benign ulcer and obtain an interval upper gastrointestinal roentgenographic series to document healing, the fact that the patient has carcinoma of the breast should not pose a significant problem. Levine et al.[10] and Thompson et al.[15] demonstrated that the reliable diagnosis of

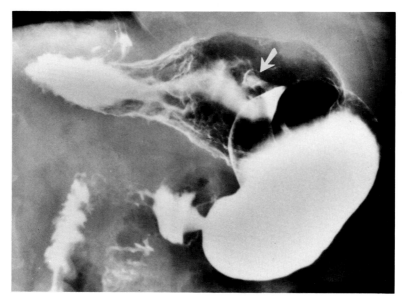

FIG 28–2.
Scirrhous metastatic carcinoma of the breast to the gastric fundus. Note small ulcer *(arrow).*

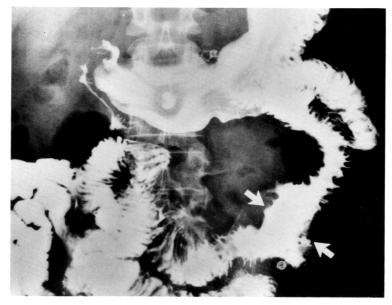

FIG 28–3.
Bull's-eye lesion of melanoma in the gastric antrum. Note large aneurysmal ulceration in the jejunum *(arrows).*

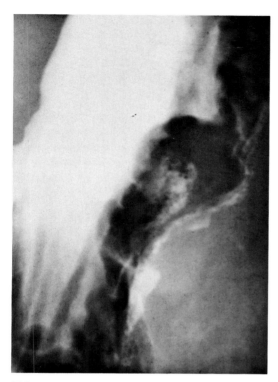

FIG 28–4.
Large ulcerating mass due to adenocarcinoma of the lung.

benign ulcer is practically 100% certain when radiographic criteria are met. In equivocal cases endoscopy and biopsy should be performed.

The major possibilities to be considered in evaluating ulcerative lesions in the patient with cancer are listed in Table 28–1. The routine upper gastrointestinal roentgenographic series remains the most widely used and reliable radiographic examination in determining whether a gastric ulcer is benign or malignant. Criteria for the diagnosis of a benign gastric ulcer are well known[16–18] and include extraluminal location, regular radiating folds to the edge of the crater, edema collar or mound, Hampton's line, a smooth and sharply defined margin, and healing on follow-up study. According to Nelson,[16] when two of these criteria are present the diagnosis of benign ulcer can be made with reasonable confidence. The upper gastrointestinal roentgenographic series, however, cannot pinpoint the cause of a benign gastric ulcer. This is particularly true in the patient with cancer who has undergone various treatment regimens or radiation protocols. Greater curvature ulceration, often due to the inges-

tion of nonsteroidal anti-inflammatory drugs, frequently is difficult to evaluate definitively on an upper gastrointestinal roentgenographic series because the criteria used to distinguish a benign from a malignant ulcer are most applicable to the classic gastric ulcer occurring on the lesser curvature of the stomach at the incisura angularis; greater curvature ulcers, even when benign, tend to be intraluminal.

Polypoid lesions, ulcerating or not, are difficult

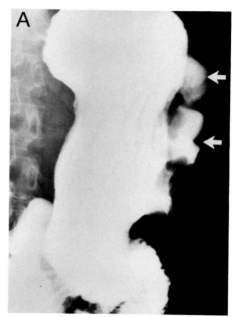

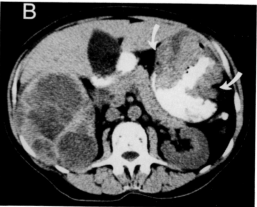

FIG 28–5.
A, large ulcer along the greater curvature of the gastric body (metastatic melanoma; *arrows*). **B,** computed tomography demonstrates large associated mass with necrosis *(arrows)*. Note large liver and right-sided renal metastases.

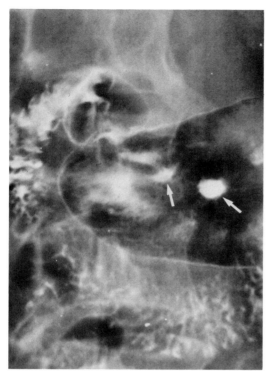

FIG 28–6.
Multiple benign gastric ulcers *(arrows)* in a patient
with leukemia.

to evaluate in the patient with cancer, because a
small hyperplastic polyp cannot be readily distinguished from a small metastasis. As polypoid lesions enlarge, the features that distinguish a submucosal metastatic lesion from a benign mucosal adenomatous polyp become more apparent. Thus a
round smooth polypoid lesion with central ulceration and obtuse (90 degrees or more) junctions
with the bowel wall is submucosal, whereas an irregular acutely angled lesion tends to be mucosal.

Because there is some degree of overlap of features of mucosal and submucosal lesions, the radiologist faces an additional dilemma in the patient with
cancer. It is difficult to distinguish a benign leiomyoma from an ulcerating submucosal metastasis, and
equally difficult to distinguish a submucosal metastasis from a new primary carcinoma or lymphoma. When multiple lesions are present, the likelihood that the lesions are metastatic or lymphomatous is increased. The endoscopist has less difficulty
evaluating submucosal lesions under these circumstances because certain lesions, such as melanoma,
have fairly characteristic pigmentation. In addition

the endoscopist can obtain biopsy tissue. However,
standard endoscopic biopsy procedures may not always achieve tissue samples adequate to establish
the diagnosis of metastasis.[19]

The presence of multiple large bull's-eye lesions is virtually diagnostic of metastatic disease,
but the appearance of smaller target lesions may
also suggest erosive gastritis (Fig 28–7). The differentiation of these entities is extremely important in
the patient with cancer in whom the leading cause
of bleeding is gastritis. Our experience has been that
aphthae generally are smaller than 5 mm in diameter, whereas bull's-eye lesions are larger than 1 cm
in diameter. Exceptions, however, do occur. Erosive gastritis can resolve in 24 to 48 hours; therefore
an interval examination that documents the disappearance of the erosions is diagnostic of benign disease. However, if one large lesion is typical of a
metastatic lesion the smaller lesions are likely to be
metastases as well. Another indication that multiple

TABLE 28–1.
**Differential Diagnosis of Ulcerative Lesions in the
Stomach**

Benign
  Single or multiple peptic ulcers
    Coincidental
    Aspirin or related compounds
    Hepatic artery chemotherapy infusion
    Zollinger-Ellison syndrome (can be malignant)
  Erosive gastritis
    Aspirin or related compounds
    Systemic chemotherapy
    General stress and debilitation
    Radiation induced
    Infection (*Candida,* cryptosporidiosis)
  Tumors with superimposed ulceration
    Benign submucosal tumor (e.g., leiomyoma)
    Benign ulcerative hyperplastic or adenomatous
      polyps
  Other
    Granulomatous disease
    Iatrogenic (e.g., nasogastric tube erosion)
Malignant
  Hematogenous metastases
    Single or multiple submucosal nodules with
      ulceration
    "Bull's-eye" or target lesions
    Infiltrative linitis plastica pattern with ulceration
  Serosal metastases
    Direct extension and invasion with breakdown
    Omental cake with extension and invasion
  New primary adenocarcinoma or lymphoma
  New primary sarcoma
  Carcinoid

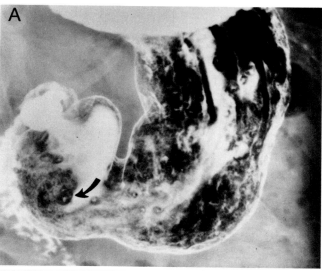

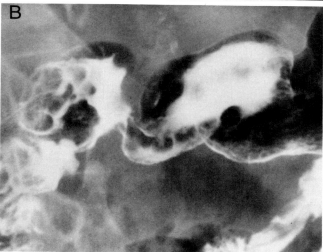

FIG 28–7.
A, metastatic melanoma with small target lesions (approximately 6 mm). One lesion, however, is larger (1 cm; *arrow).* **B,** erosive gastroduodenitis in a patient with carcinoma of the lung. Distinction from "bull's-eye" lesion is difficult: the erosions are slightly less well defined.

gastric lesions are metastatic is the presence of small bowel metastatic lesions, particularly in cases of melanoma (see Fig 28–3). There are subtle intrinsic differences between erosions and bull's-eye lesions, according to Laufer.[20] The edema surrounding aphthae tends to be more ill-defined than the sharply demarcated submucosal nodules due to metastatic implants. In addition, aphthae tend to be more localized than metastases, which have more widespread gastric involvement.

Occasional confusion occurs concerning gastric ulceration in patients with lymphoma. Lymphoma of the ulcerative type often presents with multiple ulcers and frequently is combined with the polypoid or infiltrative forms of the disease, which helps to confirm the malignant nature of the ulcerations. These ulcers usually do not meet the radiographic criteria of the benign gastric ulcer. A major exception occurs in patients receiving chemotherapy. In these patients healing malignant ulcers occasionally can assume a benign configuration on the upper gastrointestinal roentgenographic series[21] (Fig 28–8).

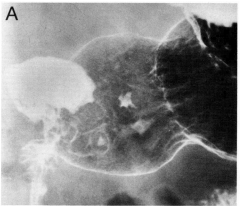

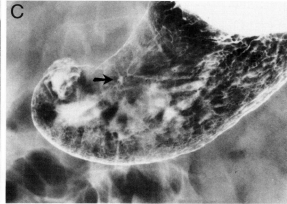

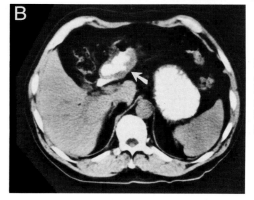

FIG 28–8.
A, antral ulcerations and target lesions due to lymphoma.
B, computed tomography shows ulcerations with minimal
mass *(arrow).* **C,** after chemotherapy there is a residual
benign appearing shallow ulcer with radiating folds
(arrow).

For radiologists and many clinicians the method of choice in the evaluation of any gastric lesion is the upper gastrointestinal series. This examination has been improved considerably over the years, particularly with the introduction of double-contrast techniques. Computed tomographic (CT) evaluation of the gastrointestinal tract also has been refined in recent years. Computed tomography is particularly useful in staging gastrointestinal neoplasms and diagnosing the complications of diverticulitis and inflammatory bowel disease. However, there are few reports on CT evaluation of gastric ulcerations. Many of these studies describe the value of CT in depicting and characterizing the various complications of penetration and perforation[22, 23]; however, the ability of CT to distinguish benign from malignant ulcers has not been studied thoroughly. In our experience, large malignant ulcers tend to be associated with large masses (see Fig 28–5). With smaller ulcers and erosions, our ability to distinguish between benign and malignant lesions is limited (see Fig 28–8). In one patient a benign ulcer on an upper gastrointestinal series had considerable mass on the CT scan (Fig 28–9); in another, with lymphoma with small bull's-eye lesions, the associated mass was minimal (see Fig 28–8). Further work in this area is needed to improve the ability to distinguish benign from malignant lesions noninvasively.

Also important is the distinction between a new primary gastric malignant lesion and metastasis in a patient with another known primary malignancy. This problem frequently occurs in patients with known adenocarcinoma of the lung or breast. Radiographic, endoscopic, and occasionally pathologic diagnosis can be difficult. However, with various immunohistologic techniques (e.g., estrogen or progesterone receptor evaluation), this dilemma can be overcome in many cases.

In summary, as in the case presented, gastric ulceration in a patient with cancer usually is benign. The diagnosis of the benign ulcer is reliable when radiologic criteria are met. The multiplicity of ulcerations is not of itself an indication that a lesion is malignant. The radiographic distinction between multiple benign erosions and small bull's-eye meta-

metastatic spread would affect the extent to which curative resection would be pursued at surgery. The CT examination with gas and contrast in the stomach showed the primary lesions again but did not reveal enlarged nodes or any liver metastases. At endoscopy the antral carcinoma was confirmed, but in addition an area of erythema and slight nodularity was noticed on the lesser curve of the distal body just about the angulus. A biopsy of the lesion was performed, and histologic examination showed a well-differentiated adenocarcinoma of the intestinal type. Review of the barium study showed that subtle abnormalities on the lesser curve had been overlooked (Fig 29–6).

A subtotal distal gastrectomy was performed of the polya type, and although the tumor was clearly through the wall of the stomach to the serosa, all but one of the resected lymph nodes were free of tumor.

Three years after the surgery the patient was seen again and complained of postprandial nausea and vomiting with some heartburn. He was sent for a barium contrast study, which showed the anatomy with a wide open stoma and a retained gastric food mass (Fig 29–7). Endoscopy revealed that the gastric mucosa was bright red and that there was a great deal of bile in the stomach, moderate esophagitis, and the bezoar. The bezoar was broken up with a basket and cleared with oral papain therapy. Biopsy of the gastric mucosa was performed, and the pathologist reported intense gastritis and severe intestinal metaplasia.

The symptoms of biliary gastritis did not resolve with medical treatment, and 6 months later, with CT showing a normal liver, the patient was operated on again and the gastrojejunal anastomosis converted to a Roux-en-Y to divert the bile away from the stomach. Six months later endoscopy showed normal gastric mucosa, with resolution of the gastritis and disappearance of the intestinal metaplasia. The patient had no dyspeptic symptoms provided he ate small frequent meals.

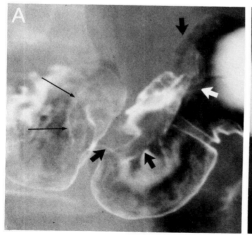
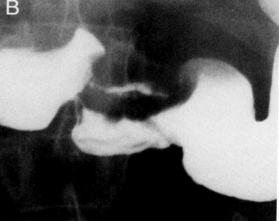

FIG 29–5.
A, double-contrast film shows the well-demarcated mass *(short arrows)* with central ulceration on the lesser curve of the antrum *(white arrow)* and producing an extrinsic impression on the duodenal bulb *(long arrows)*. **B,** single-contrast view of the tumor shows the classic sign of barium trapped in the ulcer.

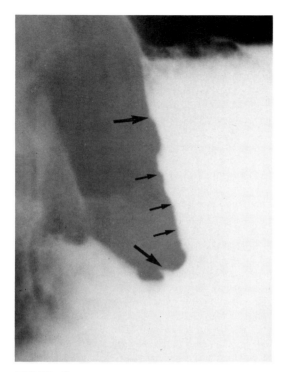

FIG 29–6.
Erect film reveals, in retrospect, a limited length of irregularity of the posterior aspect of the lesser curve. At endoscopy this was seen as a patch of slightly reddened uneven mucosa with no mass or ulceration, about 2.5 cm in diameter. It proved to be a second carcinoma, limited to the mucosa and submucosa.

DISCUSSION

1. *Ancestry*. There is considerable national variation in incidence of gastric carcinoma; the rate in Finland is several times that in the United States. It has been shown in Japanese who emigrate to the United States that the incidence of gastric carcinoma gradually falls toward that of the adopted country over the years, although this benefit is not seen in first-generation immigrants.[7] In contrast, in immigrants from countries with a high incidence of colon cancer the rate falls rapidly to that prevailing in the adopted country.

2. *Age*. Patients older than 40 years with new symptoms should be examined promptly because of the slight risk for carcinoma. However, outside of high-risk areas the likelihood of detecting curable gastric carcinoma radiologically is small.

3. *Staging*. Staging of gastric carcinoma by

CT was recommended some years ago.[8] However, especially at the cardia, mistakes in staging are readily made and surgery is usually required for symptomatic relief, regardless of CT findings, unless the disease is clinically far advanced. Many surgeons therefore do not obtain preoperative CT scans in patients with gastric carcinoma, and most radiologists will follow the surgeon's preference in the absence of strong evidence for staging.

4. *Diagnosis*. A confident radiologic diagnosis of gastric carcinoma is seldom wrong. However, in atypical cases histologic study of biopsy tissue may be helpful in distinguishing cancer from chronic benign ulcer and cancer from lymphoma or a rare granulomatous lesion. An important reason for insisting on endoscopy in a patient with gastric carcinoma is that 5% of these patients have a second primary carcinoma, usually overlooked on the barium study. The existence of the second lesion often to-

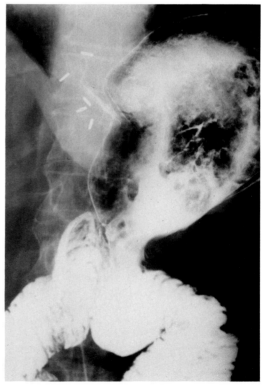

FIG 29–7.
Delayed postoperative barium study shows a retained mass of gastric residue, which was a vegetable bezoar. Endoscopy also showed intense biliary gastritis, which did not resolve until the anastomosis was converted to a Roux-en-Y.

tally changes the surgical plan for extent of resection, and a minority of "recurrent" carcinomas are due to the continued growth of the second primary lesion.

5. *Peptic ulceration*. Seventy percent of early gastric cancers have some peptic ulceration within them. Radiologic findings include small superficial ulcers with malignant changes near their margins.[9] More difficult to detect are tumors that are slightly elevated; these are best found by compression. Lesions that are flat are undetectable radiologically unless there is some neighboring fold distortion. In Japan only about 30% of early gastric carcinomas are recognized and correctly diagnosed on initial radiographic examination. When the disease is seen infrequently or a radiologist has no knowledge of having seen such lesions before, the detection rate will be low. A high index of suspicion and willingness to refer many patients for endoscopy because of trivial radiographic findings may result in early detection of a few curable gastric carcinomas.

6. *Gastric carcinoma after partial gastrectomy*. After partial gastrectomy, even for benign disease, there is an increased incidence of gastric carcinoma, higher after gastric ulcer than duodenal ulcer, probably because bile reflux causes biliary gastritis, leading to atrophy, intestinal metaplasia, and dysplasia.[10] The incidence of this development in Europe is on the order of 8% after 20 years, but even there the morbidity caused by surveillance is such that enthusiasm for follow-up has waned. In the United States the incidence of cancer development is lower and there is no indication for follow-up to detect cancer after gastric surgery for benign disease.

7. *Biliary gastritis*. Biliary gastritis causes symptoms, occasionally disabling, in some patients. These can be resolved by converting the anastomosis to a Roux-en-Y configuration, and the histologic appearance of the stomach will revert to normal. Despite the increase in operative time, some surgeons will routinely create a Roux-en-Y anastomosis for any distal gastrectomy, unless the operation is clearly for short-term palliation.

SUMMARY

Dyspepsia has a variety of causes, including several acid-related diseases such as gastroesophageal reflux and peptic gastric and duodenal ulceration. Gastric carcinoma, and several conditions not discussed here, such as cholelithiasis, chronic pancreatitis, granulomatous conditions, and Menetrier's disease, may also mimic dyspepsia.

Dyspepsia is common, and the policy of treating simple dyspepsia without radiologic investigation saves many patients from unnecessary procedures.

When investigation is required, ultrasound, in addition to endoscopy or barium radiographic study, may be useful to detect biliary, pancreatic, hepatic, or even renal disease.

Barium fluoroscopy provides a broader overview of esophageal function and disease than endoscopy does, and is satisfactory in suspected gastric and duodenal disease in mobile adults. Nevertheless, endoscopy is more sensitive for all gastric and duodenal disease, particularly for small ulcers, and is far superior when the patient's condition precludes an optimal radiologic study. If price were equal, endoscopy should be preferred in suspected peptic ulcer and barium contrast studies in heartburn. Persistent symptoms after either investigation should prompt the other.

The best barium technique is an integrated study that includes double-contrast studies, single-contrast compression, and mucosal relief methods. In particular, failure to routinely compress the antrum and duodenal bulb ensures that a minority of ulcers and nodules are missed.

Barium radiology continues to have a useful role in the investigation of dyspepsia; however, this role will increasingly be secondary, especially in gastric and duodenal disease.

REFERENCES

1. Read L, Pass TM, Komaroff AL: Diagnosis and treatment of dyspepsia. A cost-effectiveness analysis. *Med Decis Making* 1982; 2:415–438.
2. Kahn K, Greenfield S: Endoscopy in the evaluation of dyspepsia. *Ann Intern Med* 1985; 102:266–269.
3. Cotton PB, Shorvon PJ: Endoscopy and radiology in peptic ulcer disease. *Clin Gastroenterol* 1984; 13:383–403.
4. Max MH, West B, Knutson CO: Evaluation of postoperative gastroduodenal symptoms: Endoscopy or upper gastrointestinal roentgenography? *Surgery* 1979; 86:578–582.
5. Ott DJ, Chen YM, Gelfand DW, et al: Radiographic accuracy in gastric ulcer: Comparison of single-contrast and multiphasic examinations. *AJR* 1986; 147:697–700.
6. Heimbach DM, Ferguson GS, Harley JD:

Treatment of traumatic hemobilia with angiographic embolization. *J Trauma* 1978; 18:221–224.

7. Buell D, Dunn JE Jr: Cancer mortality among Japanese Issei and Nisei of California. *Cancer* 1965; 18:656–664.

8. Moss AA, Schnyder P, Marks W, et al: Gastric adenocarcinoma: A comparison of the accuracy and economics of staging by computed tomography and surgery. *Gastroenterology* 1981; 80:45–50.

9. Ichikawa H: Differential diagnosis between benign and malignant ulcers of the stomach. *Clin Gastroenterol* 1973; 2:329–343.

10. Caygill CPJ, Hill MJ, Kirkham JS, et al: Mortality from gastric cancer following gastric surgery for peptic ulcer. *Lancet* 1986; 1:929–934.

CHAPTER 30

Gastric Motility Disorders

Herbert F. Gramm, M.D.

Case Presentation

A 32-year-old white woman with nausea and vomiting was referred for an upper gastrointestinal roentgenographic series after a 12-hour fast. Diabetes mellitus had been diagnosed at age 6 years, and she has had retinopathy, nephropathy, and peripheral nephropathy for the past 5 years. A scout film of the abdomen (Fig 30–1) and upper gastrointestinal series (Fig 30–2) were performed. What are the radiographic and pathophysiologic findings?

DISCUSSION

The scout film reveals a mottled pattern representing undigested food in the gas-containing stomach (Fig 30–1). An erect spot film of the stomach shows no significant liquid residue (see Fig 30–2,A) but a dome-shaped filling defect. A subsequent prone compression film of the stomach demonstrates multiple filling defects in a nondilated, elongated stomach (see Fig 30–2,B). Fluoroscopic observation revealed ineffectual, irregularly occurring peristalsis.

The clinical and radiographic findings in this patient are characteristic of diabetic gastric neuropathy.[1] Diabetic visceral neuropathy is probably the most common of the acquired autonomic neuropathies and is a complication of type 1 diabetes mellitus. The condition usually is accompanied by other complications, as in this patient.

The radiographic manifestations of diabetic gastric neuropathy are (1) solid gastric food residue despite an 8-hour fast (see Fig 30–1), (2) ineffectual peristalsis with asynchronous waves not coordinated in time or direction (Figs 30–3 and 30–4)., (3) mildly dilated, elongated (sausage-shaped) gastric configuration (Figs 30–2,B, 30–4, and 30–5),

(4) mildly dilated, patulous duodenal bulb (see Fig 30–4), and (5) retention of solid gastric residue after emptying of the liquid contrast material, leaving a bezoarlike cast of partially opacified food in the stomach (see Fig 30–5).

Because the gastric emptying abnormalities in diabetes mellitus are primarily attributable to impaired gastric vagal innervation,[2, 3] the differential diagnosis includes those conditions mediated by vagal dysfunction (Table 30–1).

The well-known effects of vagotomy on the stomach basically are due to diminished motility and acid pepsin secretion.[4] When the effects of vagotomy are exacerbated by loss of the mixing function provided by the antrum in patients after subtotal gastrectomy, one or more bezoars may result.[5] Phytobezoars are seen after Billroth I (Fig 30–6) and Billroth II (Fig 30–7) gastrectomy. Autovagotomy secondary to tumor invasion of the vagus nerve has been associated with carcinoma of the breast,[1] lung,[6] and esophagus.[7] A large number of drugs inhibit gastrointestinal motility, and drug-induced gastric motility disorders are becoming more prevalent as the number of drugs increases.[8] Most of the drugs listed in Table 30–2 have a preferential site of action, predominantly impairing peristaltic activ-

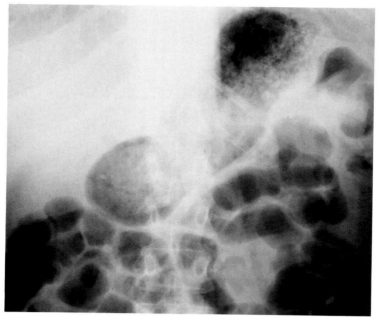

FIG 30–1.
Preliminary abdominal radiograph obtained prior to an upper gastrointestinal series demonstrates a non- dilated stomach containing some air as well as mot- tled density representing undigested food.

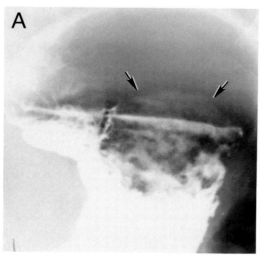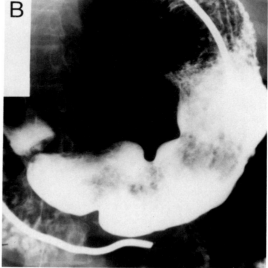

FIG 30–2.
A, erect spot film of the fundus of the stomach re- veals a small air-fluid level with a dome-shaped filling defect *(arrows)* projecting above it. **B,** prone com- pression spot film of antrum and body of the stomach demonstrates multiple filling defects in a nondilated, elongated stomach.

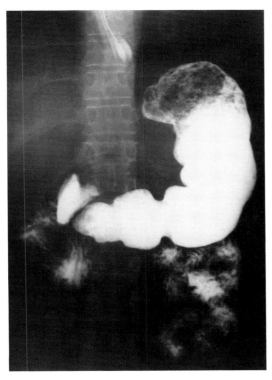

FIG 30–3.
Mildly dilated stomach with diffuse mottled filling defects and irregular peristaltic activity manifested by multiple indentations on the lesser and greater curvatures.

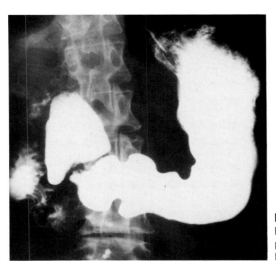

FIG 30–4.
Elongated, sausage-shaped stomach with irregular peristaltic activity. Note dilated, patulous duodenal bulb.

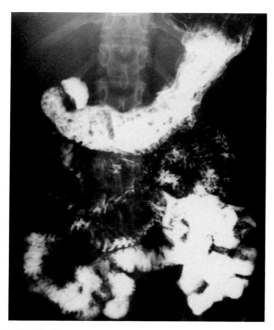

FIG 30–5.
This 30-minute follow-up film from an upper gastrointestinal series demonstrates an elongated, nondilated stomach containing a bezoarlike cast of solid food residue, with passage of most of the liquid barium into the proximal small bowel.

ity in either the stomach, the small bowel, or the large intestine; all of the listed agents have some effect on gastric emptying.

Metabolic disorders such as hypothyroidism,[9] hyperparathyroidism,[10] and hypercalcemia may be accompanied by decreased gastrointestinal motility. Patients with caloric deprivation and anorexia nervosa have delayed gastric emptying.[11] Infiltrative

TABLE 30–1.
Gastric Motility Disorders

Vagotomy
Autovagotomy
Drug induced (see Table 30–2)
Metabolic disorders
    Diabetes mellitus
    Hypothyroidism
    Hyperparathyroidism
Infiltrative conditions
Anorexia nervosa
Gastric smooth muscle and collagen diseases
Viral infections

conditions such as amyloidosis[12] and malignant neoplasm may result in gastric motility disturbance. Diseases of the gastric smooth muscle and collagen such as dystrophia myotonica,[13] progressive systemic sclerosis,[14] Ehlers-Danlos syndrome,[15] polymyositis, and dermatomyositis[16] have been implicated as causes of abnormal gastric emptying. Transient gastroparesis has been described in viral gastroenteritis and cutaneous herpes zoster.[17]

In addition to the barium meal, more sensitive and quantitative radiologic methods such as enteric-coated barium granules, barium burger, and radiopaque spheres can measure gastric emptying. However, these are not as simple, noninvasive, reproducible, or highly acceptable to patients as the radionuclide studies of gastric emptying. Many markers are used to label both liquid and solid meals[18]; we use the egg meal labeled with technetium Tc 99m.

The technique is a slight modification of that described by Kroop et al.[19] The patient is given nothing by mouth for 12 hours and does not receive any medication affecting gastrointestinal motility within 24 hours prior to the examination. After the patient has ingested labeled egg whites in the form of scrambled eggs, anterior and posterior views of the stomach are obtained for 90 minutes. With the aid of a computer, images of the activity in the stomach and small bowel are displayed on a video monitor and photographed on Polaroid film. The region of interest is outlined around the stomach in the anterior and posterior projections, and the computer calculates the amount (mean least squares) of activity in the area. The amount of radioactivity in the region of interest is proportional to the amount of the test meal remaining in the stomach. A graphic display of the counts remaining in the stomach versus time is plotted by the computer and the calculated percentage of gastric emptying is determined. A normal value should be less than 50% residual gastric activity at 60 minutes.

We have not used radioactive liquids for gastric emptying studies because liquid emptying shows less delay and less correlation with symptoms in patients with diabetic gastric neuropathy. The radionuclide gastric emptying study offers an objective assessment of the response to pharmacologic treatment with either cholinomimetic agents or dopamine antagonists for this disorder.

In summary, most patients with symptoms suggestive of a gastric emptying disorder are referred for an upper gastrointestinal roentgenographic series. Gastric outlet obstruction is readily ruled out by the lack of an air-fluid level on a

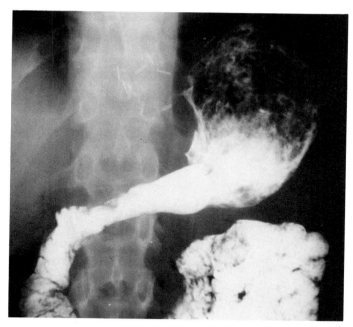

FIG 30–6.

After Billroth I gastrectomy and vagotomy this patient had a large gastric bezoar occupying the entire gas- tric remnant. Most of the barium had left the stomach on the 15-minute follow-up film.

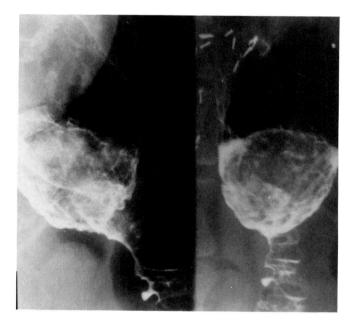

FIG 30–7.

Erect spot films of the gastric remnant and gastroje- junostomy in a patient after Billroth II gastrectomy and gastrojejunostomy. Note the large bezoar in the dependent portion of the stomach, without any signif- icant liquid barium residue, and a widely patent anastomotic site. An incidental diverticulum of the proximal jejunum is seen.

TABLE 30–2.
Drugs That Inhibit Gastric Motility

Sympathomimetic agents
  Isoproterenol
  Albuterol (salbutamol)
  Clonidine
Anticholinergic agents
  Belladonna alkaloids and their synthetic
    substitutes
Psychoactive drugs with anticholinergic effects
  Tricyclic antidepressants
  Phenothiazines
  Antiparkinsonian agents
  Tranquilizers (e.g., Diazepam)
Opioid agents
  Diphenoxylate hydrochloride and atropine
    (Lomotil)
  Methadone hydrochloride
Ganglion blockers
  Hexamethonium
  Mecamylamine
  Pentolinium
Chemotherapeutic agents
  Vincristine sulfate

horizontal beam film or fluoroscopic observation in the erect position. Advanced gastric motility disorders are easily recognized by administering a barium meal; early changes are best diagnosed by radionuclide studies, which because of their quantitative nature are also well suited for evaluating response to therapy.

REFERENCES

1. Gramm HF, Reuter K, Costello P: The radiologic manifestations of diabetic gastric neuropathy and its differential diagnosis. *Gastrointest Radiol* 1988; 3:151–155.
2. Loo FD, Palmer DW, Soergel KH, et al: Gastric emptying in patients with diabetes mellitus. *Gastroenterology* 1984; 86:485–494.
3. Feldman M, Schiller LR: Disorders of gastrointestinal motility associated with diabetes mellitus. *Ann Intern Med* 1983; 98:378–384.
4. Williams EJ, Irvine WT: Functional and metabolic effects of total and selective vagotomy. *Lancet* 1966; 1:1053–1057.
5. Goldstein HM, Cohen LE, Hagen R, et al: Gastric bezoars: A frequent complication in the postoperative ulcer patient. *Radiology* 1973; 107:341–344.
6. Allen TNK, Willson RA, Lee M: Bronchial carcinoma with autovagotomy and bezoar formation. *JAMA* 1977; 237:364–365.
7. Kirks DR, Szemes GC: Autovagotomy and gastric bezoar. *Gastroenterology* 1971; 61:96–98.
8. Hyson EA, Burrell M, Toffler R: Drug induced gastrointestinal disease. *Gastrointest Radiol* 1977; 2:183–212.
9. Kowajewski K, Kolodej A: Myoelectric and mechanical activity of stomach and intestine in hypothyroid dogs. *Am J Dig Dis* 1977; 22:235–240.
10. Eversman JJ, Farmer RG, Brown CH: Gastrointestinal manifestations of hyperparathyroidism. *Arch Intern Med* 1967; 119:605–609.
11. Dubois A, Gross HA, Ebert MH, et al: Altered gastric emptying and secretion in primary anorexia nervosa. *Gastroenterology* 1979; 77:319–323.
12. Gilat T, Spiro HM: Amyloidosis and the gut. *Am J Dig Dis* 1968; 13:619–633.
13. Kuiper DH: Gastric bezoar in a patient with myotonic dystrophy. *Am J Dig Dis* 1971; 16:529–534.
14. Cohen S, Laufer I, Snape WJ, et al: The gastrointestinal manifestations of scleroderma: Pathogenesis and management. *Gastroenterology* 1980; 79:155–160.
15. Harris RD: Small bowel dilatation in Ehlers-Danlos syndrome—An unreported gastrointestinal manifestation. *Br J Radiol* 1974; 47:623–627.
16. Horowitz M, McNeil JO, Maddern GJ, et al: Abnormalities of gastric and esophageal emptying in polymyositis and dermatomyositis. *Gastroenterology* 1986; 90:434–439.
17. Kebede D, Barthel JS, Singh A: Transient gastroparesis associated with cutaneous herpes zoster. *Dig Dis Sci* 1987; 32:318–322.
18. Horowitz M, Collins PJ, Shearman DJC: Disorders of gastric emptying in humans and the use of radionuclide techniques. *Arch Intern Med* 1985; 145:1467–1472.
19. Kroop HS, Long WB, Alavi A, et al: Effect of water and fat on gastric emptying of solid meal. *Gastroenterology* 1979; 77:997–1000.

PART IV

Small Bowel

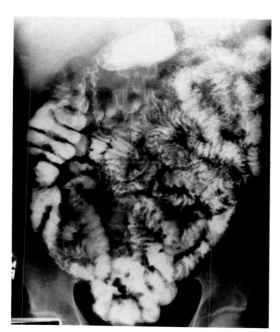

FIG 31–4.
Whipple's disease. Radiograph from a small bowel follow-through in a patient with Whipple's disease. Note severe thickening of the mucosal folds in the proximal and mild small bowel; there is almost a nodular component to the valvulae conniventes.

steatorrhea, weight loss, lymphadenopathy, and skin pigmentation. The disease is characterized pathologically by extensive infiltration of large macrophages filled with multiple glycoprotein granules that react positively to periodic acid–Schiff (PAS) stain. This PAS-positive material recently was identified as a gram-positive rod-shaped bacilli; a streptococcus seems to be responsible for the disease. The characteristic radiographic finding is an abnormal mucosal fold pattern with thickened, nodular valvulae conniventes[7, 8] (Fig 31–4). The intestinal villi can become so engorged that they produce a tiny, fine nodular pattern visible on barium studies; the changes are most prominent in the jejunum. Mild dilation, hypersecretion, segmentation, and fragmentation sometimes are demonstrated. Treatment with antibiotics cures the disease and reverses the radiographic changes.

Crohn's Disease

Although Crohn's disease (regional enteritis) usually involves the terminal ileum, it can affect any portion of the bowel. The disease commonly is

transmural. By the time it is detected radiographically there are usually extensive changes, with linear and transverse ulcerations, thickening and rigidity of the small bowel producing stenosis (string sign), and even fistulas, which are a hallmark of the disease. Another classic feature is the presence of multiple areas of relatively normal-appearing small bowel between the diseased segments (skip lesions). Crohn's disease rarely is detected early in the pathologic process; the earliest changes include irregular thickening and distortion of the valvulae conniventes as a result of submucosal inflammation and edema[1] (Fig 31–5). These changes in conjunction with the early transverse and longitudinal ulcer-

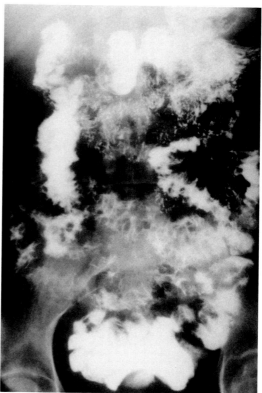

FIG 31–5.
Early Crohn's disease. Small bowel examination in a patient with Crohn's disease demonstrates diffuse nodularity of the visualized small bowel. There is evidence of some segmentation and fragmentation of the barium, mainly because of incomplete filling of the small bowel lumen. Note the absence of significant stenosis, ulceration, or fistulization. The findings are consistent with both Crohn's disease and diffuse lymphoma.

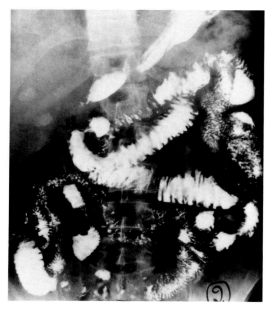

FIG 31–6.
Eosinophilic gastroenteritis. Small bowel series in a patient with proved eosinophilic gastroenteritis. The stomach is normal. In the small bowel there is thickening and distortion of the folds, especially in the jejunum.

ations can produce a nodular appearance (see Fig 31–5).

A number of inflammatory conditions, including tuberculosis, histoplasmosis, strongyloidiasis, *Yersinia* infection, and typhoid fever, may mimic the radiographic findings of Crohn's disease.[9, 10] Each of these conditions may produce various degrees of malabsorption. They rarely produce bowel symptoms in patients in North America.

Lymphoma

Intestinal lymphoma occasionally produces malabsorption. A broad spectrum of radiographic changes may be seen in the small bowel, because lymphoma mimics many entities. The abnormalities may involve a single segment, be multifocal, or be diffuse throughout most of the small bowel.[11] They may range from large polypoid intraluminal masses to diffuse multiple small nodules throughout the bowel (see Fig 31–5). The small bowel loops may be separated because of mesenteric involvement. Rarely, short constricting napkin-ring lesions are detected that cannot easily be differentiated from a primary adenocarcinoma. More commonly the le-

sions are long (6 to 10 cm) and produce thickening or obliteration of mucosal folds. A characteristic lesion is aneurysmal dilation of the bowel, which is produced by bowel necrosis and cavitation. The lesions usually are longer than 6 cm and significantly enlarge the lumen. The adjacent bowel is displaced markedly as the lymphoma extends into the adjacent mesentery.

Eosinophilic Gastroenteritis

Eosinophilic gastroenteritis is characterized by cellular eosinophilic infiltration of the small intestine, the stomach, or both, in association with episodic peripheral eosinophilia.[12, 13] The specific cause is unclear. Patients with predominant mucosal disease commonly have a history of allergy and malabsorption. The jejunum is predominantly involved, although the stomach and entire small bowel may be affected.[14, 15] Typical radiographic findings are thickening and distortion of the folds,

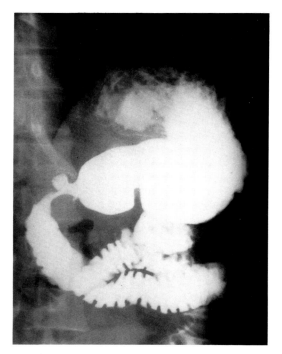

FIG 31–7.
Zollinger-Ellison syndrome. Radiograph from an upper gastrointestinal examination demonstrates a duodenal ulcer. There is dilation of the duodenum and jejunum, with marked thickening of the folds. There is also evidence of hypersecretion in the stomach, with thickened gastric folds.

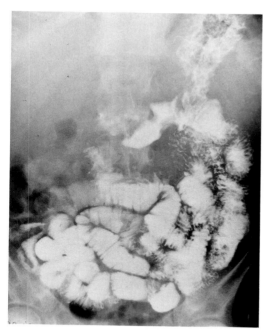

FIG 31–8.
Mastocytosis. Small bowel examination in a patient with mastocytosis. Note diffuse thickening of the valvulae conniventes with almost a nodular pattern. There is diffuse sclerosis of the bones, which is a helpful clue in the radiographic diagnosis.

especially in the jejunum (Fig 31–6). Spasm, irritability, and hypersecretion sometimes are demonstrated. The thickening of mucosal folds may be prominent enough to mimic a nodular pattern.[14, 15] When the stomach is affected the rugal folds enlarge and thicken. After treatment with steroids or removal of the sensitizing agents the radiographic findings in the small bowel may completely reverse.

Zollinger-Ellison Syndrome

Zollinger-Ellison syndrome is secondary to a non-beta islet cell tumor of the pancreas. There is evidence of hypersecretion as well as dilation of the bowel. Fulminating ulcer disease is due to markedly increased gastrin secretion by the tumor; severe diarrhea and malabsorption may occur as a result of the marked hypersecretion. Classically there is evidence of a peptic ulcer, usually in the duodenum, with thickened folds in the stomach, duodenum, and jejunum (Fig 31–7). There is evidence of hypersecretion as well as dilation of the bowel. The peptic

ulcer and abnormal stomach differentiate Zollinger-Ellison syndrome from sprue.

Other Diseases in the Differential Diagnosis

Mastocytosis (Fig 31–8), dysgammaglobulinemia (Fig 31–9), intestinal lymphangiectasia, α-betalipoproteinemia, and systemic amyloidosis (Fig 31–10) are rare entities that can produce malabsorption.[16–19] Radiographically they all produce diffuse thickening of the valvulae conniventes and small mucosal nodules. Hypersecretion is more common with intestinal lymphangiectasia.

Malabsorption also has been reported secondary to mesenteric ischemia, hypoalbuminemia, radiation enteritis, and pancreatitis, as well as scleroderma.[20–24] All of these disorders produce thickening of the valvulae conniventes.

CONCLUSION

The radiographic findings in Fig 31–1 are distorted, irregular, thickened folds in the proximal

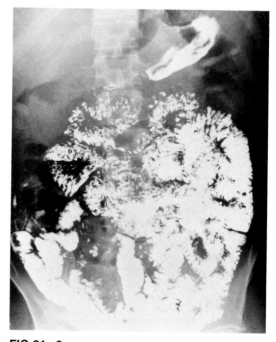

FIG 31–9.
Dysgammaglobulinemia. Small bowel follow-through demonstrates marked fold thickening, with fragmentation and segmentation. There is slight evidence of hypersecretion.

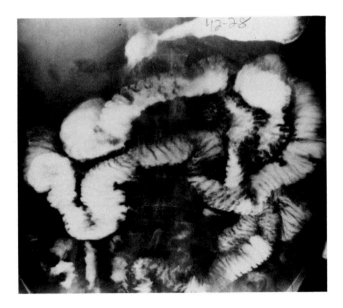

FIG 31–10.
Amyloidosis. Radiograph demonstrates uniform symmetric thickening of the valvulae conniventes throughout the small bowel. There is mild dilation and no dilution of the barium in the bowel lumen.

small bowel. The abnormality involves both the duodenum and jejunum (Fig 31–3 is from the same patient). The findings are consistent with a number of entities listed in Table 31–1. The patient gave a history of drinking water from the lakes and streams in northern Minnesota, which are known to contain *Giardia*. Stool cultures confirmed the diagnosis of giardiasis.

REFERENCES

1. Goldberg HI, Sheft DJ: Abnormalities in small intestine contour and caliber. *Radiol Clin North Am* 1976; 14:461–475.
2. Isbell RG, Carlson HC, Hoffman HN: Roentgenologic pathologic correlation in malabsorption syndromes. *AJR* 1969; 107:158–169.
3. Tully TE, Feinberg SB: A roentgenographic classification of diffuse diseases of the small intestine presenting with malabsorption. *AJR* 1974; 121:283–290.
4. Paul RE Jr: Malabsorption of the small bowel, in Taveras J, Ferrucci JT Jr (eds): *Radiology: Diagnosis, Imaging, Intervention.* Philadelphia, JB Lippincott Co, 1987, pp 1–8.
5. Beneventano TC, Wolf EL: Radiology of diffuse diseases of the small bowel, in Taveras J, Ferrucci JT Jr (eds): *Radiology: Diagnosis, Imaging, Intervention.* Philadelphia, JB Lippincott Co, 1987, pp 1–10.
6. Marshak RH, Ruoff M, Linder AE: Roentgen manifestations of giardiasis. *AJR* 1968; 104:557–560.
7. Rice RP, RouFael WM, Reeves RJ: The roentgen diagnosis of Whipple's disease (intestinal lipodystrophy). *Radiology* 1967; 88:295–301.
8. Phillips RL, Carlson HC: The roentgenographic and clinical findings in Whipple's disease. *AJR* 1975; 123:268–273.
9. Nolan DJ, Gourtsoyiannis NC: Crohn's disease of the small intestine: A review of the radiological appearances in 100 consecutive patients examined by a barium infusion technique. *Clin Radiol* 1980; 31:597–602.
10. Reeder MM, HamiHon LC: Radiologic diagnosis of tropical diseases of the gastrointestinal tract. *Radiol Clin North Am* 1969; 7:57–81.
11. Maglinte DDT: The small bowel: Neoplasms, in Taveras J, Ferrucci JT Jr (eds): *Radiology: Diagnosis, Imaging, Intervention.* Philadelphia, JB Lippincott Co, 1987, pp 1–7.
12. Goldberg HI, O'Kieffe D, Jenis EH, et al: Diffuse eosinophilic gastroenteritis. *AJR* 1973; 119:342–351.
13. Marshak RH, Linder A, Maklansky P, et al: Eosinophilic gastroenteritis. *JAMA* 1981; 245:1677.
14. Zboralske FF, Amberg JR: Detection of the Zollinger-Ellison syndrome. The radiologist's responsibility. *AJR* 1968; 104:529–543.
15. Clemett AR, Fishbone G, Levine RJ, et al:

Gastrointestinal lesions in mastocytosis. *AJR* 1968; 103:405–417.

16. Brandt LJ, Davidoff A, Bernstein L, et al: Small intestinal involvement in Waldenstrom's macroglobulinemia. *Dig Dis Sci* 1981; 26:174.

17. Olmsted WW, Madewell JE: Lymphangiectasia of the small intestine. Description and pathophysiology of the roentgenographic signs. *Gastrointest Radiol* 1976; 1:241–243.

18. Weinstein MA, Pearson KD, Agus SG: A beta lipoproteinemia. *Radiology* 1973; 108:269–273.

19. Legge DA, Carlson HC, Woolaeger EE: Roentgenologic appearance of systemic amyloidosis involving the gastrointestinal tract. *AJR* 1970; 110:406–412.

20. Seliger G, Krassner RL, Beranbaum ER, et al:

The spectrum of roentgen appearance in amyloidosis of the small and large bowel: Radiologic-pathologic correlation. *Radiology* 1971; 100:63–70.

21. Meyers MA, Kaplowitz N, Bloom AA: Malabsorption secondary to mesenteric ischemia. *AJR* 1973; 119:352–358.

22. Farthing MJG, McLean AM, Bartram CI: Radiologic features of the jejunum in hypoalbuminemia. *AJR* 1981; 136:883–886.

23. Mendelson RM, Nolan DJ: The radiological features of chronic radiation enteritis. *Clin Radiol* 1985; 36:141.

24. Horowitz AL, Meyers MA: The "hide-bound" small bowel of scleroderma. Characteristic mucosal fold pattern. *AJR* 1973; 119:332–334.

CHAPTER 32

Intermittent Abdominal Pain

Charles A. Rohrmann, Jr., M.D.

Case Presentation

A 58-year-old man was referred for evaluation of recurrent abdominal pain and distention. He reported that intermittent abdominal pain since childhood had become increasingly symptomatic during the past 6 years. Five years previously during a particularly severe episode a small bowel obstruction was diagnosed and he underwent an exploratory laparotomy. No intestinal obstruction was found.

At the time of referral the patient had cramping abdominal pain, severe bloating, and diarrhea. He had lost 10 pounds over the previous 6 months. Plain abdominal films were obtained at admission (Fig 32–1). What is the diagnosis? What should be done to confirm it?

DISCUSSION

The supine abdominal film (see Fig 32–1) demonstrates moderate to marked distention of small bowel loops with normal to moderately increased stomach and colon caliber. The upright film demonstrated many air-fluid levels in all bowel loops. Although the gas pattern is abnormal, it does not strongly support the diagnosis of small bowel obstruction because all segments of bowel have gas retention. The appearance is more that of paralytic ileus or neuromuscular dysfunction. Thus there is a disparity between the clinical presentation, the signs and symptoms of which suggest small bowel obstruction, and the radiographic picture of nonobstructive or paralytic ileus.

When analyzing a case such as this the radiologist performs an important function at the time of plain film interpretation by suggesting a nonobstructive cause for the patient's symptoms, which to the clinician can suggest an acute episode of recurrent small bowel obstruction. Because neuromuscular dysfunction of the intestinal tract can produce signs and symptoms mimicking intestinal obstruction (the pseudo-obstruction syndromes), the plain radiographs should be carefully assessed for signs suggestive of a nonobstructive cause. In addition to the generalized gas distribution in the gut, mucosal edema, intestinal pneumatosis, pneumoperitoneum, and unusual luminal gas collections can provide important clues to nonobstructive causes. The supine abdominal film in this case (see Fig 32–1), in addition to demonstrating intestinal distention, also shows scattered circular gas collections from 3 to 5 cm in diameter.

DIFFERENTIAL DIAGNOSIS

Before a differential diagnosis of chronic neuromuscular dysfunction of the small intestine can be developed, chronic recurrent mechanical obstruction

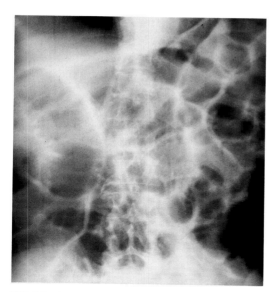

FIG 32–1.
Supine abdominal plain film shows gaseous distention of large and small intestine. The distention of the small bowel is greater than that of the colon. Note the circular collections of gas in the left upper and midportions of the abdomen. These are gas-containing small intestinal diverticula.

must be excluded. This differentiation can be made on clinical grounds, but is frequently difficult, and careful radiologic investigation should be undertaken to confirm or clarify the diagnostic possibilities. Therefore determination of the presence or absence of true mechanical obstruction should be the initial objective; this can be accomplished with barium enema and small bowel examinations. During these procedures a search should be made for evidence of neuromuscular dysfunction as well. The entire gastrointestinal tract should be examined. Esophageal motor dysfunction, gastric distention, megaduodenum, small intestinal mucosal thickening or diverticula, and colonic sacculations are important findings and are strong evidence in support of an underlying disease such as scleroderma, muscular dystrophy, or diabetes as the cause for the neuromuscular dysfunction. In addition, some disorders such as progressive systemic sclerosis affect the lungs, and the chest radiograph should be assessed for typical findings. Because certain types of intestinal pseudo-obstruction also have urinary manifestations, excretory urography may be revealing.

In our patient the esophagogram (Fig 32–2) showed moderate dilation of the esophagus. Fluo-

roscopy emphasized the absence of peristaltic activity. The upper gastrointestinal and small bowel (Fig 32–3) roentgenographic series demonstrated a normal stomach but dilated duodenum, jejunum, and ileum, with multiple large-necked diverticula. The first of these diverticula arose from the descending duodenum; they were more numerous in the jejunum but less prevalent in the ileum. The barium small bowel examination confirmed the circular gas collections seen on the plain film as representing small bowel diverticula. The transit time of contrast to the colon was prolonged. A barium enema demonstrated normal colonic caliber and length, with sigmoid diverticulosis. The chest radiograph was normal.

The important radiographic findings of esophageal dysmotility, esophageal dilation, small intestinal dilation with diverticulosis, and prolonged small intestinal transit time, combined with the clinical

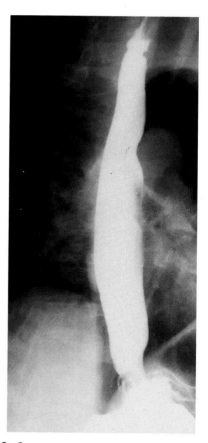

FIG 32–2.
Prone right anterior oblique barium esophagogram shows aperistalsis and dilation.

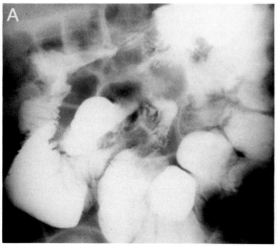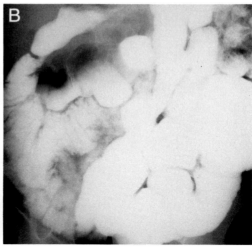

FIG 32–3.
Two views of the small bowel after an upper gastrointestinal roentgenographic series. **A,** large duodenal and proximal jejunal diverticula with wide-mouthed communications to the intestinal lumen. **B,** subsequent film with greater filling of the jejunum and ileum demonstrates numerous large diverticula affecting both intestinal segments.

impression of recurrent small bowel obstruction, suggest a type of chronic intestinal neuromuscular dysfunction.

CLASSIFICATION OF CHRONIC INTESTINAL NEUROMUSCULAR DYSFUNCTION

Chronic intestinal motor dysfunction usually is one manifestation of an underlying disease process affecting multiple body systems. Such cases are termed *secondary* because they are the result of a multisystem disease process that interferes with the coordinated peristaltic function of the intestine (Table 32–1).[1–3] For example, progressive systemic sclerosis and amyloidosis alter intestinal smooth muscle function by destroying and replacing it with either fibrous tissue or amyloid deposits. In Chagas' disease *Trypanosoma cruzi* toxin destroys the myenteric plexus. Medications such as cytoxin, vincristine, tricyclic antidepressants, and phenothiazines also may produce a chronic intestinal motor dysfunction because of impairment of intestinal peristalsis.[3] The various muscular dystrophies may cause smooth muscle dysfunction resulting in intestinal motor dysfunction.[4] Myotonic muscular dystrophy can cause esophageal spasm, dilation, and disordered peristalsis with gastric dilation and be-

zoar formation. Small bowel dilation and megacolon with stasis of intestinal contents also has been described. Only recently has Duchenne-type progressive muscular dystrophy been shown to have diffuse intestinal manifestations resulting in esophageal and intestinal dysfunction.[5] Radiologic manifestations include esophageal dysmotility, with diverticulum formation and gastric, small intestinal, and colonic stasis. Pathologically the gastrointestinal tract demonstrates extensive smooth muscle fibrosis similar to that found in progressive systemic sclerosis.[5]

In *primary* intestinal neuromuscular disorders no underlying disease process is present. These primary disorders also have been termed chronic idiopathic intestinal pseudo-obstruction.[3, 6, 7] This heterogenous group of disorders is classified in Table 32–2. Chronic idiopathic intestinal pseudo-obstruction is a syndrome with many causes, including disorders of smooth muscle function; some are related to dysfunction of the myenteric plexus. Histologic abnormalities are identifiable with appropriate staining methods.[8] Abnormalities of the smooth muscle include autosomal dominant and recessive forms of familial visceral myopathy, which also has been termed hereditary hollow visceral myopathy.[9–12] The pathologic findings in visceral myopathy include muscle cell degeneration with vacuole formation, cell loss, and fibrosis. The involved areas

TABLE 32–1.

Disorders Associated With Chronic Intestinal Neuromuscular Dysfunction

Collagen Diseases
   Progressive systemic sclerosis
   Dermatomyositis; polymyositis
   Systemic lupus erythematosus
   Ehler's-Danlos syndrome
Endocrine Disorders
   Hypothyroidism
   Diabetes mellitus
   Pheochromocytoma
   Hypoparathyroidism
Neuromuscular disorders
   Myotonic dystrophy
   Parkinson's disease
   Familial autonomic dysfunction
   Psychosis
   Duchenne's muscular dystrophy
   Jejunal diverticulosis
Miscellaneous
   Jejunoileal bypass
   Amyloidosis
   Celiac sprue
   Ceroidosis
   Chagas' disease
   Sclerosing mesenteritis
   Drugs

show muscular thinning, predominately affecting the longitudinal layer.[8, 12, 13] Differentiation from progressive systemic sclerosis is possible because the muscle cells in progressive systemic sclerosis do not undergo vacuolar degeneration and the circular layer is more involved than in visceral myopathy.[8, 14] Several disorders of the myenteric plexus have been identified in patients with chronic idiopathic intestinal motor dysfunction.[15] Pathologic abnormalities include neuronal degeneration, reduction in numbers of neurons, presence of intranuclear inclusions, and axonal degeneration with Schwann cell proliferation.[8]

SMALL INTESTINAL DIVERTICULOSIS

Although much of the literature regarding small intestinal diverticulosis refers to the finding as jejunal diverticulosis,[16] most patients also have involvement of the duodenum or ileum.[17] Therefore the designation small intestinal diverticulosis seems more appropriate. Most cases of small intestinal di-

verticulosis are asymptomatic and are found incidentally during barium examination of the small intestine, surgery, or autopsy.[16–18] The prevalence of small intestinal diverticulosis is approximately 2% and is less common than duodenal diverticulosis (10%) or colonic diverticulosis (up to 40% of persons older than 40 years). When found in the small intestine, diverticula occur seven times more frequently in the jejunum than in the ileum and are more common in men than in women.[17] Even though intestinal diverticula are incidental findings and unrelated to clinical symptoms in most patients, there are nonobstructive complications, including steatorrhea, megaloblastic anemia, inflammation, perforation, and hemorrhage.[17]

The patient described had extensive small intestinal diverticulosis as a primary radiographic manifestation. The presence of esophageal aperistalsis and widening suggested a diffuse process as a cause for the symptoms and indicated intestinal motor dysfunction rather than mechanical obstruction of the small intestine. Although diverticulosis of the small intestine classically has been associated with progressive systemic sclerosis, analysis of a selected group of patients with this finding and severe symptoms demonstrated histologic abnormalities consistent with visceral neuropathy or visceral myopathy as well as progressive systemic sclerosis.[18] In some patients small intestinal diverticulosis is a consequence of abnormal structure of either the smooth muscle or myenteric plexus. The smooth muscle layers demonstrate fibrotic replacement, with focal wall weakening. In disorders of the myenteric plexus uncoordinated peristaltic activity results in

TABLE 32–2.

Classification of Chronic Idiopathic Intestinal Pseudo-obstruction

Smooth muscle dysfunction
   Familial visceral myopathy
      Autosomal dominant
      Autosomal recessive
   Sporadic visceral myopathy
Myenteric plexus dysfunction
   Developmental failure
   Familial visceral neuropathy
      Autosomal recessive
      Autosomal dominant
   Sporadic visceral neuropathy
      Degenerative
      Paraneoplastic
      With mental retardation

areas of high intraluminal pressure. These structural deficiencies or peristaltic abnormalities can cause protrusion of mucosa and submucosa through the muscular gaps created by blood vessels at the mesenteric border. These diverticula are one manifestation of an abnormal intestinal motility pattern and structure. When intestinal function deteriorates severely the syndrome of intestinal pseudo-obstruction can become clinically apparent. If chronic intermittent obstructive symptoms are present, radiologic definition of small intestinal diverticula could be of pivotal importance in suggesting a systemic disease as a cause for the symptoms. Dilation of the intestine, with retention of fluid, the occurrence of pneumatosis intestinalis, and pneumoperitoneum, combined with findings in the esophagus (dysmotility) and stomach (hypomotility), support diagnosis of a generalized disorder as cause for the dysmotility syndrome. No distinctive radiographic appearance of the diverticula has been correlated with a specific underlying disease. In addition to signaling the possibility of a disorder causing neuromuscular dysfunction, small intestinal diverticulosis can produce mechanical complications, including obstruction from enteroliths, volvulus, inflammation, or neoplastic degeneration.[17]

The radiographic differentiation of progressive systemic sclerosis, the visceral myopathies, and the visceral neuropathies in a patient with small intestinal diverticulosis is possible if mucosal characteristics specific for progressive systemic sclerosis[19, 20] are defined. In addition, identification of hyperperistaltic activity as found in some patients with visceral neuropathies can be diagnostically helpful.[14] Figure 32–4 emphasizes the use of the radiographic findings to determine whether the disease process is diffuse, as in progressive systemic sclerosis, or localized, as in sclerosing mesenteritis or some types of Parkinson's disease.

The radiologist can play a pivotal role in the evaluation and management of chronic, intermittent, or recurrent abdominal pain. Differentiating true obstruction from a nonobstructive enteropathy should be the primary objective of radiologic consultation. The radiologist should be particularly alert to the possibility of intestinal motor dysfunction in patients whose pain syndrome is of long duration with onset at an early age, in instances of diffuse gastrointestinal or multisystem complaints, and in patients with no prior surgery or in whom surgery has not demonstrated intestinal obstruction. Plain film radiography and barium contrast examination of the entire intestinal tract to define the extent of disease and to identify mucosal characteristics or motility patterns remain valuable contributions to a useful differential diagnosis.

Diffuse Manifestations
Progressive systemic sclerosis
Visceral neuropathy
Visceral myopathy
Paraneoplastic neuropathy

Localized Manifestations
Sclerosing mesenteritis
Cathartic abuse
Parkinson's disease

Specific Mucosal Characteristics
Progressive systemic sclerosis

No Specific Mucosal Characteristics
Visceral neuropathy
Visceral myopathy
Paraneoplastic neuropathy

Amotile
Visceral myopathy

Dysmotile
Visceral neuropathy
Paraneoplastic neuropathy

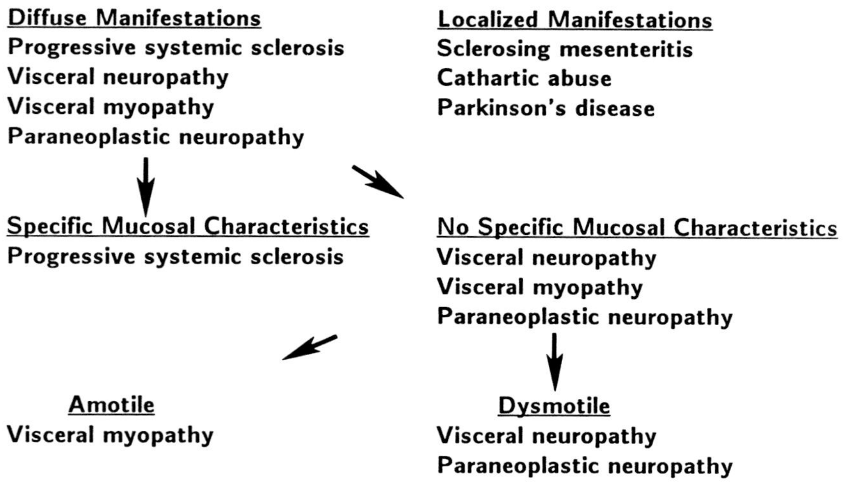

FIG 32–4.
Barium contrast examination of all intestinal segments can assist in refining the differential diagnosis in patients with chronic intestinal neuromuscular dysfunction. If the findings are diffuse, diseases such as progressive systemic sclerosis, visceral neuropathy, or visceral myopathy are suggested. Localized manifestations could suggest a disease process such as sclerosing mesenteritis. Search should be made for typical mucosal characteristics or abnormal motility pattern suggesting a specific disorder.

CHAPTER 34

Ulcerated Duodenal Mass

Howard J. Ansel, M.D.

Case Presentation

A 54-year-old man had abdominal pain and vomiting; occult blood was present in his feces. His symptoms, which had been present for several months, had improved slightly with treatment for peptic ulcer disease, but had returned. Therefore the upper gastrointestinal tract was examined. Figure 34–1 is a lateral view of the stomach and duodenum. What is the finding? What is the differential diagnosis?

DISCUSSION

Figure 34–1 shows a circumferential mass with central ulceration in the second portion of the duodenum. The duodenal bulb and more distal duodenum appear normal.

The differential diagnosis of an ulcerated lesion within the duodenum is broad; of prime concern is the possibility that the lesion is malignant. The most common primary tumor of the duodenum is adenocarcinoma (Fig 34–2), which frequently arises at or proximal to the level of the papilla. The mass may be polypoid or may be primarily infiltrating and stenosing. It usually is associated with some element of obstruction and bleeding.[1]

Sarcomatous lesions of the small bowel occur less frequently than adenocarcinoma. Of the sarcomas, leiomyosarcoma is the most common, frequently appearing as a large subserosal mass with areas of central cavitation. The radiograph in the case presented demonstrates a large area of ulceration, but there is no large extraluminal component to the mass.[2]

Primary lymphoma of the duodenum is rare; a lesion that crosses the pylorus probably represents lymphoma. At times lymphoma involving periduo-denal nodes may present with extrinsic mass effect on the duodenum, causing widening of the duodenal sweep. In our patient the stomach does not appear to be involved and no extrinsic mass involves the duodenum.[3]

Villous adenocarcinomas are generally polypoid and frondlike. They are seen as a filling defect within the duodenum rather than as an ulcerating mass (Fig 34–3). There is a high incidence of malignancy within villous tumors of the upper gastrointestinal tract.[4]

Carcinoma of the ampulla of Vater is seen as a polypoid or ulcerating mass in the second portion of the duodenum. Because of the potential for obstruction of the common bile duct, these patients often have jaundice. When detected, ampullary carcinomas often involve only the ampullary side of the duodenum.

Carcinoma of adjacent structures may invade the duodenum directly. This is especially true of carcinoma of the pancreas, in which an infiltrating and ulcerating mass may be encountered (Fig 34–4). Carcinoma of the head and uncinate process usually involves the second and third portions of the duodenum, whereas carcinoma of the body more frequently involves the third and fourth portions. In

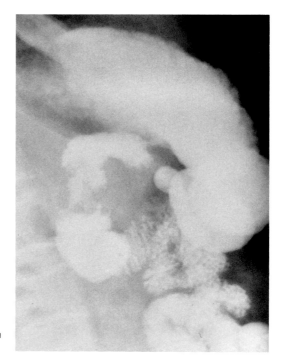

FIG 34–1.
Lateral view from an upper gastrointestinal
examination demonstrates an annular ulcerated lesion
of the second portion of the duodenum.

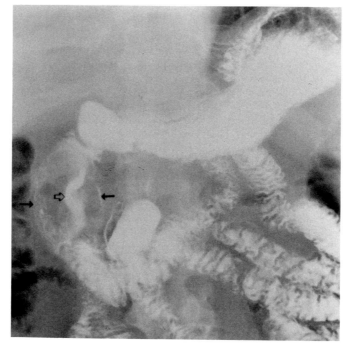

FIG 34–2.
A polypoid mass *(black arrows)* with central serpigi-
nous ulceration *(arrowhead)* fills the second portion
of the duodenum in this patient with adenocarcinoma
of the duodenum. A duodenal diverticulum is noted
distally.

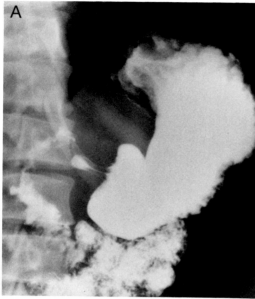

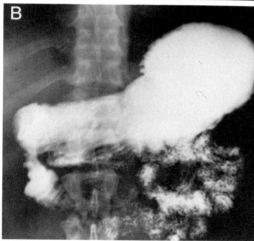

FIG 35–1.

A and B, radiographs from an upper gastrointestinal series demonstrate marked deformity of the descending duodenum, with mild narrowing of the lumen, thickened mucosal folds, and asymmetric involvement with a pseudodiverticulum.

A primary malignant process of the duodenum could produce mucosal abnormalities in the descending segment. Duodenal adenocarcinoma usually presents as a short, annular constricting lesion and generally is located distal to the bulb[1–4, 6, 7] (Fig 35–3). However, the lesion in this patient is larger than would be expected for a duodenal carci-

noma. Moreover, a carcinoma involving the entire descending duodenum probably would produce ulceration and obstruction, not seen in this case. Primary lymphoma usually extends over a longer segment of the duodenum than does an adenocarcinoma, and ulceration is common[1–4] (Fig 35–4). The absence of significant ulceration makes lymphoma an unlikely diagnostic consideration. Hematogenous metastases and submucosal lesions probably would not be as large or would be associated with mucosal ulceration.

Malignancies that secondarily involve the duodenum usually cause asymmetric radiographic findings[1–4] (Fig 35–5). Displacement of the duodenal wall is commonly seen before obstruction (see Fig 35–5), and circumferential narrowing from extrinsic metastases is rare. If stenosis is present, associ-

TABLE 35–1.

Differential Diagnosis of Duodenal Stenosis or Obstruction in the Adult

Congenital
    Annular pancreas
    Duodenal duplication cyst
    Intraluminal diverticulum or web
Malignancy
    Intrinsic
        Primary adenocarcinoma
        Lymphoma
        Metastasis (hematogenous)
        Intramural sarcoma
    Extrinsic
        Pancreatic adenocarcinoma
        Lymph node metastases (lymphoma, gastrointestinal tumor)
        Contiguous invasion from gallbladder, right colon, or right kidney carcinoma
Inflammatory disorders
    Intrinsic
        Postbulbar ulcer
        Duodenitis
        Crohn's disease
        Tuberculosis
        Strongyloidiasis
    Extrinsic
        Pancreatitis: Phlegmon, pseudocyst, abscess
        Abscess from infection in adjacent organ (perinephric or pericholecystic abscess)
Trauma
    Duodenal hematoma
Abdominal aortic aneurysm
    Large aneurysm: Preoperative
    Aortoduodenal fistula: Postoperative
Supermesenteric artery syndrome

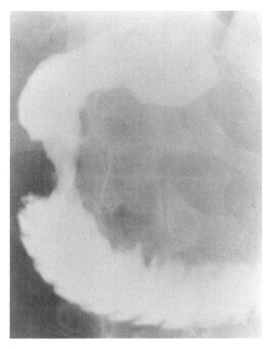

FIG 35–2.
Annular pancreas. Note mild narrowing of descending duodenum due to annular pancreas.

ated mucosal ulceration is usually seen. The lack of displacement caused by extrinsic mass and the absence of mucosal ulceration in this case eliminate secondary malignancy as a diagnostic possibility.

The predominant mucosal abnormalities in this patient strongly indicate an inflammatory process. Acute postbulbar peptic ulceration can be identified on an upper gastrointestinal series. Such ulcers usu-

ally occur on the medial aspect of the duodenum, with a lateral incisura causing some degree of narrowing[8, 9] (Fig 35–6). Occasionally an acute ulcer is associated with diffuse mucosal irregularity, spasm, or obstruction. These findings can be confusing and may suggest another process, such as a malignant lesion or pancreatitis. Peptic ulcers occurring in the postbulbar region can produce duodenal

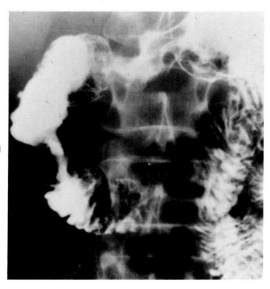

FIG 35–3.
Duodenal carcinoma. Lateral radiograph from an upper gastrointestinal series demonstrates a short constricting ("apple core") lesion of the descending duodenum. Note abrupt shelving margins and ulceration of mucosa, classic findings of duodenal carcinoma.

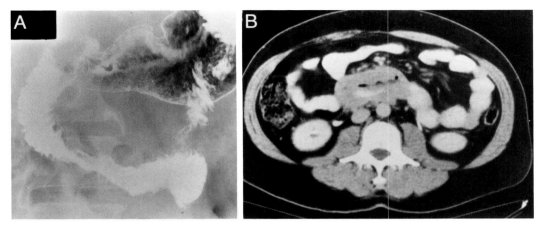

FIG 35−4.
Primary duodenal lymphoma. **A,** radiograph from an upper gastrointestinal series demonstrates an area of stenosis extending over the entire third portion of the duodenum. Note extensive ulceration. **B,** computed tomography scan at the level of the third portion of the duodenum shows thickening of the duodenal wall due to marked infiltration of the wall by lymphoma. Note air and oral contrast material in the narrow duodenal lumen.

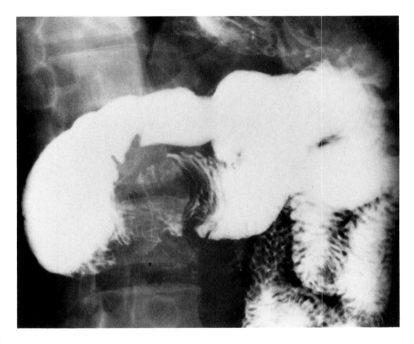

FIG 35−5.
Metastatic colon carcinoma. Anteroposterior radiograph in a patient with prior colon cancer demonstrates marked extrinsic compression of the third portion of the duodenum as a result of enlarged metastatic lymph nodes. Note intact mucosa and absence of circumferential narrowing, findings suggestive of a submucosal or serosal process.

stenosis as they heal[8] (see Fig 35–6). Typically this results in a short area of stenosis. The abnormalities in this case are too extensive for chronic peptic ulcer disease.

A more diffuse inflammatory process such as duodenitis could be considered in this case. The four most common radiographic features of duodenitis are thickened folds (folds >4 mm), mucosal nodularity, bulbar deformity, and duodenal erosions.[10] Thickened folds and nodularity are the most sensitive findings. Some radiographic features of this case are compatible with duodenitis; however, the degree of luminal narrowing and the presence of pseudodiverticula are not characteristic of duodenitis and suggest a different diagnosis.

Crohn's disease is a possibility; the radiographic features of duodenal Crohn's disease are listed in Table 35–2.[1–4, 11–15] The early findings in the duodenum are more subtle and less specific than those of advanced disease.[13] As is the case elsewhere in the intestinal tract, aphthous ulcers are the earliest finding and are best detected on double-contrast studies.[15] With progression of the disease mucosal folds become edematous and thickened, producing a disorganized or even nodular appearance (Fig 35–7,A). Mucosal coating may be poor,

and mild narrowing due to spasm may be noted. As the disease progresses, effacement of the mucosa can be seen and may be associated with small regions of outpouching (pseudodiverticula). Pseudodiverticula are a radiographic hallmark of Crohn's disease, representing asymmetric involvement of the bowel wall. Perforation of these small diverticula may lead to fistula formation in other areas of the intestine, but rarely in the duodenum. Cobblestone ulceration, also common in the small bowel and colon, is rarely seen in the duodenum. In the presence of mucosal disruption, multiple areas of involvement help differentiate active Crohn's disease from a malignant process. Eventually the duodenum becomes rigid and stiff, resulting in a smooth, tapered stenosis that can cause partial gastric outlet obstruction (Fig 35–7,B). Surgical intervention may be required for obstruction at this level or elsewhere in the small bowel. Crohn's disease initially may involve only the duodenal bulb and adjacent descending duodenum and may progress proximally to involve the stomach. When this occurs, distortion of the antrum and proximal duodenum produces a tubular or funnel-shaped structure, the pseudo-post-Billroth I sign (Fig 35–7,C).[11] Consequently the radiographic features of this case are most con-

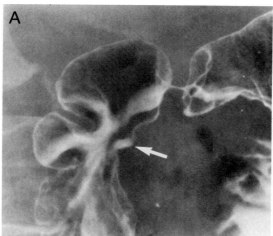

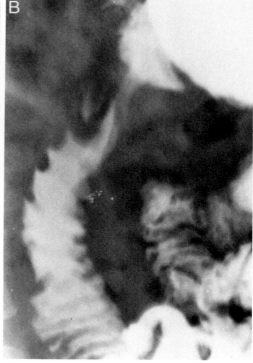

FIG 35–6.
Postbulbar ulcer. **A,** classic example of lateral duodenal wall incisura due to postbulbar ulcer on medial wall *(arrow).* **B,** radiograph from an upper gastrointestinal series in a patient with an acute postbulbar ulcer. Note marked narrowing and distortion of the duodenal mucosal folds without evidence of postbulbar ulcer, which was demonstrated on endoscopy.

TABLE 35–2.

Roentgenologic Findings in Duodenal Crohn's Disease

Early
  Blunted, thickened, disorganized mucosa
  Moderate narrowing and spasm
Late
  Effacement, loss of mucosal pattern
  Pseudodiverticula
  Ulceration, cobblestone appearance
  Stenosis
    Moderate to severe: Obstruction
    Associated with spasm: String sign
    Strictures, single or multiple
    Located at apex of duodenal bulb
    Skip areas
  Pseudo-post-Billroth I sign, most characteristic
  Fistula, usually from colon or small bowel

sistent with early Crohn's disease of the duodenum. However, for completeness let us consider the remaining conditions listed in Table 35–1.

Tuberculosis rarely involves the duodenum, found in only 0.5% of autopsies in patients with tuberculosis.[4] The distal antrum and pylorus usually are involved in contiguity with the duodenum. The radiographic pattern of nodular hyperplastic thickening of folds, diffuse ulceration, and luminal narrowing caused by the constricting inflammatory mass may be indistinguishable from Crohn's disease.[16] Thus the findings in Figure 35–1 could be caused by tuberculosis. Strongyloidiasis involving the duodenum also may simulate Crohn's disease.[17] Diffuse mucosal inflammation and ulceration and abnormal peristalsis may result in atony and duodenal dilation. Healing with fibrosis may cause stenosis.

Inflammatory processes may secondarily involve the duodenum. For example, pancreatitis can cause circumferential mucosal thickening and lumi-

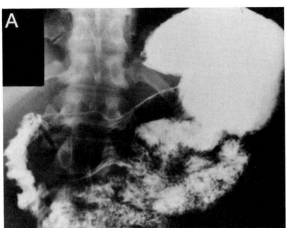
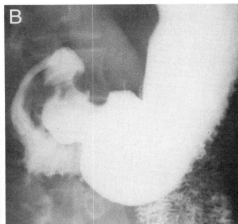
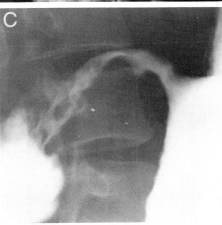

FIG 35–7.
Crohn's disease. **A,** anteroposterior radiograph in a patient with early duodenal Crohn's disease. The mucosal folds are markedly thickened without any definite ulceration. There is mild narrowing of the duodenal lumen. The duodenal bulb was normal on other radiographs. **B,** oblique radiograph in a patient with a severe stricture of the postbulbar duodenum due to Crohn's disease. The patient had long-standing Crohn's disease of the small bowel. **C,** oblique radiograph from an upper gastrointestinal examination shows severe Crohn's disease involving the stomach and proximal duodenum. The antrum, pylorus, and duodenal bulb blend into one continuous tubular structure, with normal stomach and duodenum proximal and distal to the diseased segment. The severe stricture and ulceration of the duodenum are identical to severe Crohn's disease in the small bowel and colon.

nal narrowing in the duodenum.[1-4, 18] These findings can be indistinguishable from those seen with a primary duodenal mucosal process (Fig 35−8,A and B).[19] The postinflammatory fibrosis of chronic pancreatitis can lead to stenosis, usually of the second portion of the duodenum (see Fig 35−8,A). Occasionally pancreatitis can affect the more distal duodenum, mimicking a primary neoplastic or inflammatory disorder in this region (see Fig 35−8,B). Other inflammatory disorders, such as a pericholecystic abscess, also can produce inflammatory changes in the descending duodenum. The prolonged history in this patient and the lack of symptoms suggestive of pancreatitis or cholecystitis mititate against these diagnoses.

Although a duodenal hematoma can cause narrowing of the lumen, the absence of radiographic features of an intramural, submucosal process makes this diagnosis unlikely. These lesions usually efface and narrow the lumen asymmetrically.[1-4]

An abnormality related to the vascular system is not a good possibility in this case. Aortic aneurysms typically involve the third portion of the duodenum, not the second, and they narrow the lumen only after they are quite large.[20] Dilation of the duodenum is seen with supermesenteric artery syndrome. However, this dilation ends abruptly in the

horizontal segment.[1, 4] The diagnosis is confirmed by positioning the patient in the left lateral decubitus or prone position, which allows duodenal emptying. The findings in this case are not compatible with compression from an aortic aneurysm or by the superior mesenteric artery.

In summary, the radiographic findings (see Fig 35−1) in this patient are most compatible with a primary inflammatory process involving the duodenum. The most likely diagnoses are Crohn's disease, strongyloidiasis, and tuberculosis. What can be done to define the radiographic diagnosis further? Because the duodenum usually becomes involved after the small bowel in Crohn's disease, a small intestinal examination should be done. Follow-up films of the small intestine (Fig 35−9) demonstrated features suggestive of Crohn's disease in the distal ileum.

This is an unusual case because the first symptoms and radiographic findings of Crohn's disease were localized to the upper gastrointestinal tract. The overall incidence of duodenal involvement in patients with Crohn's disease is 7% to 10%.[1-4, 11-15] In the majority of patients Crohn's disease develops in the duodenum only after small bowel or colon disease has been present for a number of years. However, in one series of 23

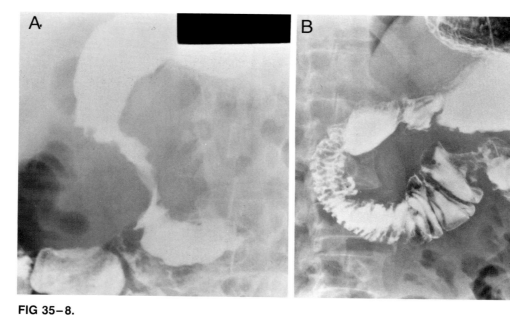

FIG 35−8.
Pancreatitis. **A,** postbulbar duodenal stenosis due to severe pancreatitis. **B,** oblique radiograph from an upper gastrointestinal examination shows an annular constricting lesion of the fourth portion of the duodenum due to acute pancreatitis. Ten days later a follow-up radiograph was normal.

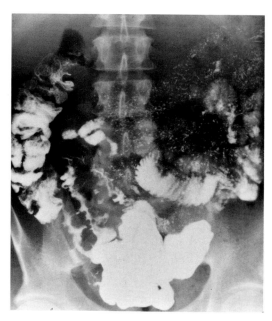

FIG 35–9.
Crohn's disease. Radiograph from small bowel follow-through series performed on the same day as that in Figure 35–1 shows obvious changes of Crohn's disease of the terminal ileum.

patients, six were referred for radiographic evaluation with a clinical diagnosis of peptic ulcer disease.[13] Five of these six patients had radiographic small bowel findings of Crohn's disease. One patient had isolated duodenal features of Crohn's disease; Crohn's disease was identified in the terminal ileum 2 years later.

This case of duodenal Crohn's disease stresses the importance of differentiating among mucosal, submucosal, and serosal processes. Limiting the differential diagnosis to the mucosa permits the clinician to select the most likely possibilities and perform the most appropriate procedure to confirm the suspected diagnosis.

REFERENCES

1. Kemp Harper RA: *Radiology of the Duodenum.* Chicago, Year Book Medical Publishers, 1967, pp 122–211.
2. Eaton SB Jr, Ferrucci JT Jr: *Radiology of the Pancreas and Duodenum.* Philadelphia, WB Saunders Co, 1973, pp 88–168.
3. Eisenberg R: Duodenal narrowing/obstruction, in *Gastrointestinal Radiology: A Pattern Approach.* Philadelphia, JB Lippincott Co, 1983, pp 385–402.
4. Ferrucci JT: The postbulbar duodenum, in Tavers JM, Ferrucci JT (eds): *Radiology: Diagnosis, Imaging, Intervention,* vol 4. *Gastrointestinal Radiology.* Philadelphia, JB Lippincott Co, 1987, pp 1–17.
5. Glazer GM, Margulis AR: Annular pancreas: Etiology and diagnosis using endoscopic retrograde cholangiopancreatography. *Radiology* 1979; 133:305–306.
6. Bosse G, Neely JA: Roentgenologic findings in primary malignant tumors of the duodenum. *AJR* 1969; 107:111–118.
7. Rudan N, Nola P, Popovic S: Primary adenocarcinoma of the duodenum. Report of 2 cases. *Cancer* 1984; 54:1105–1109.
8. Bilbao MK, Frische LH, Rosch J, et al: Postbulbar duodenal ulcer and ring-stricture: Cause and effect. *Radiology* 1971; 100:27–35.
9. Thompson WM, Norton G, Kelvin FM, et al: Unusual manifestations of peptic ulcer disease. *Radiographics* 1981; 1:1–16.
10. Gelfand DW, Dale WJ, Ott DJ, et al: Duodenitis: Endoscopic-radiologic correlation in 272 patients. *Radiology* 1985; 157:577–581.
11. Nelson SW: Some interesting and unusual manifestations of Crohn's disease ("regional enteritis") of the stomach, duodenum and small intestine. *AJR* 1969; 107:86–101.
12. Legge DA, Carlson HC, Judd ES: Roentgenologic features of regional enteritis of upper gastrointestinal tract. *AJR* 1970; 116:355–360.
13. Thompson WM, Cockrill H, Rice RP: Regional enteritis of the duodenum. *AJR* 1975; 123:252–261.
14. Marshak RH, Maklansky D, Kurzban JD, et al: Crohn's disease of the stomach and duodenum. *Am J Gastroenterol* 1982; 77:340–343.
15. Levine MS: Crohn's disease of the upper gastrointestinal tract. *Radiol Clin North Am* 1987; 25:79–91.
16. Rohner HG, Müller-Wallra FR, Wienbeck M: Tubercular stenosis of the duodenum. *Leber Magen Darm* 1982; 12:245–248.
17. Louisy CL, Barton CJ: The radiological diagnosis of *Strongyloides stercoralis* enteritis. *Radiology* 1971; 98:535–541.
18. Makrauer FL, Antonioli DA, Banks PA: Duodenal stenosis in chronic pancreatitis. *Dig Dis Sci* 1982; 27:525–532.
19. Renert WA, Pitt MJ, Capp MP: Acute pancreatitis. *Semin Roentgenol* 1973; 8:405–414.
20. Thompson WM, Jackson DC, Johnsrude IS: Aortoenteric and paraprosthetic-enteric fistulas: Radiologic findings. *AJR* 1976; 127:235–242.

CHAPTER 36

Radiologic Detection of Meckel's Diverticulum

Dean D. T. Maglinte, M.D.
John C. Lappas, M.D.
Frederick M. Kelvin, M.D.

Case Presentation

A 17-year-old boy was examined repeatedly because of severe unexplained anemia requiring multiple admissions to the community hospital. Results of diagnostic methods including barium contrast, radionuclide, arteriographic, and computed tomographic studies were interpreted as normal. Figure 36–1 includes 15- and 30-minute overhead radiographs from the more recent of two conventional small bowel examinations that yielded normal results. What observation should have been made and what should have been done to confirm the diagnosis?

DISCUSSION

The 15-minute overhead radiograph (see Fig 36–1,A) shows a saccular collection of contrast in the pelvis that differs from the rest of the barium-filled loops. As is common in many peroral small bowel examinations, no fluoroscopy and compression radiographic study was performed until the cecum was filled. At 30 minutes (see Fig 36–1,B), after the cecum was filled, compression radiography of the distal ileum (i.e., spot-filming of the terminal ileum) was performed. The results were considered normal; the saccule seen on the 15-minute radiograph was obscured by other segments of pelvic ileum.

The patient was referred to our institution, where enteroclysis (see Fig 35–1,C and D) readily demonstrated a saccule with effaced folds and a narrow neck, consistent with a Meckel's diverticulum.

A congenital small bowel diverticulum with ulcerations in its neck was found at surgery.

Until recently the difficulty in the preoperative demonstration of a symptomatic Meckel's diverticulum was well recognized by radiologists and clinicians. Despite the relative frequency of this anomaly, failure to establish the diagnosis by routine small bowel examination was almost universal. Stenosis of the ostium, filling with intestinal contents or feces, muscular contractions, rapid emptying, and small size have been cited as reasons for failure to demonstrate the abnormality.[1, 2] Problems encountered in a conventional peroral small bowel follow-through examination include failure to demonstrate loops of small bowel in a state of adequate distention and separate from other adjacent loops and failure to visualize the fold pattern in the distal small bowel.[3] The deleterious effect of gastrointestinal secretions on barium suspension and the vari-

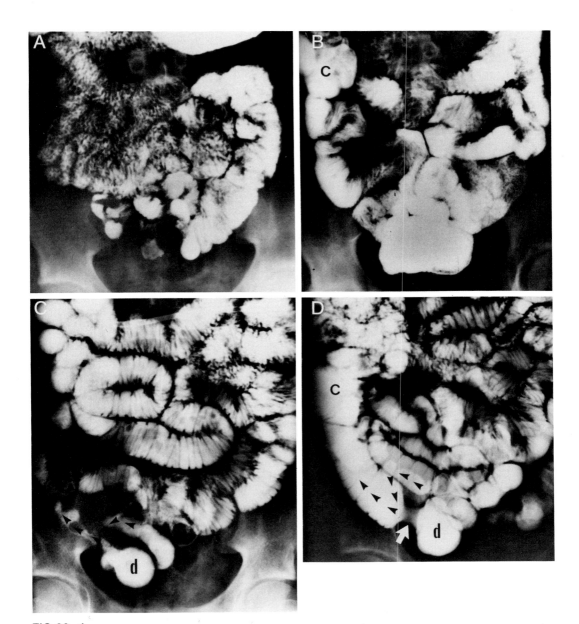

FIG 36–1.
A, 15-minute overhead radiograph from conventional small bowel examination. A small saccule in the pelvis is beginning to fill with contrast. **B,** 30-minute overhead radiograph from the same study shows barium in the cecum *(C)*. Spot film of the terminal ileum at this time was considered normal. The saccule seen in **A** is now obscured by filled loops of pelvic ileum. **C,** an early enteroclysis radiograph shows the saccule *(d)* starting to fill with contrast. The direction of contrast flow at fluoroscopy *(arrowheads)* shows that an abnormal saccule is present. **D,** further filling and distention of all segments shows the diverticulum *(d)* connected by a narrow neck *(arrow)* to the distal ileum *(arrowheads)*. Ulcerations were present at the neck of the diverticulum and ectopic gastric mucosa were found at surgery. *C* = cecum.

ability in gastrointestinal peristalsis also limit the effectiveness of the peroral small bowel examination.

Frequently not appreciated is that the number of errors in the diagnosis of Meckel's diverticulum and other lesions of the mesenteric small bowel can be reduced by less reliance on the overhead serial radiograph and substitution of fluoroscopy and compression radiography two to three times during the examination.[4] In the case presented, fluoroscopy and compression radiography performed at 15 minutes (see Fig 36–1,A) may have lead to the correct diagnosis. By the time fluoroscopy and spot filming of the terminal ileum were performed, the cecum was filled and the diverticulum obscured by adjacent loops of small bowel and therefore not appreciated.

Enteroclysis involves infusion of contrast through a tube, with the tip lying in the distal duodenum or proximal jejunum, while the radiologist attempts to compress all segments of small bowel. This procedure eliminates most of the inherent limitations of the conventional study. The diverticulum in our patient was demonstrated readily (see Fig 36–1,C and D) by the radiologist, who was present during the entire procedure.

It is possible, although distinctly uncommon, to demonstrate a Meckel's diverticulum on an overhead radiograph during conventional small bowel radiography if there is little or no overlap of small bowel loops. Occasionally Meckel's diverticula are shown by reflux filling of the distal ileum during a barium enema study. The diagnosis, however, has been inconstant and unreliable. In adults enteroclysis more consistently diagnoses Meckel's diverticulum and other small bowel diverticula than does any other method.[5–7]

The accuracy of the small bowel follow-through series in the diagnosis of Meckel's diverticulum can be improved with the fluoroscopic small bowel meal. Fluoroscopy and compression radiography are performed two to three times during the procedure, sometimes augmented by gas-enhanced double-contrast follow-through or peroral pneumo-colon examination, to assess poorly distended segments or poorly visualized folds.[4] This concept of a dedicated small bowel follow-through study was suggested initially in 1982 by Maglinte et al.[8] in an analysis of lesions missed on small bowel examinations. Most of the reports of small bowel lesions missed during follow-through examinations refer to conventional barium studies in which fluoroscopy was based on observations derived from overhead abdominal radiographs. Elimination of overhead serial radiographs and the substitution of serial fluoro-

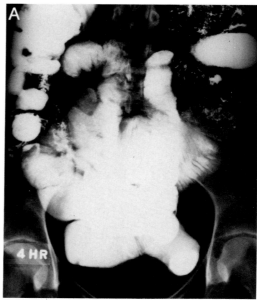

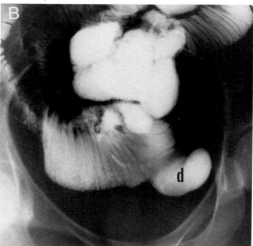

FIG 36–2.
Fluoroscopic small bowel meal in the demonstration of a Meckel's diverticulum. **A,** 4-hour overhead radiograph of a small bowel follow-through study shows filling of loops of ileum and partial filling of colon. No diagnosis is possible. **B,** compression radiograph with tube angulation of filled pelvic segments readily demonstrates a Meckel's diverticulum *(d)*. A mucosal triangular plateau indicating the junction of the diverticulum to a loop of ileum is well shown. An intrauterine contraceptive device superimposed on the compressed pelvic loop of ileum was not seen on the overhead radiograph.

radiography will improve detection of Meckel's diverticulum and other lesions by peroral small bowel examination[4] (Fig 36–2).

Enteroclysis facilitates compression of adequately distended segments of the entire small bowel, particularly the pelvic loops of the ileum, thereby allowing demonstration of their fold pattern and testing the distensibility of each segment. Frequent intermittent fluoroscopy and compression during infusion of contrast allows careful evaluation of suspected loops. Errors of diagnosis secondary to incomplete filling of the small bowel and the unreliable timing of the serial films after barium ingestion are avoided (Fig 36–3). The variability of position of a diverticulum because of its mobile tip is minimized by continuous distention at enteroclysis.

Meckelian diverticula account for 90% of all omphalomesenteric duct abnormalities, the most common type of congenital anomaly of the gastrointestinal tract,[9] occurring in 1% to 3% of the general population.[10] Vitelline duct remnants may become symptomatic or may remain silent. The frequency with which they produce disease ranges from 22%[11] to 34%.[9] Silent diverticula may remain undiscovered throughout life. The clinical presentations produced by Meckel's diverticula are listed in Table 36–1. Men are affected about three times as often as women. Seventy-five percent of these diverticula are 1 to 5 cm in diameter; the remainder are larger. Most are in the distal small bowel.

Plain abdominal radiographs generally are of no value in demonstrating a Meckel's diverticulum, although occasionally a large diverticulum may accumulate gas, increasing the likelihood of detection. Small persistent gas collections in a diverticulum sometimes are seen retrospectively, but usually are dismissed at the time as gas in an adherent loop of small bowel. Enteroliths within a Meckel's diverticulum, although rare, may be seen on plain radiographs.[12] Faceted single or multiple calculi have been described, and approximately 25% are sufficiently calcified to be identified radiographically (Fig 36–4). Contrast studies will differentiate the Meckel's diverticulum enterolith from colonic en-

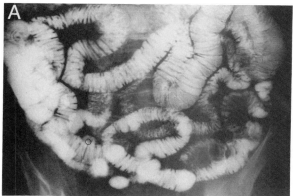
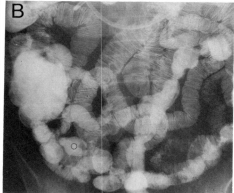
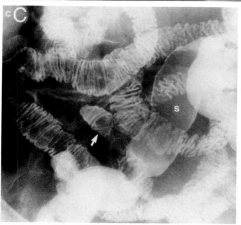

FIG 36–3.
A high index of suspicion and compression radiography of all filled segments of the small bowel is the most important radiologic maneuver in the demonstration of a Meckel's diverticulum. **A,** prone radiograph (without compression) during single-contrast phase of enteroclysis does not show the Meckel's diverticulum *(open dot)*. Compression at this time did not suggest the diagnosis because of incomplete filling. **B,** the diverticulum *(open dot)* not shown during initial fluoroscopy was suspected in this double-contrast noncompression prone radiograph with the small bowel better distended. **C,** meticulous compression of the segment in question unequivocally demonstrates a Meckel's diverticulum *(arrow)* in this 65-year-old man with anemia. S = sigmoid; C = cecum.

TABLE 36–1.

Clinical Presentation of Meckel's Diverticulum*

Symptoms Group and Frequency	Onset of Symptoms	Symptoms	Complications	Comments
Ulceratng (40%)†	Infancy or childhood	Pain, melena	Perforation	Greatest number of ulcers are in the ileal mucosa at neck of diverticulum.
Obstructing (32%)	Any age, usually childhood	Symptoms of low obstruction	Volvulus or intussusception, gangrene or perforation	Intussusception is associated with Meckel's in 5–10% of cases. The presence of a Meckel's diverticulum in a hernial sac (Littre's hernia) accounts for about 15% of obstructive group.
Inflammatory (17%)	Infancy or childhood	Appendicitis-like, acute or chronic	Perforation	In 15% of cases in this group, inflammation and perforation are results of foreign body in the diverticulum (fish bones, vegetable remains, gallstones).
Umbilical (5%)	First few weeks of life	Leakage at umbilicus	Infection prolapse	Extent of umbilical sinus determined radiographically by injection of contrast at sinus.
Neoplastic (6%)	Middle life	Intestinal neoplasms	Perforation or obstruction	Leiomyoma, sarcoma, carcinoid and adenocarcinoma reported.

*Modified from Ghahremani GG: Radiology of Meckel's diverticulum. *CRC Crit Rev Diagn Imaging* 1986; 26:1–43.
†Percentages have been computed from several large series and are only approximations.

teroliths, appendicoliths, gallstones, ureteral calculi, calcified nodes, or stones in a bladder diverticulum.

The spectrum of radiologic findings in Meckel's diverticulum has been reviewed recently.[13] The variable appearance of this entity on contrast examination reflects the morphology of the anomaly, that is, a blind sac attached to the antimesenteric border of the distal small bowel (Fig 36–5). The identification of the congenital nature of the sac rests on the demonstration of the junctional fold pattern, the site of exit of the omphalomesenteric duct. Identification of the mucosal triangular plateau, the junctional fold pattern of the distended ileum and diverticulum, or the triradiate fold pattern, the junctional fold pattern with the loops partially collapsed, mandates the diagnosis of Meckel's diverticulum; no other abnormality in the small bowel produces these findings. Demonstration of the saccular outpouching or an abnormal collection of barium should lead to a search for the junctional fold pattern, although sometimes this may be difficult to display; too much barium in the diverticulum or too dense a barium mixture may obscure the fold pattern. Adequate compression during infusion or the use of double-contrast methods will avert this error.

Superimposition of two intestinal loops can produce a pseudo–triangular plateau (Fig 36–6). This pitfall can be avoided by proper positioning and adequate compression. A pseudosaccule can be produced by axial projection of a loop of bowel, especially when fixed by adhesions. Double-contrast methods and correct positioning will clarify the nature of the sac. A communicating duplication or an acquired diverticulum should not be confused with a Meckel's diverticulum. A communicating duplication, a rare anomaly, has an axis parallel to the axis of the bowel loop and lies, as does an acquired diverticulum, on the mesenteric border. There is no mucosal triangular plateau (Fig 36–7). Acquired diverticula are usually multiple, larger, and predominantly in the jejunum.

Idiopathic localized dilation of the ileum (ileal dysgenesis) in adults is usually mistaken preoperatively for a Meckel's diverticulum. This uncommon lesion appears as an aperistaltic saccular segment in direct continuity with the normal ileal lumen.[14] Most patients have symptoms of obstruction; bleeding is another initial feature. Careful fluoroscopy will show absence of peristalsis in the dilated segment, whereas the caliber and motility of the adja-cent segments are normal. Ileal dysgenesis is differentiated from a Meckel's diverticulum by the absence of a junctional fold pattern and the direct continuity of the dilated lumen with the normal adjacent ileum.

Blind pouches following side-to-side intestinal anastomosis also can be mistaken for a Meckel's diverticulum if the surgical history is unknown.[15–17] The blind pouch syndrome should be considered in a patient with anemia, episodes of diarrhea, intermittent crampy abdominal pain, weight loss, and history of previous side-to-side or end-to-side intestinal anastomosis. Contrast study will show the pouch and the anastomotic site. There will be no junctional fold pattern. Division of the circular muscles during side-to-side anastomosis results in stasis secondary to motility disturbances, with subsequent dilation of the proximal segment and formation of a blind pouch. Hypertrophy of the pouch, inflammation, and ulceration ensue, typically 5 to 15 years after the surgery. Recently this type of surgical anastomosis has been replaced by end-to-end anastomosis to restore bowel continuity and to prevent the blind pouch syndrome.

Radiographically, Meckel's diverticulum presenting as intussusception or volvulus will appear as intussusception or a twist, but the diverticulum usu-

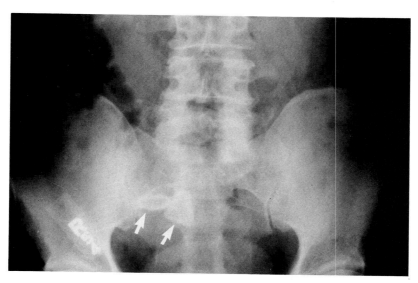

FIG 36–4.
Meckel's stones resulting from stasis secondary to a narrow neck with associated chronic diverticular inflammation are sometimes sufficiently calcified to be identified on plain films. Multiple Meckel's enteroliths *(arrows)* are characteristically triangular, flat, and have a radiolucent center. A solitary Meckel's stone may be difficult to distinguish from an appendicolith or urinary tract calculus. Extreme mobility and connection to the small bowel on contrast study are diagnostic features.

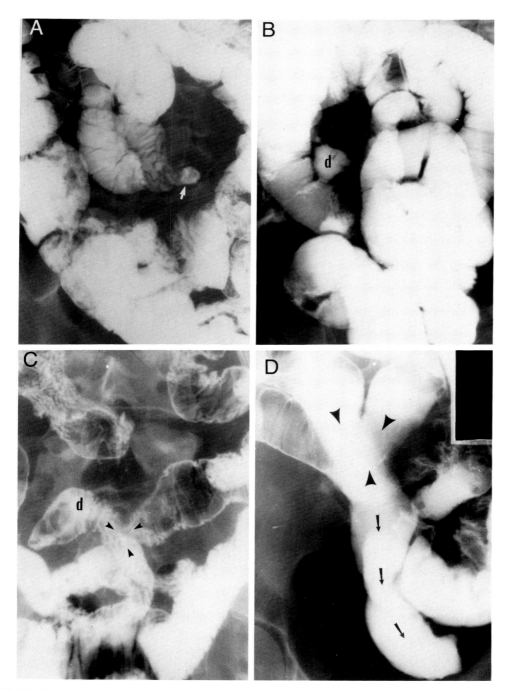

FIG 36–5.

Varied radiographic appearance of Meckel's diverticula. In all four patients barium contrast, radionuclide, angiographic, and endoscopic studies failed to show a cause for unexplained gastrointestinal bleeding; the diagnoses were confirmed at surgery. **A,** a small distorted Meckel's diverticulum *(arrow)* in an elderly man with anemia. The distortion and suggestion of a filling defect inside the diverticulum suggests a symptomatic diverticulum. **B,** a deformed Meckel's diverticulum *(d)* in a 6-year-old boy with anemia. **C,** a moderate sized diverticulum *(d)* containing a defect in the fundus corresponding to ectopic gastric mucosa. Note the triradiate junctional fold pattern *(arrowheads).* **D,** a large diverticulum can easily be mistaken for a pelvic segment of ileum if the continuity of all loops of ileum are not critically assessed. Identification of the junctional fold pattern *(arrowheads)* confirms the diagnosis of a Meckel's diverticulum.

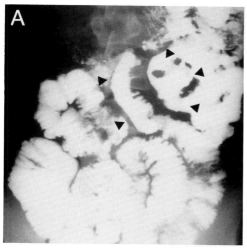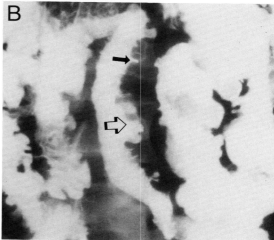

FIG 37–1.
A, conventional small bowel follow-through barium examination demonstrates segments of abnormal appearing bowel *(arrowheads)* that are abnormally separated from adjacent segments. These segments are slightly narrowed and irregular. **B,** fluoroscopic spot film demonstrates marked thickening of the fold pattern in some areas and loss of fold pattern in others, resulting in an undulating, nodular contour. The involvement of the bowel is not symmetric, resulting in pseudodiverticular outpouchings *(open arrow)* and linear ulcers *(closed arrow).*

of the barium may be seen with large amounts of gastrointestinal secretions.

A dilated small bowel or thick folds and an absent fold pattern are suggestive of several disorders. In the case presented the bowel is not dilated but thick folds and loss of fold pattern are present. A corollary to dilation is the detection of narrowing (less than 1 cm when the bowel is distended). Narrowed segments are commonly encountered in Crohn's disease, for example.

When evaluating small bowel containing an abnormal fold pattern it is helpful to determine whether the stomach is also involved. Gastric involvement along with small bowel involvement occurs in Zollinger-Ellison syndrome, lymphoma, Crohn's disease, Menetrier's disease, eosinophilic enteritis, and amyloidosis. In the case presented the stomach is not involved.

The extent of the small bowel abnormality should be established. Involvement of just a few segments of bowel (localized) or more extensive small bowel involvement (generalized) may be important in determining the cause. In this case several segments of bowel, mainly jejunum, are involved.

The appearance of the folds themselves should be noted. Folds thicker than 3 mm that are straight, perpendicular to the bowel wall, and regular in appearance, with one thick fold looking similar to its neighbor, are indicative of hemorrhage and edema (Fig 37–2). Irregular folds that are abnormally oriented to the bowel wall and that vary in thickness, from slight to almost complete effacement, are indicative of cellular infiltrative processes such as Crohn's disease and lymphoma (Fig 37–3).

Finally, it is helpful to determine whether nodules are present in addition to fold thickening. The presence of 1 to 3 mm nodules suggests nodular lymphoid hyperplasia (Fig 37–4), whereas nodules larger than 3 mm are more suggestive of lymphoma than Crohn's disease.

DIFFERENTIATION OF CROHN'S DISEASE AND LYMPHOMA

Features of Crohn's Disease

The early radiographic changes in Crohn's disease include aphthous ulcers, which may occur anywhere in the gastrointestinal tract, and fine mucosal granularity.[2] Aphthous ulcers are typically 1 to 3 mm in diameter with a surrounding halo of edema.[3] Although their radiographic appearance is characteristic, they can be confused with nodular lymphoid hyperplasia in children and young adults, particularly in the terminal ileum. Aphthous ulcers are difficult to detect in the small bowel and are most often

TABLE 37–1.

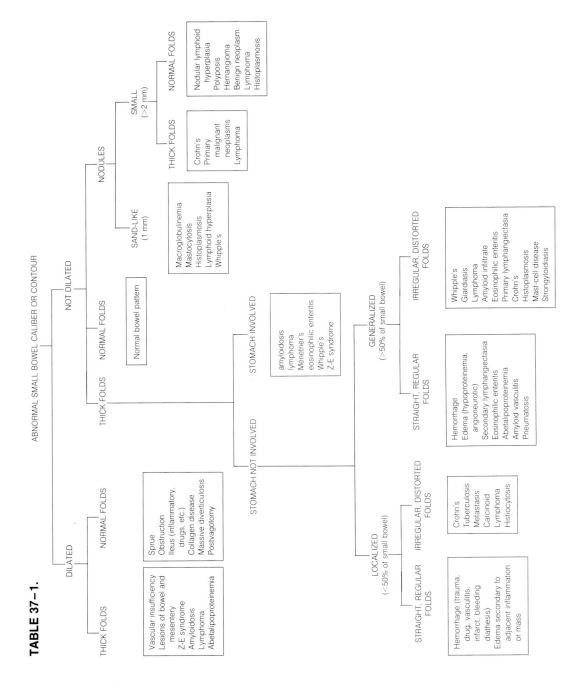

ABNORMAL SMALL BOWEL CALIBER OR CONTOUR

DILATED

NOT DILATED

THICK FOLDS

Vascular insufficiency
Lesions of bowel and
  mesentery
Z-E syndrome
Amyloidosis
Lymphoma
Abetalipoproteinemia

NORMAL FOLDS

Sprue
Obstruction
Ileus (inflammatory,
  drugs, etc.)
Collagen disease
Massive diverticulosis
Postvagotomy

THICK FOLDS

NORMAL FOLDS

Normal bowel pattern

NODULES

SAND-LIKE
(1 mm)

Macroglobulinemia
Mastocytosis
Histoplasmosis
Lymphoid hyperplasia
Whipple's

SMALL
(>2 mm)

THICK FOLDS

Crohn's
Primary
malignant
neoplasms
Lymphoma

NORMAL FOLDS

Nodular lymphoid
  hyperplasia
Polyposis
Hemangioma
Benign neoplasm
Lymphoma
Histoplasmosis

STOMACH INVOLVED

amyloidosis
lymphoma
Ménétrier's
eosinophilic enteritis
Whipple's
Z-E syndrome

STOMACH NOT INVOLVED

LOCALIZED
(<50% of small bowel)

STRAIGHT, REGULAR
FOLDS

Hemorrhage (trauma,
  drug, vasculitis,
  infarct, bleeding
  diathesis)
Edema secondary to
  adjacent inflammation
  or mass

IRREGULAR, DISTORTED
FOLDS

Crohn's
Tuberculosis
Metastasis
Carcinoid
Lymphoma
Histiocytosis

GENERALIZED
(>50% of small bowel)

STRAIGHT, REGULAR
FOLDS

Hemorrhage
Edema (hypoproteinemia,
  angioneurotic)
Secondary lymphangiectasia
Eosinophilic enteritis
Abetalipoproteinemia
Amyloid vasculitis
Pneumatosis

IRREGULAR, DISTORTED
FOLDS

Whipple's
Giardiasis
Lymphoma
Amyloid infiltrate
Eosinophilic enteritis
Primary lymphangiectasia
Crohn's
Histoplasmosis
Mast-cell disease
Strongyloidiasis

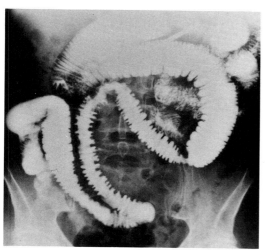

FIG 37–2.
Jejunal fold thickening that is regular with folds oriented perpendicular to the lumen is seen when hemorrhage or edema infiltrate the bowel. In this patient intestinal hemorrhage developed secondary to anticoagulant overdose.

found when spot films of the terminal ileum are obtained after a double-contrast barium enema (Fig 37–5).

Linear ulcerations occur in more advanced Crohn's disease and may be longitudinal or transverse (Fig 37–6). "Cobblestoning" results from the combination of linear and transverse ulceration with intervening edematous mucosa (Fig 37–7). Ulceration may extend transmurally, producing fistulas

between bowel loops or from bowel into the mesentery, vagina, bladder, skin, or colon (Fig 37–8). Frank abscess or phlegmon may form after transmural ulceration.

Small bowel fold thickening may occur in Crohn's disease, and the edematous valvulae conniventes often have a distorted, irregular appearance. The pattern of fold thickening is not specific for Crohn's disease, however; ischemia, radiation,

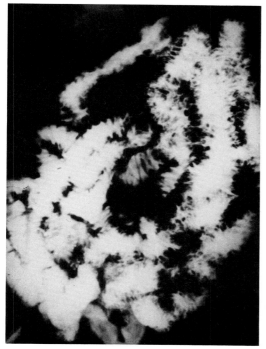

FIG 37–3.
Fold thickening throughout the small bowel, characterized by irregular, distorted folds oriented at various angles to the bowel wall. Many cellular infiltrative processes can produce this appearance; in this case amyloid infiltrate was present.

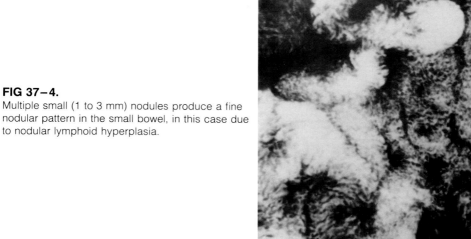

FIG 37–4.
Multiple small (1 to 3 mm) nodules produce a fine nodular pattern in the small bowel, in this case due to nodular lymphoid hyperplasia.

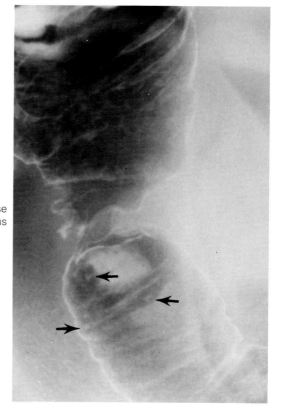

FIG 37–5.
Small aphthous ulcers *(arrows)* are present in the ileum adjacent to an anastomosis with the ascending colon. This patient with Crohn's disease had undergone an ileocecal resection the previous year.

loss of fold pattern along one wall of the bowel, with or without formation of outpouchings of relatively uninvolved areas on the opposite wall, suggests Crohn's disease.

The radiographic features are most suggestive of Crohn's disease (see Fig 37–1,A and B). There is loss of fold pattern along one wall of some segments, with small linear ulcerations perpendicular to the lumen. Asymmetric outpouchings are seen on the opposite wall. Separation of segments is diffuse rather than masslike. In this case the diagnosis of Crohn's disease was confirmed at surgery.

Other Diagnostic Possibilities

Other diagnostic possibilities should be considered when the radiographic features on small bowel follow-through studies suggest Crohn's disease or lymphoma. Thickened folds occur in many pathologic processes, including radiation enteritis and ischemia. Ischemia may be diffuse (thrombosis), focal (emboli), or multifocal (vasculitis). Angulation and tethering of bowel loops can occur in a variety of disorders other than Crohn's disease, including carcinoid, serosal metastases, and endometriosis. Intrinsic small bowel masses such as adenocarcinoma can separate bowel loops; leiomyosarcoma may excavate, simulating the endoexoenteric form of lymphoma. The inflammatory changes of Crohn's disease are nonspecific in many instances. Acute infectious processes (e.g., pelvic abscess, appendicitis, *Yersinia* enteritis) and chronic inflammatory diseases (e.g., tuberculosis, histoplasmosis, actinomycosis) can mimic the radiographic features of Crohn's disease.

OTHER IMAGING METHODS

Small bowel follow-through examination is not the only method capable of imaging the small intestine. Enteroclysis offers better mucosal detail, which may be important in identifying the early changes of Crohn's disease,[13, 14] and better defines the proximal extent, true diameter, and length of many strictures.[14, 15] However, enteroclysis involves greater patient discomfort and provides no information regarding the esophagus, stomach, and duodenum. Nevertheless, enteroclysis is probably the best method for detecting the subtle changes of both Crohn's disease and lymphoma. Computed tomography, ultrasound, and magnetic resonance imaging may demonstrate lymphadenopathy and hepatosplenomegaly associated with small bowel lymphoma and allow direct visualization of abscesses and mesenteric disease processes in Crohn's disease and lymphoma.[16–21] None of the three provides delineation of mucosal detail, however. Finally, instillation of gas through a rectal tube at the time of small bowel follow-through examination provides an air contrast view of the colon and terminal ileum (peroral pneumocolon). Double-contrast imaging generally is limited to the distal portion of the small bowel on both peroral pneumocolon and conventional air contrast barium enema examinations.[22]

In the case presented a conventional small bowel follow-through examination was performed. The patient ingested 500 ml of a 50% wt/vol barium sulfate solution. Multiple compression spot films of the small bowel were obtained during fluoroscopy, and additional overhead radiographs were taken at 30-minute intervals.

A 14- × 17-inch radiograph obtained 30 minutes after ingestion of barium (see Fig 37–1,A) demonstrates barium-filled jejunum and ileum of normal caliber with the exception of a few segments that are slightly narrowed, with irregular contours. The normal fold pattern has been replaced by thickened folds and loss of fold pattern. Several segments are abnormally separated from each other.

A fluoroscopic spot film (see Fig 37–1,B) demonstrates that in the areas with no discernible fold pattern the contour of the bowel wall is nodular and undulating. There is eccentric involvement of bowel segments, with relative straightening of one wall and pseudodiverticular outpouching of the opposite wall. Also present are linear collections of barium extending perpendicular to the bowel lumen and into the bowel wall, suggesting linear ulcerations.

REFERENCES

1. Goldberg HI, Sheft DJ: Abnormalities in small bowel contour and caliber: A working classification. *Radiol Clin North Am* 1976; 14:461–475.
2. Glick SN, Teplick SK: Crohn disease of the small intestine: Diffuse mucosal granularity. *Radiology* 1985; 154:313–317.
3. Ekberg O, Lindstrom C: Superficial lesions in Crohn's disease of the small bowel. *Gastrointest Radiol* 1979; 4:389–393.
4. Marshal RH, Lindner AE: *Radiology of the Small Intestine*, ed 2. Philadelphia, WB Saunders Co, 1976, pp 197–198.

5. Bartram CF: *Radiology in Inflammatory Bowel Disease.* New York, Marcel Dekker, 1983, pp 119–125.

6. Pringot J, Bodart P: Inflammatory diseases, in Margulis AR, Burhenne HJ (eds): Alimentary Tract Radiology, ed 3. St. Louis, CV Mosby Co, 1989, pp 764–777.

7. Glick SN: Crohn's disease of the small intestine. *Radiol Clin North Am* 1987; 25:25–46.

8. Zorroza J, Dodd GD: Lymphoma of the gastrointestinal tract. *Semin Roentgenol* 1980; 15:272–287.

9. Goldberg HI, Jeffrey RB: Recent advances in the radiographic evaluation of inflammatory bowel disease. *Med Clin North Am* 1980; 64:1059–1081.

10. Goldberg HI, Caruthers SB, Nelson JA, et al: Radiographic findings of the national cooperative Crohn's disease study. *Gastroenterology* 1979; 77:925–937.

11. Sartoris DJ, Harel GS, Anderson MF, et al: Small bowel lymphoma and regional enteritis: Radiographic similarities. *Radiology* 1984; 152:291–296.

12. Glick SN, Teplick SK, Goodman LR, et al: Development of lymphoma in patients with Crohn disease. *Radiology* 1984; 153:337–339.

13. Herlinger H: The small bowel enema and the diagnosis of Crohn's disease. *Radiol Clin North Am* 1982; 20:721–742.

14. Ekberg O: Crohn's disease of the small bowel examined by double contrast technique: A comparison with oral technique. *Gastrointest Radiol* 1977; 1:355–359.

15. Saunders DE, Ho CS: The small bowel enema: Experience with 150 examinations. *AJR* 1978; 127:743–751.

16. Goldberg HI, Gore RM, Margulis AR, et al: Computed tomography in the evaluation of Crohn's disease. *AJR* 1983; 140:277–282.

17. Frager DH, Goldman M, Beneventano TC: Computed tomography in Crohn's disease. *J Comput Assist Tomogr* 1983; 7:819–824.

18. Megibow AJ, Balthazar FJ, Naidich DP, et al: Computed tomography of gastrointestinal lymphoma. *AJR* 1983; 141:541–552.

19. James S, Balfe DM, Lee JKT, et al: Small bowel disease: Categorization by CT examination. *AJR* 1987; 148:863–868.

20. Corsina WF, Arger PH, Levine MS, et al: Gastrointestinal tract focal mass lesions: Role of CT and barium evaluations. *Radiology* 1986; 158:581–587.

21. Kerber GW, Greenberg M, Rubin JM: Computed tomography evaluation of local and extraintestinal complications of Crohn's disease. *Gastrointest Radiol* 1984; 9:143–148.

22. Wolf KJ, Goldberg HI, Wall SD, et al: Feasibility of the peroral pneumocolon in evaluating the ileocecal region. *AJR* 1985; 145:1019–1024.

CHAPTER 38

Internal Hernias

Morton A. Meyers, M.D.
Cheryl H. Grandone, M.D.

Case Presentation

Since childhood this 23-year-old woman has had periodic vomiting, cramps, and abdominal distention shortly after large meals. Clinical examination revealed left-sided tenderness with a palpable mass. What is the differential diagnosis? What radiographic methods are available to confirm the diagnosis?

DISCUSSION

The early radiograph from a small bowel series shows a circumscribed oval mass of herniated jejunal loops immediately lateral to the ascending duodenum (Fig 38–1,A). The 2-hour delayed film demonstrates stasis of barium within these loops and depression of the distal transverse colon (Fig 38–1,B).

Combining the information rendered by the clinical history, physical examination, and radiographic findings, the correct diagnosis of internal hernia must be considered.

Although the pattern of pain demonstrated by the patient may resemble peptic ulcer disease, examination of radiographs from the upper gastrointestinal series does not confirm gastric or duodenal disease. The pattern of pain also may be mimicked by gallbladder disease or abdominal angina. Ultrasonography of the gallbladder or oral cholecystography would be useful to rule out potential disease in this area; however, these examinations were not included. Clinical examination also supports a left-sided, not right-sided, mass, as would be expected with gallbladder disease. The age of the patient rules out abdominal angina as a likely differential diagnosis.

Given the clinical history of periodic vomiting and abdominal distention, causes for intermittent intestinal obstruction must be considered. Although external hernias and adhesions account for the majority of small bowel obstructions, physical examination did not reveal an external hernia, nor did history indicate previous surgery, which may render adhesions. Less common conditions such as adult hypertrophic pyloric stenosis, superior mesenteric artery syndrome, and annular pancreas are additional considerations. The contrast examination, however, does not demonstrate the appropriate radiographic pattern of gastric or duodenal disease indicative of these entities.

Internal hernias account for 0.5% to 3% of all cases of intestinal obstruction,[1, 2] with a high rate of mortality, exceeding 50% in most series.[2–4]

The small bowel examination provides the most useful diagnostic hallmarks: (1) abnormal location and disturbed arrangement of loops of small intestine, (2) crowding of loops secondary to encapsulation within a hernial sac, as seen on serial radiographs, and (3) segmental dilation with prolonged stasis within herniated loops.[5–7]

Based on their anatomic location of origin, internal hernias may be conveniently classified as (1) paraduodenal, (2) through the foramen of Winslow,

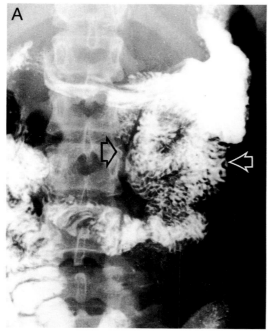
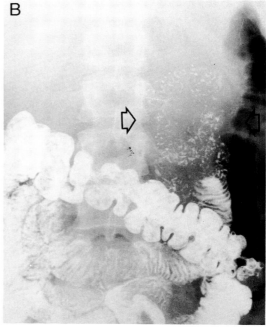

FIG 38–1.

Small left paraduodenal hernia. **A,** small bowel series shows a circumscribed ovoid mass of herniated jejunal loops lateral to the ascending duodenum *(arrows).* **B,** two-hour film reveals status of barium within these loops *(arrows)* and depression of the dis- tal transverse colon. At surgery the hernial sac con- tained only a few feet of jejunum. This was readily re- duced and the peritoneal defect repaired. (From Meyers MA: *Radiology* 1970; 95:29–37. Used by permission.)

(3) pericecal, (4) intersigmoid, or (5) transmesen- teric or transmesocolic. Figure 38–2 summarizes the relative incidence of internal hernias at various locations.

The majority of internal hernias result from congenital anomalies of intestinal rotation and peri- toneal attachment.[2, 9–11] Acquired defects of the mes- entery or peritoneum secondary to abdominal surgery or trauma also may serve as hernial rings.[12, 13] The retroperitoneal group of internal hernias is seen more frequently in adults; the transmesenteric types are more commonly present in the pediatric age group.[2, 10, 14]

PARADUODENAL HERNIAS

The patient presented has a left-sided paraduo- denal hernia, the most common type of internal her- nia. Of the paraduodenal hernias, 75% occur on the left and 25% on the right. The fossa of Landzert, a left paraduodenal fossa, is present in 2% of autopsy cases.[15] It is situated at some distance to the left of the ascending, or fourth, portion of the duodenum and is caused by the raising up of a peritoneal fold by the inferior mesenteric vein as it runs along the lateral side of the fossa and then above it (Fig 38–3). The small intestine may herniate through the orifice posteriorly and downward toward the left, lateral to the ascending limb of the duodenum, ex- tending into the descending mesocolon and left por- tion of the transverse colon. The hernial orifice is paraduodenal, but the herniated loops may present at a distance.

The clinical manifestations of paraduodenal hernia may range from chronic or intermittent mild digestive complaints to acute intestinal obstruction. A history of periodic cramps, vomiting, and disten- tion, frequently dating back to childhood, as in our patient, may be elicited. The postprandial pain often is relieved by postural changes.

The preoperative diagnosis of a paraduodenal hernia can be established by radiologic evaluation. Barium contrast studies are best performed during a

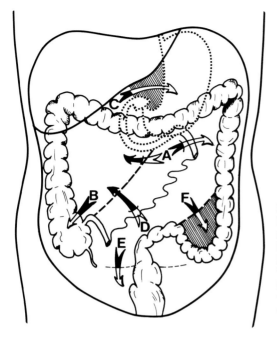

FIG 38–2.
Location and relative incidence of internal hernias according to the collective review by Hansmann and Morton[8]: paraduodenal hernias *(A)*, 53%; pericecal hernias *(B)*, 13%; hernias through the foramen of Winslow *(C)*, 8%; transmesenteric hernias *(D)*, 8%; hernias into pelvic structures *(E)*, 7%; transmesosigmoid hernias *(F)*, 6%. (From Ghahremani GG, Meyers MA: *Curr Probl Radiol* 1975; 5:1–30. Used by permission.)

symptomatic period. Examination and results in intervals between recurrent internal herniation may be negative, as in our patient, or may demonstrate mild degrees of dilation, stasis, or edematous folds. Serial filming and diligent fluoroscopy are essential.

In our patient with a small left paraduodenal hernia a circumscribed mass of a few loops, most typically jejunal, is seen in the left upper quadrant immediately lateral to the ascending duodenum. The herniated loops may depress the distal transverse colon and indent the posterior wall of the stomach. Stasis of barium within the hernial contents and mild dilation of the duodenum may be associated findings. Encapsulation within the hernial sac prevents separation or displacement of the individual loops from the rest of the hernial contents during serial radiographs. Lateral films may be particularly useful for detection of retroperitoneal displacement of the hernial contents, showing loops projecting over the spine. On barium enema examination the descending colon may be anterior, to the left, or posterior to a left paraduodenal hernia (Fig 38–4).

Arteriographic visualization of vessels and their branches supplying the small bowel loops can assist in the radiologic diagnosis of paraduodenal hernia. In a left-sided paraduodenal hernia the proximal jejunal arteries show an abrupt change of course along the medial border of the hernial orifice, where they are redirected posteriorly behind the inferior mesenteric vessels to accompany the herniated loops. A line connecting the points at which these arteries suddenly change their course indicates the medial border of the hernial orifice beyond which the small intestinal loops herniate.[5, 16]

Computed tomography may contribute to the diagnosis of the nonobstructed left-sided paraduodenal hernia by demonstrating herniated loops between the stomach and the body of the pancreas (Fig 38–5), with perhaps medial displacement of the duodenojejunal junction.[17, 18] These findings generally are readily differentiated from other causes of intestinal malrotation or obstruction.[19–21]

Without a specific radiologic diagnosis a small internal hernia may not be evident at laparotomy. The hernia may reduce spontaneously or after traction at surgery. The usual exploratory laparotomy is often inadequate for evaluation of all significant peritoneal fossae and possible mesenteric defects that represent potential sites of herniation.

The less common right paraduodenal hernia usually involves the mesenteric parietal fossa (fossa of Waldeyer), immediately behind the superior mesenteric artery and inferior to the transverse duodenum. The small bowel is entrapped behind the ascending mesocolon and the right half of the transverse mesocolon (Fig 38–6). The ascending colon

A

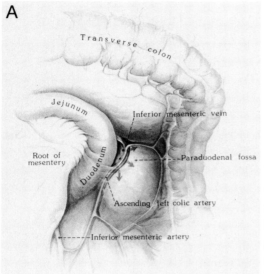

B

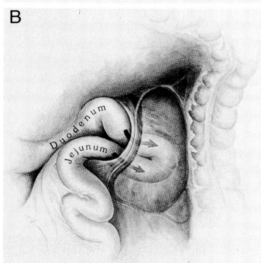

C

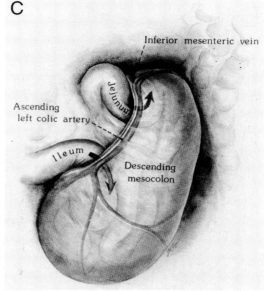

FIG 38–3.
A–C, development of a left paraduodenal hernia.
The small bowel loops herniate via the fossa of
Landzert into the descending mesocolon. Note the
position of the inferior mesenteric vein and ascending
left colic artery in the anterior margin of the neck of
the sac. (From Meyers MA: Internal abdominal
hernias, in *Dynamic Radiology of the Abdomen:
Normal and Pathologic Anatomy,* ed 3. New York,
Springer-Verlag, 1988, pp 423–448. Used by
permission.)

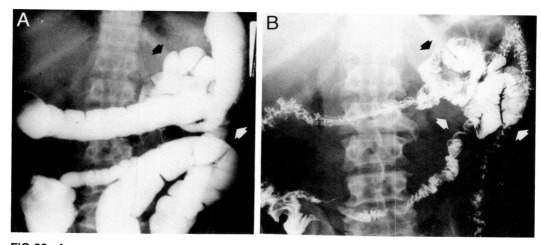

FIG 38–4.
Left paraduodenal hernia. Filled **(A)** and post-evacuation **(B)** barium enema study demonstrates refluxed proximal ileal loops forming a circumscribed ovoid mass *(arrows),* with stasis within the left paraduodenal fossa. (From Ghahremani GG, Meyers MA: Herniation of the colon, in Greenbaum El (ed): *Radiographic Atlas of Colon Disease.* Chicago, Year Book Medical Publishers, 1980. Used by permission.)

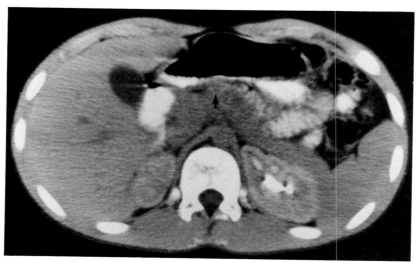

FIG 38–5.
Left paraduodenal hernia. Computed tomographic scan in a 13-year-old boy identifies a single loop of jejunum *(arrow)* between the stomach and the body of the pancreas. (From Day DL, Drake DG, Leonard AS, et al: *Gastrointest Radiol* 1988; 13:27–29. Used by permission.)

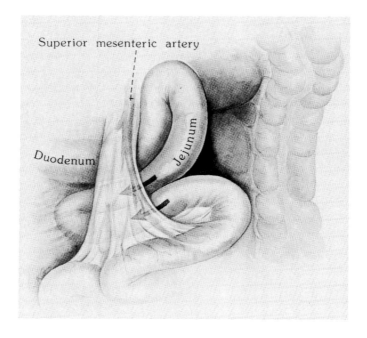

FIG 38–6.

Development of a right paraduodenal hernia via the fossa of Waldeyer toward the ascending mesocolon. Note the position of the superior mesenteric artery anterior to the hernia and in the leading edge of the sac. (From Meyers MA: Internal abdominal hernias, in *Dynamic Radiology of the Abdomen: Normal and Pathologic Anatomy,* ed 3. New York, Springer-Verlag, 1988. Used by permission.)

always lies lateral to the right paraduodenal hernia, and the cecum is found in its normal position (Fig 38–7).

HERNIAS THROUGH THE FORAMEN OF WINSLOW

Internal hernias may occur through the foramen of Winslow. The potential opening is situated beneath the free edge of the lesser omentum, cephalad to the duodenal bulb and deep to the liver. The foramen, which provides communication between the greater peritoneal cavity and the lesser peritoneal sac, may open to some extent when the trunk is flexed. Predisposing causes include a common or abnormally long mesentery or persistence of the ascending mesocolon, permitting excessive mobility of bowel and enlargement of the foramen.

Alteration in intra-abdominal pressure may tend to provoke herniation, which may be facilitated by an elongated right lobe of the liver directing the mobile intestinal loops toward the foramen of Winslow.

The onset is usually acute, with severe progressive pain and signs of bowel obstruction. Some re-

lief of pain may be achieved with forward bending or the knee-chest position.

The characteristic plain film findings are demonstration of a circumscribed collection of gas-containing intestinal loops high in the abdomen medial and posterior to the stomach, associated with mechanical small bowel obstruction (Fig 38–8). Distinction from other conditions that can present with gas in the lesser sac (e.g., perforated peptic ulcer or abscess) is possible by identification of the presence of a mucosal pattern and fluid levels within the herniated bowel. The fluid levels do not conform precisely to the anatomic recesses of the lesser omental cavity.

Barium studies readily confirm the diagnosis of hernia into the foramen of Winslow. The characteristic displacement of the stomach to the left and anteriorly may be associated with displacement of the duodenum to the left. A small bowel series documents the site of obstruction corresponding to the anatomic location of the foramen of Winslow. A barium enema may reveal obstruction, with a tapered point near the hepatic flexure if the herniation contains the cecum and ascending colon (Fig 38–9).

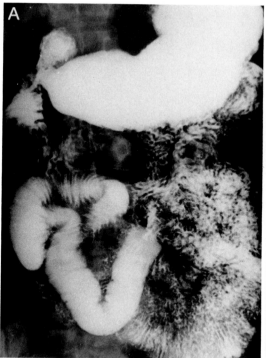 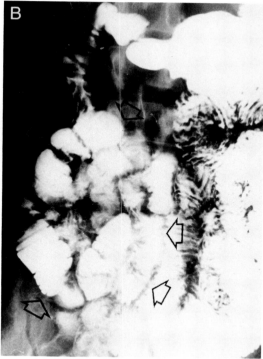

FIG 38–7.
A, paraduodenal hernia. The afferent and efferent limbs, which lie close together, both appear obstructed. **B,** later the small intestinal loops within the circumscribed ovoid hernial sac *(arrows)* into the ascending mesocolon are still dilated but with a small degree of obstruction. The alternation sites of narrowing represent adhesions between loops. (From Meyers MA: *Radiology* 1970; 95:29–37. Used by permission.)

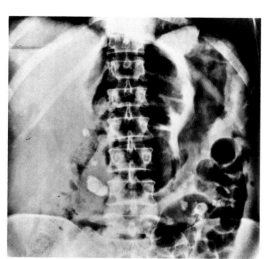

FIG 38–8.
Cecal herniation through the foramen of Winslow. Plain film demonstrates gas-containing cecum with identifiable interhaustral septa within the lesser sac, displacing the stomach toward the left.

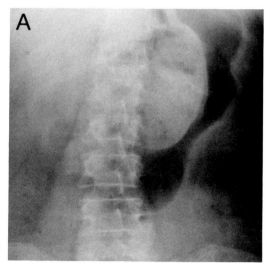

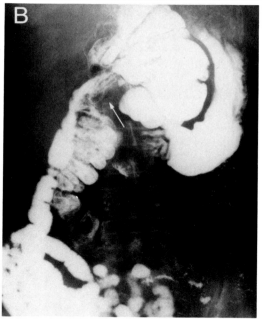

FIG 38–9.
Hernia through the foramen of Winslow. **A,** plain film shows mottled gas density consistent with large bowel impressing on the lesser curvature of the stomach. **B,** small bowel follow-through study confirms herniation of the cecum and ascending colon into the lesser sac. Note compression of the ascending colon at the foramen of Winslow *(arrow).* (From Goldberger LE, Berk RN: *Gastrointest Radiol* 1980; 5:169–172. Used by permission.)

PERICECAL HERNIAS

Peritoneal fossae in the ileocecal region as well as congenital and acquired defects in the mesentery of the cecum or appendix may lead to development of a pericecal hernia. In most cases a portion of ileum passes through defects in the mesentery of the cecum to occupy the right paracolic gutter (Fig 38–10). Lateral and oblique projections during contrast examination are particularly valuable for demonstration of the fixed position of herniated loops posterolateral to the cecum. Transitory transmigration of the small intestine anteriorly over the ascending colon may mimic internal hernias through a persistent ascending mesocolon.

INTERSIGMOID HERNIAS

The intersigmoid fossa, a peritoneal pouch formed between the two loops of the sigmoid colon and its mesentery, serves as a potential site for an

PART V

Colon–Appendix

CHAPTER 39

Obstructing Lesion in the Sigmoid Colon

Janis Gissel Letourneau, M.D.

Case Presentation

A 60-year-old man had dull lower abdominal discomfort, cramping, and mild constipation. His stool tested positive for occult blood. A double-contrast barium enema revealed a constricting lesion at the rectosigmoid junction (Fig 39–1). What is the differential diagnosis?

DISCUSSION

This patient had relatively nonspecific symptoms. The presence of occult blood in the stool is also nonspecific and can occur with both benign and malignant intestinal disease. However, in this clinical setting it is necessary to rule out the most serious of potential diagnostic considerations, colonic carcinoma. The differential diagnosis of this particular lesion is broad, despite its characteristic features.

Radiographic techniques for evaluating these lesions are relatively limited. A barium enema with single-contrast or double-contrast technique provides valuable data when a circumferential stenotic lesion is present. Water-soluble contrast medium should be used when a perforation is suspected or when operative intervention is anticipated in the near future. However, the value of water-soluble contrast medium is impaired by its limited capability to demonstrate mucosal detail. Both barium and water-soluble contrast enemas can be facilitated by the use of parenterally administered glucagon to relieve any element of spasm that might contribute to luminal narrowing. Although computed tomographic scanning is usually not the primary radiographic tool for excluding colonic carcinoma as a diagnostic consideration, it is used with variable success for preoperative assessment in these patients.[1-3] Computed tomography is of greater value in the assessment of suspected sigmoid diverticulitis.[4] In this setting pericolonic disease is readily apparent.

Stenosis of the sigmoid colon has many causes. Limiting the extensive differential diagnosis depends on characterization of the stricture, including its length, margins, mucosa, and the presence or absence of contiguous mass effect.[5-7] The most common cause of stenosis in the sigmoid colon is adenocarcinoma. Such lesions typically are relatively short, with abrupt margins and some disruption of the normal mucosal pattern. Larger lesions causing stenosis tend to be circumferential or annular. Although retrograde flow of barium may be severely impaired and even absent, the patient may not give a history of frank constipation or abdominal cramping. In cases with significant obstruction to flow of the contrast medium it may be difficult to define the proximal margin of the "apple-core" lesion (Fig 39–2).

Other malignant processes can cause narrowing of the sigmoid colon. Lymphoma can present in a variety of forms within the colon, including multi-

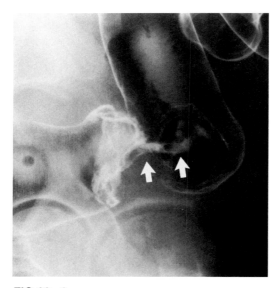

FIG 39–1.
Relatively short stricture in the sigmoid colon *(arrows)*. The distal margin of the lesion is well seen, is abrupt, and demonstrates mucosal irregularity.

ple polyps, solitary polypoid lesions with or without ulceration, segmental aneurysmal dilation, and localized annular constrictive lesions[5, 7] (Fig 39–3). Metastatic serosal foci from intraperitoneal seeding of carcinoma also can cause luminal compromise.[8] Because of the location of the mesenteric reflection, these implants typically occur on the superior border of the sigmoid colon. The desmoplastic response induced by the metastases can cause transverse pleat-

ing of the mucosa. The extrinsic nature of these lesions and the integrity of the mucosa should serve to differentiate them from primary colon cancer.

Diverticulitis is the next most common cause for obstruction in the sigmoid colon. Rupture of a colonic diverticulum causes perforation of luminal contents and development of a localized inflammatory process or, rarely, diffuse intra-abdominal infection. Diverticuli form in areas of weakness of the bowel wall, at the sites of penetration of the vasa vasorum, and represent small outpouchings of mucosa and submucosa through the muscularis. It is presumed they develop because of increased intraluminal pressure due to slow colonic evacuation, stasis, and spasm. Luminal compromise by a pericolonic inflammatory process can be exaggerated by significant sigmoid spasm. Spasm also can alter the appearance of the margin of such a stenosis, making it appear more abrupt and hence more malignant. Administration of glucagon in patients with diverticulitis often helps to elucidate the benign features of the stenosis. Typically, contrast enemas reveal a variably long stenosis with gradually tapered margins. The mucosa may be difficult to assess but should be intact. Extraluminal transverse and longitudinal tracking of contrast may be seen within the pericolonic mass, and significant extrinsic mass effect may be present (Fig 39–4). Fistulas to adjacent structures may be seen.[5, 7] Computed tomography can be helpful in assessing the extent of such pericolonic involvement.[4]

Narrowing of the sigmoid colon also can be seen after an ischemic event.[9, 10] In the acute set-

FIG 39–2.
Typical "apple-core" lesion, representing an adenocarcinoma, in the sigmoid colon. Almost complete obstruction to flow of retrograde contrast is seen.

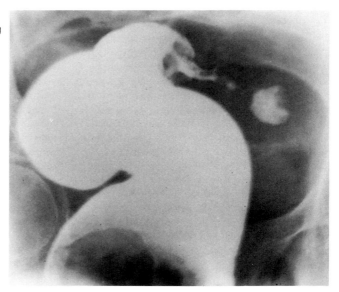

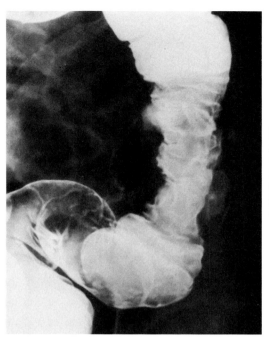

FIG 39-3.
Area of narrowing near the junction of the descending and sigmoid colon. There is some nodularity to the lesion. The margins of the lesion are not characteristic for a benign or malignant process. This was found to be non-Hodgkin's lymphoma.

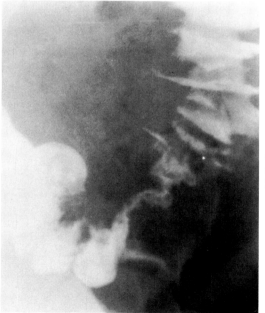

FIG 39-4.
Irregular long segment of narrowing of the sigmoid colon with tapered margins. Transverse tracking of contrast medium and associated spasm were seen in this patient with diverticulitis.

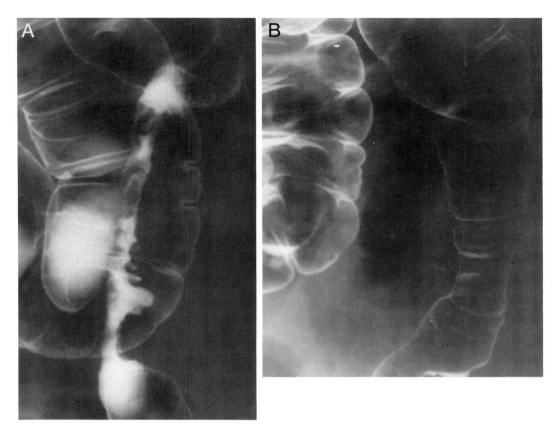

FIG 39–5.
A, long area of luminal narrowing with apparent colonic wall edema representing acute ischemic colitis. **B,** restoration of the lumen occurred over 3 months.

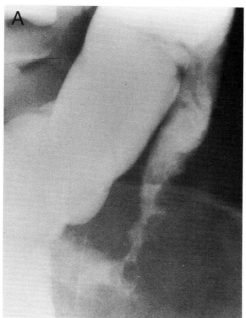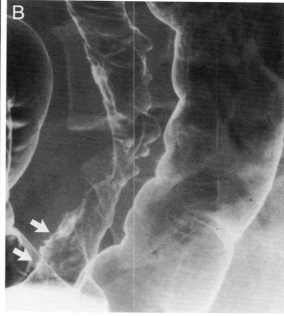

FIG 39–6.
A, mucosal irregularity with ulceration and luminal narrowing in a patient with Crohn's disease of the descending colon. **B,** healing of the inflammatory process has left a residual stricture with pseudodiverticuli. Some minimal mucosal ulceration persists *(arrows).*

ting the stenosis may have features of a malignant neoplasm, with mucosal irregularity and sharp margins. However, with healing progressive fibrosis causes development of a smooth stricture with tapered margins (Fig 39–5).

A variety of inflammatory processes also can cause stenosis of the sigmoid colon. Strictures can be seen in ulcerative colitis. These are usually single but may be multiple. Once the inflammatory process is quiescent the mucosa in these stenotic regions is smooth. The margins of the stricture are tapered. Because carcinoma is more frequent in these patients and infiltrating adenocarcinoma may produce a similar smooth, tapered lesion, biopsy of such strictures is advisable.[5, 7] Colonic involvement with Crohn's disease may produce lesions that are difficult to distinguish from carcinoma (Fig 39–6). The deep ulceration seen with Crohn's disease produces mucosal irregularity. Associated spasm and bowel wall infiltration may contribute to abrupt margination of the stenosis; usually, however, the multifocal nature of the disease reveals its identity.[5, 7] Infectious colitides, such as amebiasis, schistosomiasis, and shigellosis, can produce stricturing of the sigmoid colon[11, 12]; these usually have typically benign features. Tuberculosis, because of its chronic, indolent nature, can lead to strictures with mucosal irregularity that mimic malignant lesions.[13] Nonspecific benign ulcers of the colon occur rarely, and their healing can cause colonic narrowing. These are most common in the right colon but can be seen in the distal colon. The strictures that follow healing of these ulcers can have benign or malignant radiographic features.[14]

Stricture of the sigmoid colon also can follow pelvic external beam or implantation radiation.[15] Typically it is a late complication of radiation therapy, occurring months to years after treatment. It appears to be related to radiation injury to the small vessels supplying the affected bowel. This injury results in mucosal atrophy and fibrosis, which in turn produce bowel wall thickening and luminal narrowing. Straightening and angulation of the bowel also are seen, and are most apparent when the small intestine is affected. Fixation of the colon can cause a stricture with an abrupt margin (Fig 39–7); coincident mucosal ulceration can mimic a malignant annular lesion.

Occasionally retractile mesenteritis occurs as a limited process affecting only the colonic mesentery. Associated thickening and retraction of the mesentery can cause luminal narrowing with either

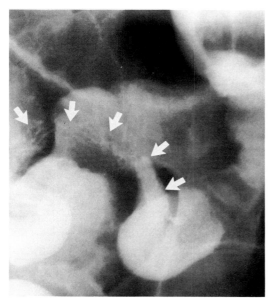

FIG 39–7.
Stricture of the sigmoid colon with indeterminant features *(arrows)* is seen after external beam radiation treatment. Its length makes a primary malignant process unlikely.

benign or malignant characteristics.[16] Adhesive bands are relatively uncommon in the sigmoid colon and occur as a result of previous abdominal or pelvic surgery or pelvic infection. These produce short, smooth stenoses with normal mucosa.[17]

In the case presented (see Fig 39–1), the abrupt margins of the lesion and its mucosal irregularity exclude many of the potential differential diagnostic considerations. Diagnostic possibilities include colonic adenocarcinoma, lymphoma, diverticulitis, ischemic colitis, and postradiation colitis. Because of the absence of diverticuli in other areas of visualized bowel, diverticulitis is unlikely. Ischemic and postradiation colitis can be excluded on a historical basis, leaving adenocarcinoma and lymphoma as the most likely considerations. A colon cancer was found at sigmoidoscopy and was surgically resected.

Many different pathologic processes, benign and malignant, can result in stenosis of the sigmoid colon. Although only a few diseases commonly cause luminal narrowing in this region, other less common entities must be considered. Evaluation of the specific characteristics of the lesions can help to limit the differential diagnosis and further direct the diagnostic evaluation.

REFERENCES

1. Freeny PC, Marks WM, Ryan JA, et al: Colorectal carcinoma evaluation with CT: Preoperative staging and detection of postoperative recurrence. *Radiology* 1986; 158:347–353.
2. Mayes GB, Zornoza J: Computed tomography of colon carcinoma. *Am J Roentgenol* 1980; 135:43–46.
3. Thoeni RF, Moss AA, Schnyder P, et al: Detection and staging of primary rectal and rectosigmoid cancer by computed tomography. *Radiology* 1981; 141:135–138.
4. Hulnick DH, Megibow AJ, Balthazar EJ, et al: Computed tomography in the evaluation of diverticulitis. *Radiology* 1984; 152:491–495.
5. Dreyfuss JR, Janower ML. *Radiology of the Colon.* Baltimore, Williams & Wilkins Co, 1980.
6. Johnson CD, Carlson HC, Taylor WF, et al: Barium enemas of carcinoma of the colon: Sensitivity of double- and single-contrast studies. *Am J Roentgenol* 1983; 140:1143–1149.
7. Marshak RH, Lindner AE, Maklansky D: *Radiology of the Colon.* Philadelphia, WB Saunders Co, 1980.
8. Ginaldi S, Lindell MM Jr, Zornoza J: The striped colon: A new radiographic observation in metastatic serosal implants. *Am J Roentgenol* 1980; 134:453–455.
9. Brandt LJ, Katz HJ, Wolf EL, et al: Simulation of colonic carcinoma by ischemia. *Gastroenterology* 1985; 88:1137–1142.
10. Mitty HA, Efremidis S, Kuler R: Colonic stricture after transcatheter embolization for diverticular bleeding. *Am J Roentgenol* 1979; 133:519–521.
11. Cardosa JM, Kimura K, Stoopen M, et al: Radiology of invasive amebiasis of the colon. *Am J Roentgenol* 1977; 128:935–941.
12. Farman J, Rabinowitz JG, Meyers MA: Roentgenology of infectious colitis. *Am J Roentgenol* 1973; 119:375–381.
13. Balthazar EJ, Bryk D: Segmental tuberculosis of the distal colon: Radiographic features in 7 cases. *Gastrointest Radiol* 1980; 5:75–80.
14. Gardiner GA, Bird CR: Nonspecific ulcers of the colon, resembling annular carcinoma. *Radiology* 1980; 137:331–334.
15. Meyer JE: Review: Radiography of the distal colon and rectum after irradiation of carcinoma of the cervix. *Am J Roentgenol* 1981; 136:691–699.
16. Williams RG, Nelson JA: Retractile mesenteritis: Initial presentation as colonic obstruction. *Radiology* 1978; 126:35–37.
17. Brody PA, Schudt DR, Magnuson A, et al: Complete colonic obstruction secondary to adhesions. *Am J Roentgenol* 1979; 133:917–918.

CHAPTER 40

Ulcerative and Granulomatous Colitis: Radiologic Differentiation and Management

Hugh J. Williams, Jr., M.D.
Frederick M. Kelvin, M.D.

Case Presentation

A 26-year-old man with a 2-year history of diarrhea of fluctuating severity was seen during an episode of severe exacerbation. Double-contrast examination of the colon was performed (Fig 40–1). Proctosigmoidoscopy revealed a few punctate rectal ulcerations; other findings were normal. Stool culture and microscopy findings were negative. What is your diagnosis?

DISCUSSION

Double-contrast colon examination (Fig 40–1) demonstrates a diffuse abnormality of the colon from the cecum to the mid–transverse colon. There is diffuse ulceration of this portion of the colon, including punctate and linear ulcers. The wall of the involved colon is irregularly scarred and the lumen narrowed. Haustral markings are absent. In addition a few punctate ulcerations involve the right lateral wall of the rectum. The remainder of the colon appears normal. Disease involvement to this extent allows us, for practical purposes, to limit the differential diagnosis to inflammatory diseases of the colon. Although the causes of colitis are numerous, there are two predominant categories: colitis with a known cause (related to infection, radiation, ischemia, or toxins) and idiopathic colitides, such as ulcerative and granulomatous colitis. Significant differences in clinical management require that colitis with a known cause be differentiated from idiopathic colitis. The colon can respond morphologically to a multitude of insults in a limited number of ways, and there is tremendous overlap in the radiographic features of the many colitides. Differentiation among these groups therefore cannot be made by radiographic techniques alone. Reliable differentiation may be achieved, however, by synthesizing the results from radiographic studies with the clinical findings, including history, stool microscopy and culture, endoscopy, and sometimes colonic or rectal biopsy results. After the diagnosis of idiopathic inflammatory disease has been established, radiographic distinction between ulcerative colitis and granulomatous colitis usually can be achieved.

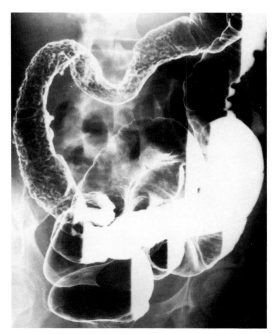

FIG 40–1.
Left lateral internal radiograph from a double-contrast barium examination.

DIFFERENTIATION OF ULCERATIVE AND GRANULOMATOUS COLITIS

Pathologically, ulcerative colitis and granulomatous colitis affect the colon in different and usually distinctive ways. Ulcerative colitis is essentially a superficial inflammation of the colon, primarily involving the mucosa, whereas granulomatous colitis involves both the mucosa and submucosa at an early stage and the reaction tends to become transmural. Radiographically, the double-contrast examination[1] is the most useful imaging method for demonstrating the morphologic changes caused by ulcerative and granulomatous colitis, usually permitting their differentiation. Distinguishing features of ulcerative and granulomatous colitis are well presented in the literature,[2–4] and many are discussed here.

Early Mucosal Changes

Of the many distinguishing features of ulcerative and granulomatous colitis seen on double-contrast studies, some are more useful than others. We have found changes expressed early in the course of both diseases to be the most valuable in allowing differentiation. Granularity is the earliest radiographically detectable change in ulcerative colitis and is the result of mucosal edema and hyperemia (Fig 40–2,A). In granulomatous colitis the earliest change is the aphthous ulcer, which results from central ulceration of the mucosa overlying a hypertrophied submucosal lymphoid follicle (Fig 40–2,C). These early changes are relatively specific for the two main types of idiopathic colitis, with only sporadic cases of granularity in granulomatous colitis[5] and aphthous ulcers in ulcerative colitis[6] reported in the literature.

The identification of granularity and aphthous ulcers is essential for early double-contrast study detection and differentiation of inflammatory disease in patients experiencing an initial bout of colitis; however, their utility does not stop there. These early radiographic manifestations of colitis also may herald the extension of existing disease by appearing at the leading edge of already well-established but advancing colitis (Fig 40–3) or by their presence at a colonic location remote from existing disease. Reactivation of quiescent disease also may be signalled by the appearance of granularity or aphthous ulcers. Knowledge of these different presentations is important, as patients will be referred for radiographic examination at various stages of disease expression. Even when there is extensive disease, making differentiation difficult, the presence of granularity or aphthous ulcers somewhere in the colon usually allows the correct diagnosis. In the case presented (see Fig 40–1) the small collection of aphthous ulcers in the transverse colon is diagnostic of granulomatous colitis.

Differences in Distribution

Differences in disease distribution are also useful in distinguishing ulcerative from granulomatous colitis. For practical purposes, colonic involvement by these diseases can be thought of as occurring in two orientations: longitudinally (along the length of the colon) and circumferentially. Classically, longitudinal continuity of disease is characteristic of ulcerative colitis. Disease begins in the rectum and advances proximally and continuously for a variable distance. The rectum is involved in all cases. In contrast, longitudinal discontinuity of disease, with skip areas, best describes the distribution of granulomatous colitis. The rectum is involved in approximately one half of these patients.

Knowledge of the classic presentations of ulcerative and granulomatous colitis is important, but

further evaluation is required to differentiate between ulcerative and granulomatous colitis and to determine the extent of colonic involvement.

Proctosigmoidoscopy is more sensitive than the double-contrast examination in the detection of inflammatory changes and detects these changes at an earlier stage of activity. In fact, 15% to 20% of patients with colitis with a normal-appearing rectosigmoid colon on the double-contrast study have mild disease activity at endoscopy.[6] Therefore the double-contrast enema should not be considered a substitute for proctosigmoidoscopy in disease detection. Conversely, although proctosigmoidoscopy usually precedes the double-contrast examination, normal endoscopic findings should not preclude performance of this radiographic study. In a significant number of patients with colitis, diseased colon segments may lie entirely above the proctosigmoidoscopic level and require double-contrast examination for detection. This includes as many as 40%[6] to 70%[11] of patients with granulomatous colitis with a normal rectum and distal colon and 5% to 20% of patients with ulcerative colitis,[2, 6] depending on the extent of distal colon and rectum healing that has occurred prior to endoscopy (so-called ulcerative colitis variants). It may be reasonably argued, however, that the patient with typical changes of ulcerative colitis endoscopically, in which the proximal extent of disease is visualized, need not undergo the double-contrast examination.

Double-contrast radiography is better than proctosigmoidoscopy for distinguishing between ulcerative and granulomatous colitis. Its advantage lies primarily in its ability to provide information from the entire colon, thereby allowing the distinction. This is particularly important in patients with inflammatory changes exclusively above the endoscopic level but can also be valuable in those with endoscopically indeterminate rectosigmoid colitis, who may harbor more diagnostic features above the endoscopic field of view. In one study, if only the region of the rectosigmoid colon was considered on the double-contrast examination, regardless of inflammatory changes proximally, the double contrast study was more specific than proctosigmoidoscopy in differentiating between active ulcerative colitis and granulomatous disease.[6] In that study, classification of ulcerative colitis by endoscopy was difficult, being misclassified as granulomatous disease in 6%. Fewer than 1% of ulcerative colitis patients were misclassified by the double contrast examination. All patients with endoscopic misclassifications had characteristic features of ulcerative colitis radio-

graphically, both within and above the endoscopic range. This phenomenon did not exist for the classification of granulomatous colitis. Neither method misclassified granulomatous colitis as ulcerative disease.[6] Signs of more chronic inflammatory disease, such as loss of colon wall distensibility, shortening of the colon, and luminal narrowing, also are better evaluated with the double-contrast study.

The extent of colon involvement by inflammatory disease is better determined with the double-contrast examination in all cases except ulcerative proctitis. However, compared with colonoscopy, the double-contrast study underestimates the extent of colonic involvement in ulcerative colitis by approximately one third the total length of the colon.[12] Armed with this knowledge, the clinician can use double-contrast radiography to develop a rough estimate of actual colon involvement. This information is important for determining the future risk for carcinoma. Because this risk is low in granulomatous colitis and there is no useful correlation between changes seen on double-contrast radiography, clinical symptoms, and the course of the disease,[13] underestimating the extent of colon involvement in granulomatous disease is less important.

The philosophies governing the long-term management of ulcerative and granulomatous colitis are decidedly different. Management of ulcerative disease revolves around early recognition of malignancy or its precursor, dysplasia. Epithelial dysplasia occasionally can be recognized on the double-contrast study, but these precancerous lesions cannot be consistently identified with this technique,[14] especially in the presence of active inflammation. Periodic total colonoscopy with multiple random or directed biopsy procedures probably is the most effective surveillance technique for early malignant disease in patients with ulcerative colitis who do not undergo prophylactic proctocolectomy. The double-contrast enema may be helpful in directing colonoscopic biopsy to an abnormality detected during the study. Because slightly more than half of radiographically detected malignant lesions in ulcerative disease appear indistinguishable from benign strictures,[15] the finding of a stricture on double-contrast radiography indicates the need for endoscopic biopsy. However, because the incidence of carcinoma in granulomatous colitis is less than in the ulcerative form, routine surveillance in this disease is infrequent. Further, the correlation between the radiologic severity and clinical severity of granulomatous colitis is poor,[13] and routine double-contrast radiography to assess the status of the disease usually is not indicated. Instead, emphasis is placed on the identification of inflammatory complications, such as fistulas, abscesses, and obstructing strictures. A single-contrast, rather than double-contrast, colon examination probably is more appropriate for identifying colonic fistulas. Computed tomography, US, and MRI offer a cross-sectional perspective of the colon and surrounding tissues that may provide valuable information for the management of colitis. These techniques, however, are only capable of evaluating the extramucosal manifestations of colitis and rely primarily on the presence of well-established disease for their effectiveness. They are unable to detect the earliest changes of ulcerative and granulomatous colitis, such as granularity and aphthous ulcers. Because of this, cross-sectional techniques should not be considered a substitute for the double-contrast examination or endoscopy when the goal is primary disease detection and differentiation. CT and US are important, however, for detection of the complications associated with colitis, particularly in granulomatous disease. The role of MRI in this disease remains to be established.

CT is the most widely used cross-sectional technique in the evaluation of colitis. In a study of patients who had had disease for, on average, 8 or more years, Gore et al.[16] found that the most common CT abnormality allowing disease detection was mural thickening. The average wall thickness was significantly greater in granulomatous than in ulcerative colitis (13 mm and 7.8 mm, respectively), permitting accurate differentiation between the two diseases (Fig 40−8). In addition, the wall thickening was homogeneous in granulomatous colitis and inhomogeneous, as a result of fat infiltration of the submucosa, in ulcerative colitis. The presence of changes involving the mesentery, such as fibrofatty proliferation, phlegmon, and abscess, also was helpful in distinguishing granulomatous from ulcerative colitis. In this study CT did not alter the original diagnosis established by barium studies and endoscopy in any patients, and those with indeterminate colitis could not be further categorized. At present, therefore, there is little or no indication for CT in the evaluation of known or suspected ulcerative colitis.

Like CT, US is capable of detecting the colonic changes of colitis, especially in granulomatous disease, because of the greater degree of mural thickening. US also can identify disease complications, particularly abscess formation.[17] The scans, however, may be degraded by the presence of intestinal gas, and the technique is impractical for imaging the entire colon. Its predominant role is in the detection and drainage of abscesses complicating granulomatous colitis, although occasionally it is the first technique to recognize mural thickening, particularly in granulomatous disease.

The role of MRI in evaluating colitis is still evolving, and eventually MRI may prove to have advantages over CT. Its superior soft tissue contrast resolution most likely will enhance identification of even small abscesses.[18] Other advantages include the ability to scan directly in the axial, coronal, and sagittal planes, which should better display the relationship of abscesses, fistulas, and sinus tracts to the colon and surrounding abdominal tissues. The lack

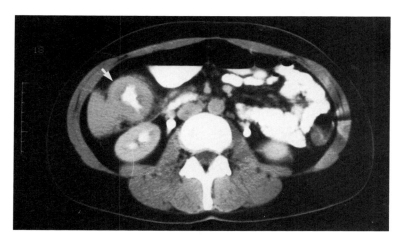

FIG 40−8.
(Same patient as in Fig 40−7) computed tomographic scan shows marked homogeneous thickening of the ascending colon wall (approximately 13 mm) consistent with granulomatous colitis *(arrow).*

of an intraluminal contrast agent and long scan acquisition time are hurdles to overcome before this technique becomes practical in these patients.

In one of the newest radiologic techniques for evaluating colitis, leukocytes are labeled in vitro with indium 111 and subsequently reinjected into the donor. The labeled leukocytes migrate to sites of inflammation, and abdominal and pelvic images are acquired with a gamma scanning device to assess the location and intensity of indium activity within the colon (Fig 40–9). Compared with the barium enema or colonoscopy, this appears to be an accurate, noninvasive method of assessing the extent and severity of inflammation in patients with ulcerative or granulomatous colitis. One weakness of the technique is its inability to distinguish between the two diseases.[19] This tends to make indium scanning superfluous when endoscopy or double-contrast radiography or both subsequently will be required to differentiate between the two colitides. As with cross-sectional techniques, indium scanning is capable of detecting abscesses complicating colitis.[20] The main role of indium scanning probably will be in the assessment of the extent of inflammatory disease in patients with disease too active to permit endoscopy or double-contrast examination.

Abdominal and pelvic abscesses are a well-rec-ognized complication of granulomatous colitis. They occur both spontaneously and postoperatively in a variety of locations, including the mesentery and the pelvic and abdominal musculature, as well as intraperitoneally and intrahepatically. Traditionally it was believed that abscesses in this disease required open surgical drainage; more recently, however, percutaneous abscess drainage has proved effective.[21, 22] In granulomatous colitis percutaneous abscess drainage can perform several functions: In patients with severe underlying bowel disease requiring surgical therapy, it allows a single-stage operation rather than the standard two-stage procedure (i.e., initial surgical drainage of the abscess followed some time later by a second operation for bowel resection). In these cases the acute problem of the abscess is resolved and surgery is reserved for treatment of the underlying diseased bowel. This temporizing before surgery allows improvement in the patient's nutritional status and facilitates recovery. When the degree of bowel disease does not warrant surgery, percutaneous abscess drainage may result in resolution of the abscess without need for further surgical intervention, even in complicated abscesses with fistulas to the bowel.[21] Apparently the iatrogenic creation of a cutaneous fistula along the catheter path after percutaneous abscess drainage, previously a concern, has not proved to be a problem.

The method used for detection of abscesses in granulomatous colitis is a matter of personal preference; cross-sectional and nuclear medicine techniques are capable of this function. CT, however, should be regarded as the method of choice in guiding percutaneous drainage of these abscesses. CT allows accurate planning of an access route to the abscess cavity, and use of intestinal contrast agents usually facilitates distinction between fluid in fixed and scarred loops of bowel from the abscess cavity. Avoidance of puncturing bowel loops decreases the chance of creating enterocutaneous fistulas. For convenience, we prefer to use CT for detection as well as drainage of abscesses, in a single operation.

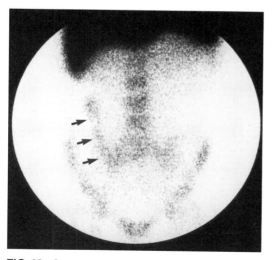

FIG 40–9.
Indium-111 scan (same patient as in Figs 40–7 and 40–8). Accumulation of tracer in the region of the ascending colon and cecum *(arrows)* indicates active inflammation. Good anatomic correlation of disease extent with that seen on double-contrast study and computed tomographic scan.

REFERENCES

1. Laufer I: Air contrast studies of the colon in inflammatory bowel disease. *Crit Rev Diagn Imaging* 1977; 9:421–447.
2. Kelvin FM, Oddson TA, Rice RP, et al: Double contrast enema in Crohn's disease and ul-

cerative colitis. *Am J Roentgenol* 1978; 131:207–213.

3. Gardiner R, Stevenson GW: The colitides. *Radiol Clin North Am* 1982; 25:797–817.

4. Caroline DF, Evers K: Colitis: Radiographic features and differentiation of idiopathic inflammatory bowel disease. *Radiol Clin North Am* 1987; 25:47–66.

5. Joffe N: Diffuse mucosal granularity in double-contrast studies of Crohn's disease of the colon. *Clin Radiol* 1981; 32:85–90.

6. Williams HJ, Stephens DH, Carlson HC: Double-contrast radiography: Colonic inflammatory disease. *Am J Roentgenol* 1981; 137:315–322.

7. Margulis AR, Goldberg HI, Lawson TL, et al: The overlapping spectrum of ulcerative and granulomatous colitis: A roentgenographic pathologic study. *Am J Roentgenol* 1971; 113:325–334.

8. Hildell J, Lindstrom C, Wenckert A: Radiographic appearances in Crohn's Disease. II. The course as reflected at repeat radiography. *Acta Radiol Diagn* 1979; 20:944–955.

9. Farmer RG, Hawk WA, Turnbull RB Jr: Clinical patterns in Crohn's disease: A statistical study of 615 cases. *Gastroenterology* 1975; 68:627–635.

10. Holdstock G, DuBoulay CE, Smith CL: Survey of the use of colonoscopy in inflammatory bowel disease. *Dig Dis Sci* 1984; 29:731–734.

11. Laufer I, Hamilton J: The radiological differentiation between ulcerative and granulomatous colitis by double contrast radiography. *Am J Gastroenterol* 1976; 66:259–269.

12. Gabrielsson N, Granquist S, Sandelin P, et al: Extent of inflammatory lesions in ulcerative colitis assessed by radiology, colonoscopy, and endoscopic biopsies. *Gastrointest Radiol* 1979; 4:395.

13. Goldberg HI, Caruthers SB Jr, Nelson JA, et al: Radiographic findings of the National Cooperative Crohn's Disease Study. *Gastroenterology* 1979; 77:925–937.

14. Hooyman JR, MacCarty RL, Carpenter HA, et al: Radiographic appearance of mucosal dysplasia associated with ulcerative colitis. *AJR* 1987; 149:47–51.

15. James EM, Carlson HC: Chronic ulcerative colitis and colon cancer: Can radiographic appearance predict survival patterns? *Am J Roentgenol* 1978; 130:825–830.

16. Gore RM, Marn CS, Kirby DF, et al: CT findings in ulcerative, granulomatous, and indeterminate colitis. *Am J Roentgenol* 1984; 143:279–284.

17. Kaftori JK, Percy M, Kleinhaus U: Ultrasonography in Crohn's disease. *Gastrointest Radiol* 1984; 9:137–142.

18. Wall SD, Fisher MR, Amparo EG, et al: Magnetic resonance imaging in the evaluation of abscesses. *Am J Roentgenol* 1985; 144:1217–1221.

19. Stein DT, Gray GM, Gregory PS, et al: Location and activity of ulcerative and Crohn's colitis by indium 111 leukocyte scan: A prospective comparison study. *Gastroenterology* 1983; 84:388–393.

20. Froelich JW: Nuclear medicine imaging of inflammatory bowel disease. *Radiol Clin North Am* 1987; 25:47–66.

21. Casola G, VanSonnenberg E, Neff CC, et al: Abscesses in Crohn's disease: Percutaneous drainage. *Radiology* 1987; 163:19–22.

22. Safrit HD, Mauro MA, Jaques PF: Percutaneous abscess drainage in Crohn's disease. *Am J Roentgenol* 1987; 148:859–862.

CHAPTER 41

Thumbprinting

Howard J. Ansel, M.D.

Case Presentation

A 40-year-old man was admitted to the hospital with bloody diarrhea. Except for a mastoid infection recently treated with antibiotics, he was in good health. Abdominal films were obtained (Fig 41–1). What is the finding? What is the differential diagnosis? What is the likely outcome?

DISCUSSION

The roentgenologic sign of smooth marginal indentations along the bowel wall depicted in this case is termed "thumbprinting." Although most frequently attributed to vascular disease of the bowel, thumbprinting is found in a variety of other conditions and generally indicates localized infiltration of the bowel wall. Whether infiltration is by blood, neoplasm, or edema fluid, the radiographic picture may be similar.

Ischemia of the bowel is the most frequent cause of thumbprinting. Ischemia results in endothelial damage to mural blood vessels; as spaces develop between the endothelial cells blood escapes into the interstitium of the bowel wall. The resulting localized hematomas protrude into the bowel lumen, causing the uniform polypoid defects of thumbprinting. This form of ischemia generally is self-limiting, and the bowel heals over time. Later follow-up radiographs of the bowel may show complete healing, with return to a normal configuration or healing with stricture. In some instances infarction occurs.[1–4]

The radiographic distribution of thumbprinting in bowel ischemia frequently corresponds to the distribution of a specific feeding vessel and rarely is generalized throughout the entire colon. It is not unusual for the rectum to be involved by ischemic change. In one study[5] 19% of 52 patients had rectal involvement averaging 42 cm in length. Involvement of the mesenteric wall of the bowel by thumbprinting has been reported to suggest ischemia as a cause. Bowel ischemia may be the result of major vessel occlusion, small vessel disease, venous occlusion, or low flow states.[1] Although ischemia may result from embolic and atherosclerotic occlusive disease, it also should be considered in young women taking oral contraceptives[6] and in patients with arteritis, sickle cell disease, or blood hypercoagulability.

Ischemia leads to intramural hematoma, but primary hemorrhage into the bowel wall also must be considered as a cause of thumbprinting. Such hemorrhage may be the result of direct trauma, excessive anticoagulation (Fig 41–2), or bleeding disorders such as Schönlein-Henoch purpura and hemophilia (Fig 41–3). In these situations conservative management frequently results in rapid return of the bowel to normal.[5]

Thumbprinting, probably secondary to ischemic change, has been reported in patients with obstructing colonic lesions, such as colonic carcinoma and diverticulitis. In patients with thumbprinting that resolves the colon should be evaluated to exclude such lesions.

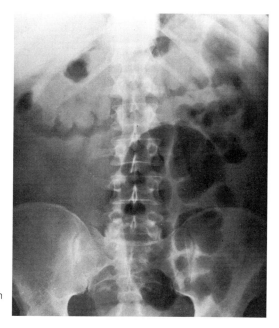

FIG 41–1.
Regular, smooth, scalloped appearance along the superior border of the transverse colon is present in this young man with bloody diarrhea.

Colitis also is signalled by thumbprinting (Fig 41–4). Ulcerative colitis, granulomatous colitis, pseudomembranous colitis, and infectious colitis are potential causes. In these cases thumbprinting is the result of edema and inflammatory change within the bowel wall. In some situations the radiographic pic-

ture may be indistinguishable from that of ischemic change; ulceration may be present in both instances. With ischemia the ulceration is the result of mucosal death and sloughing and may not be apparent until after the thumbprinting begins to resolve. Typically, ulcerative colitis involves the rectum and a continu-

FIG 41–2.
Extensive thumbprinting is present throughout the colon in this patient with uncontrolled anticoagulation. The diffuse involvement may suggest colitis, but no ulceration is seen. The involvement is more extensive than is usualy seen with ischemic disease.

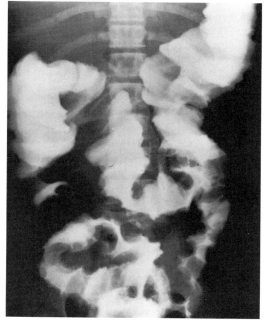

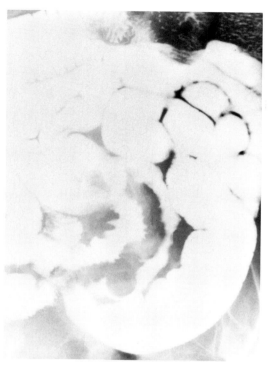

FIG 41−3.
Wall thickening manifested by separation of bowel loops and thumbprinting in the small bowel in a patient with hemophilia.

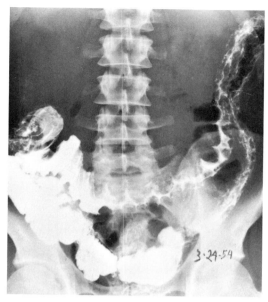

FIG 41−4.
Edema and ulceration in a patient with ulcerative colitis.

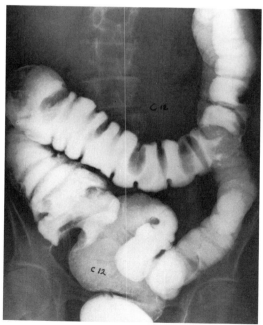

FIG 41−5.
Scattered large thumbprints in the transverse and ascending colon in a patient with lymphoma. In this case the defects are attributed to deposits of tumor within the bowel.

ous length of distal colon. The amount of involvement may be extensive, and in severe cases includes the entire colon. Crohn's disease often demonstrates skip areas as well as areas of deep ulceration, fistula formation, and terminal ileal involvement. The infectious colitides such as amebiasis, strongyloidiasis, schistosomiasis, and cytomegalovirus in the immune-compromised patient also may demonstrate thumbprinting of the colon. These conditions typically have more extensive ulceration and may mimic ulcerative colitis. Both amebiasis and tuberculosis may have a tendency for cecal involvement, with truncation of the cecum suggesting the diagnosis. The terminal ileum frequently is involved in tuberculosis.[7, 8]

The radiographic picture of pseudomembranous colitis is variable. The abdominal film may appear normal or suggest severe toxic colon. In toxic colon thumbprinting may be present. As in the case presented, these patients typically have a history of previous antibiotic exposure. Unlike our patient, however, *Clostridium difficile* or its toxin is present

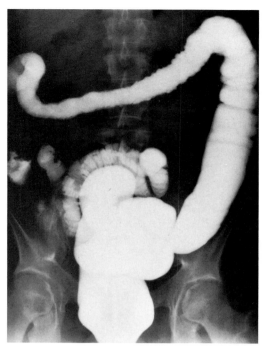

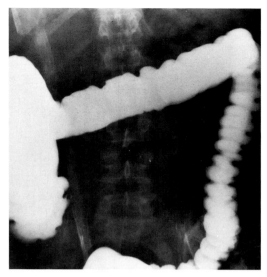

FIG 41–7.
(Same patient as in Fig 41–6) Films taken several months later show that the colon has healed. However, the transverse colon is distorted and the normal haustral pattern is lost.

FIG 41–6.
In the case presented, a repeated barium enema study a short time after the ischemic event shows diffuse ulceration throughout the transverse colon.

in the feces and pseudomembranes coat the bowel mucosa at endoscopy in these individuals.[9, 10]

Neoplastic lesions, especially lymphoma of the bowel (Fig 41–5), also may present with thumbprinting. These lesions tend to be less symmetric, less numerous, and may be associated with an extracolonic mass. The intraluminal component may be ulcerated or have a more polypoid appearance than typical thumbprinting.

Hematogenous metastases to bowel may present as nodular defects along the bowel wall, usually on the antimesenteric side. These lesions may be ulcerated and are frequently less numerous and less symmetric than other causes of thumbprinting.[11]

Pneumatosis cystoides intestinalis may mimic thumbprinting. Usually these gas-filled cysts in the bowel wall are easily differentiated from fluid-filled lesions.[12]

Conservative management with follow-up examination frequently is the best way to manage possible intestinal ischemia. The patient should be closely observed to exclude the possibility of bowel necrosis or perforation. In most instances, however,

the colon heals and reverts to normal. The clinical picture may suggest one of the colitides; biopsy findings or examination of the feces for infectious causes may lead to the diagnosis and institution of appropriate therapy. If the patient's condition does not improve over time, lymphoma should be considered. Computed tomography and evaluation of the remainder of the gastrointestinal tract may be helpful in confirming this diagnosis.

In the case presented, the cause of thumbprinting was bowel infarction. The thumbprinting resolved, followed by extensive ulceration (Fig 41–6) and finally by healing with fibrosis (Fig 41–7). Shortly after the last examination the patient had a myocardial infarction.

REFERENCES

1. Wittenberg J, Athanasoulis CA, Shapiro JH, et al: A radiographic approach to the patient with acute extensive bowel ischemia. *Radiology* 1973; 106:13–24.
2. Scott JR, Miller WT, Urso M, et al: Acute mesenteric infarction. *Am J Roentgenol Radium Ther* 1971; 113:269–279.
3. Eisenberg RL, Montgomery CK, Margulis AR: Colitis in the elderly: Ischemic colitis mimick-

ing ulcerative and granulomatous colitis. *AJR* 1979; 133:1113–1118.

4. Wittenberg J, Athanasoulis CA, Williams LF Jr, et al: Ischemic colitis radiology and pathophysiology. *Am J Roentgenol Radium Ther* 1975; 123:287–300.

5. Wittenberg J: Ischemic colitis, in Dreyfuss JR, Janower ML (eds): *Radiology of the Colon.* Baltimore, Williams & Wilkins Co, 1980, pp 293–316.

6. Ghahremani GG, Meyers MA, Farman J, et al: Ischemic disease of the small bowel and colon associated with oral contraceptives. *Gastrointest Radiol* 1977; 2:221–228.

7. Lichtenstein JE: Radiologic-pathologic correlation of inflammatory bowel disease. *Radiol Clin North Am* 1987; 25:3–24.

8. Margulis AR: Radiology of ulcerating colitis. Annual oration in memory of Robert S. Stone, M.D. *Radiology* 1972; 105:251–263.

9. Stanley RJ, Melson GL, Tedesco FJ, et al: Plain-film findings in severe pseudomembranous colitis. *Radiology* 1976; 118:7–11.

10. Stanley RJ, Melson GL, Tedesco FJ: The spectrum of radiographic findings in antibiotic-related pseudomembranous colitis. *Radiology* 1974; 111:519–524.

11. O'Connell BJ, Thompson AJ: Lymphoma of the colon. The spectrum of radiologic changes. *Gastrointest Radiol* 1978; 2:377–385.

12. Marshak RH, Lindner AE, Maklansky D: Pneumatosis cystoides coli. *Gastrointest Radiol* 1977; 2:85–89.

CHAPTER 42

Tender Right Lower Quadrant Mass: Rule Out Appendiceal Abscess

Michael P. Federle, M.D.

Case Presentation

A 21-year-old man had a 5-day history of abdominal pain and fever. On admission he had a palpable tender right lower quadrant mass, a temperature of 39°C, and peripheral leukocytosis (14,000 cells/mm^3). The clinical diagnosis was subacute appendicitis with an "appendix mass." The radiology department was consulted for further evaluation. Abdominal computed tomography (CT; Fig 42–1) was recommended. What are the findings? What is the differential diagnosis? What further steps should be taken?

DISCUSSION

Periappendiceal abscesses or phlegmons occur in 1% to 13% of patients with acute appendicitis.[1–3] Periappendiceal abscess and acute appendicitis have different clinical presentations, and management differs as well. Acute appendicitis is basically a clinical diagnosis supported by an appropriate history, physical findings, and laboratory test results. Plain radiography has a limited role in establishing the diagnosis, whereas ultrasonography recently has been documented to improve the accuracy of diagnosis significantly, particularly in young women.[4]

A patient with a periappendiceal abscess typically has had symptoms for 5 to 7 days before seeking medical care. Some have a palpable right lower quadrant mass, the appendix mass. The nature and significance of the appendix mass have aroused much clinical interest and controversy. Until recently, cross-sectional imaging was rarely used in evaluation of such masses; clinical and radiographic evaluation were inadequate for distinguishing true abscesses from nonliquefied phlegmons (Fig 42–2). A periappendiceal phlegmon represents inflamed edematous omentum and mesentery along with adherent loops of bowel. An abscess may be small and localized by a capsule or diffusely distributed within the abdomen and pelvis. The failure to distinguish phlegmons and abscesses is probably the basis for the widely divergent opinions concerning the natural history and proper management of the appendix mass.

Computed tomography directly images the periappendiceal area and can distinguish a phlegmon from a liquefied abscess. As a result the differential diagnosis can be narrowed, directly influencing management decisions.

Conservative therapy (bed rest, fluids, parenteral antibiotics) will result in clinical improvement in 72% to 96% of patients with periappendiceal in-

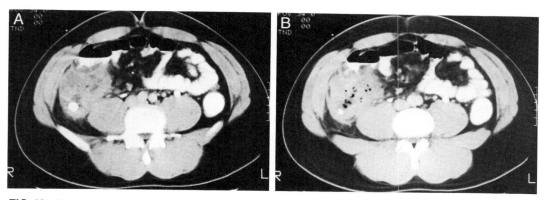

FIG 42–1.
A and **B.** computed tomographic scans of the right lower quadrant in a 21-year-old man with palpable tender right lower quadrant mass.

flammatory masses.[1, 2, 5] Some surgeons prefer immediate surgical exploration, with drainage and appendectomy; others emphasize the high frequency of postoperative complications and prefer initial primary antibiotic therapy. Early surgery results in morbidity in 24% to 36% of patients[6, 7] because of incomplete drainage requiring re-exploration, wound infections (43% in Arnbjornsson's[8] series), and fistula formation. Because of adhesions and phlegmonous masses, inadvertent enterotomies and extensive bowel resections often result.[6]

DIFFERENTIAL DIAGNOSIS

A confident clinical diagnosis usually is made with an appropriate patient history and a palpable tender right lower quadrant mass. However, inflammatory and neoplastic conditions, including right-sided diverticulitis, typhlitis, Crohn's disease, pelvic inflammatory disease, foreign body perforation, perforated neoplasm, and mesenteric adenitis, may exactly mimic appendiceal abscess in clinical and certain radiographic features.

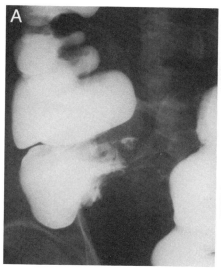
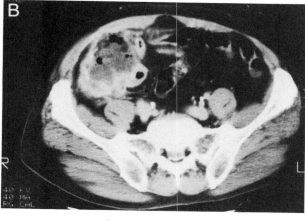

FIG 42–2.
Periappendiceal abscess. **A,** classic barium enema findings of a mass indenting the cecum and terminal ileum, with no filling of the appendix. Phlegmon cannot be distinguished from abscess. **B,** computed tomographic scan demonstrates a liquefied, gas-containing, encapsulated abscess, which was drained percutaneously.

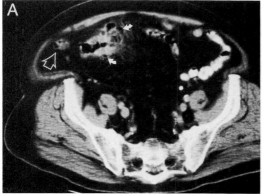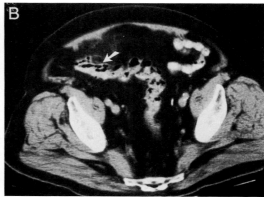

FIG 42–3.
Palpable tender right lower quadrant mass in a 57-year-old man. Sigmoid diverticulitis. **A,** the mass is identified as a thick-walled segment of bowel with extraluminal gas and infiltrated mesenteric fat *(arrows)*. The cecal tip, with diverticula, is identified as a sepa-rate structure *(open arrow)*. **B,** contiguous section shows the sigmoid colon *(arrow)*, with numerous diverticula, leading into the inflammatory mass later confirmed at surgery to represent sigmoid diverticulitis.

Diverticulitis of the cecum or of an elongated sigmoid colon may closely simulate appendicitis and may cause a palpable right lower quadrant mass. A barium (or Hypaque) enema or CT is indicated when diverticulitis is likely, especially in older patients, and usually will establish the correct diagnosis (Fig 42–3). CT and a barium enema study can demonstrate colonic wall thickening, luminal narrowing, diverticula, and extravasation of gas or contrast media.[9] CT has the advantage of directly visualizing the full extent of inflammatory masses, but the colonic disease and the status of the appendix itself usually are more recognizable after contrast enemas. In some cases of cecal diverticulitis, however, an accurate distinction cannot be made. This does not necessarily negate the value of CT, nor does it affect initial examination of the patient.

Colonic, appendiceal, or ileal neoplasms may perforate, resulting in a pericecal abscess that is indistinguishable from an appendiceal abscess (Fig 42–4). Ancillary findings such as an intraluminal

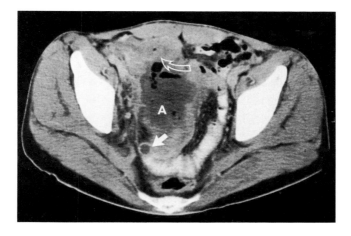

FIG 42–4.
Perforated ileal non-Hodgkin's lymphoma. A pelvic and right lower quadrant abscess *(A)* is noted, and an obstructed right ureter *(arrow)* and thickened bowel loops *(open arrow)*. This cannot be reliably distinguished from an appendiceal abscess.

mass or lymphadenopathy, or an atypical presentation such as anemia or heme-positive stools in an older individual should prompt further evaluation. Initial therapy of antibiotics, bed rest, and possibly percutaneous abscess drainage may be unchanged, but further tests are mandatory and should include a barium enema.

CT is of proved value in diagnosing other causes of right lower quadrant inflammatory masses. In cases of foreign body perforations, CT may demonstrate the foreign body along with the inflammatory mass. Typhlitis, inflammation and infiltration of the cecum, is becoming increasingly common as a result of infections in immunocompromised patients, for example, those with leukemia or acquired immune deficiency syndrome (AIDS). The diagnosis should be suspected in patients with neutropenia with fever, abdominal pain, and diarrhea and is supported by CT findings of a dilated, fluid-filled, thick-walled cecum.[10] Demonstration of a coexisting pericecal abscess usually requires immediate surgery, whereas typhlitis alone usually responds to medical management. Inflammatory masses develop at some point in many patients with Crohn's disease, and the right lower quadrant is the most frequent site. CT is indicated to establish the nature of the mass and may demonstrate thickened edematous mesenteric fat ("creeping fat"), mesenteric adenopathy, thickened loops of adherent bowel, or an abscess.[11] Only an abscess requires interventional therapy. CT-guided percutaneous abscess drainage is an attractive alternative to surgery in such cases. Clinical evaluation and sonography

are crucial in distinguishing pelvic inflammatory disease, and complications such as tubo-ovarian abscess, from appendicitis. CT has an ancillary role in patients with uncertain diagnosis or extensive abscesses. Sonography and clinical evaluation also are mainstays in diagnosis of mesenteric adenitis, usually diagnosed in children with sonographic demonstration of right lower quadrant mesenteric nodes.

The CT appearance of periappendiceal abscess has been described in several recent reports.[12-15] In my experience with more than 75 cases, CT can play an important role in treatment of these abscesses by categorizing them into three groups.

Group 1 includes phlegmon or small abscesses. Perforation of the appendix may be localized and walled off from the rest of the peritoneal cavity by adjacent omentum, mesentery, and small bowel segments. This phlegmonous mass can be recognized on CT as a heterogeneous, contrast-enhancing structure incorporating or displacing bowel loops (Fig 42-5). Surgery is not necessary or therapeutic in such cases. Approximately 45% of patients who have undergone surgery because of "appendiceal abscess" had no evidence of drainable pus but only a phlegmon at surgery. Attempts to drain or resect such a phlegmon have resulted in an unacceptably high rate of complications, prolonged hospital stay, and unnecessary resections of bowel. Even simple appendectomy frequently is impossible in this setting. Small (<3 cm) abscesses can be functionally grouped with phlegmons, and small abscesses resolve completely with antibiotic therapy alone and do not recur during a follow-up period of 4 to 6

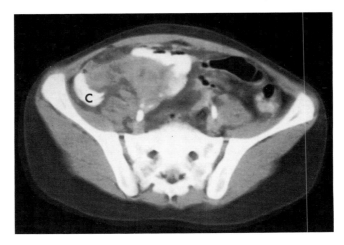

FIG 42-5.
Periappendiceal phlegmon. Heterogeneous nonencapsulated right lower quadrant mass envelops and displaces small bowel segments and cecal tip *(C)*. Mass resolved with antibiotic therapy alone.

weeks. A few phlegmons will evolve into abscesses in spite of antibiotic therapy and are then treated as such.

Group 2 includes localized abscesses. A localized abscess consists of a collection of fluid and sometimes gas surrounded by a contrast-enhancing wall. An appendiceal origin of the abscess is suggested by focal thickening and mass effect on the wall of adjacent cecum and terminal ileum. Appendicoliths are noted more commonly on CT (20% to 25%) than on plain radiographs (7% to 14%) because of the tomographic nature and contrast sensitivity of CT.

Periappendiceal abscesses are treated like other abdominal abscesses, with percutaneous drainage.[16] CT is used to reach an initial diagnosis and also to determine a safe access route for needle and catheter, and often to follow the succession of guidewires, dilators, and catheters (scoutview-guided abscess drainage). In a recent series of 28 appendiceal abscesses, 93% were successfully drained percutaneously without morbidity or recurrence. One patient had unsuccessful drainage related to perforation of the abscess wall by the guidewire in a procedure guided by sonography rather than CT. Another patient, with diabetes, had an extensive gas-forming retroperitoneal abscess. Catheters were placed percutaneously in an attempt to improve patient status prior to definitive surgery. In 46% of percutaneously drained abscesses, fistulas to the cecum and appendix were demonstrated on abscess sinograms obtained 3 days after initial drainage (Fig 42–6). These fistulas were of little clinical significance, however; they produced low output (<50 ml/day), and 12 of the 13 fistulas closed within 2 weeks, and one remained open for 3½ weeks. Patients were routinely discharged from the hospital after clinical resolution of symptoms (decreased pain and normalization of temperature and white blood cell count), regardless of the presence of a fistula.

Group 3 includes extensive and poorly defined

FIG 42–6.
Small periappendiceal abscess. **A,** appendicolith *(arrow)* adjacent to a thickened wall of cecum *(C).* **B,** small loculated abscess *(A)* resolved with antibiotics without drainage.

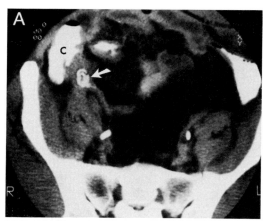

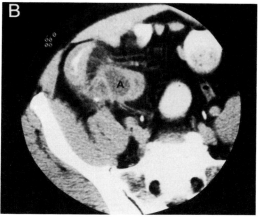

periappendiceal abscesses. In a minority of patients with appendiceal perforation, extensive abscesses develop, with interloop, pelvic, or retroperitoneal involvement (Fig 42–7). These patients are poor candidates for percutaneous catheter drainage and usually require immediate surgery. However, CT may be of value. Sometimes extensive spread of pus throughout the retroperitoneum (due to perforation of a retrocecal appendix) requires a flank incision for drainage rather than a laparotomy (celiotomy). Other patients with extensive abscesses may benefit from CT-guided percutaneous catheter drainage as a temporizing measure rather than a definitive alternative to surgery.

There is considerable controversy as to the necessity and timing of appendectomy in patients with palpable inflammatory masses.[1–3, 5–8] If surgery is performed early and an abscess or phlegmon is found, appendectomy is considered dangerous unless the appendix is easily and freely accessible. The standard surgical procedure has been to drain abscesses or to treat all appendiceal masses with antibiotics and to consider an interval appendectomy after 4 to 6 weeks, when the inflammation has subsided. The incidence of recurrent appendicitis has been estimated at 10% to 20%.[1–3, 5–8] In one third of cases the appendix will be free of inflammation at

interval surgery, and in others the appendix cannot be found. It is presumed that perforation and fulminant abscess formation result in destruction of the appendix. Our current hospital policy is interval appendectomy in children and young adults at 4 to 6 weeks, after resolution of the acute phlegmon or abscess, unless early surgery is indicated for drainage of an extensive abscess and the appendix is easily located and excised.

Finally, we reemphasize the importance of adequate long-term follow-up. Patients with conservative or percutaneous catheter management of presumed appendiceal inflammatory masses should be monitored for recurrent mass or appendicitis. If access to medical care is limited, as by foreign travel, interval appendectomy may be preferred. When any doubt exists as to the diagnosis of appendiceal abscess, a standard contrast enema study must be performed. This is particularly important in excluding underlying tumor in older patients.

The abdominal CT scan in the patient presented demonstrates a retrocecal mass containing fluid and gas, contained by a contrast-enhancing wall. A calcified appendicolith is also noted (Fig 42–8). Appendiceal abscess was diagnosed, and the abscess confirmed by thin-needle aspiration. After consultation with the surgeons, a 12 F sump cathe-

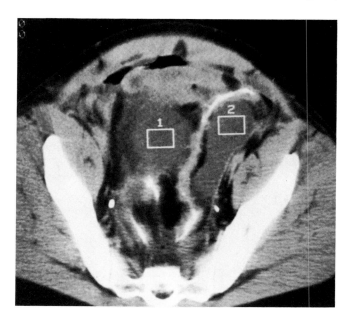

FIG 42–7.
Poorly encapsulated abscesses. Several loculations of pus *(cursors)* are present in the pelvis and between loops of bowel. Extensive abscesses lacking a safe access route for percutaneous drainage are best treated surgically.

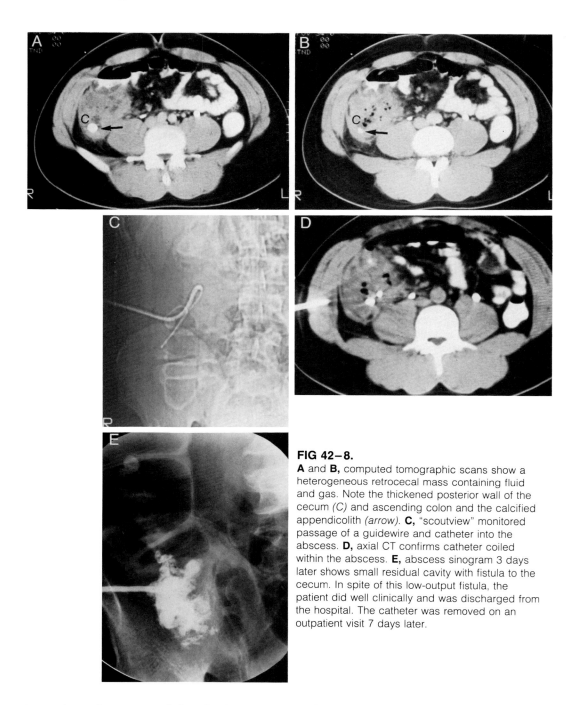

FIG 42–8.
A and **B,** computed tomographic scans show a heterogeneous retrocecal mass containing fluid and gas. Note the thickened posterior wall of the cecum *(C)* and ascending colon and the calcified appendicolith *(arrow).* **C,** "scoutview" monitored passage of a guidewire and catheter into the abscess. **D,** axial CT confirms catheter coiled within the abscess. **E,** abscess sinogram 3 days later shows small residual cavity with fistula to the cecum. In spite of this low-output fistula, the patient did well clinically and was discharged from the hospital. The catheter was removed on an outpatient visit 7 days later.

ter was inserted percutaneously into the abscess cavity using CT guidance and a standard guidewire exchange method. Initial drainage was 150 ml pus; within hours the patient had decreased pain and a rapid decrease in temperature and leukocytosis. A routine abscess sinogram performed after 3 days demonstrated a small residual abscess cavity and a fistula to the cecum (Fig 42–8,E). The patient felt well and was discharged on hospital day 7 with a catheter in place. He returned as an outpatient on day 10, showed no residual abscess cavity or fistula, and the catheter was removed. He was scheduled to return to surgical clinic after 4 weeks for discussion of possible interval appendectomy.

REFERENCES

1. Thomas RD: Conservative management of the appendix mass. *Surgery* 1973; 73:677–680.
2. Bradley EL, Isaacs J: Appendiceal abscess revisited. *Arch Surg* 1978; 113:130–132.
3. Jordan JS, Kovalcik PJ, Schab CW: Appendicitis with a palpable mass. *Ann Surg* 1981; 198:227–229.
4. Puylaert JBCM: Acute appendicitis: US evaluation using graded compression. *Radiology* 1986; 158:355–360.
5. Mosegaard A, Nielsen OS: Interval appendectomy. *Acta Chir Scand* 1979; 1458:109–111.
6. Paull DL, Bloom GP: Appendiceal abscess. *Arch Surg* 1982; 117:1017–1019.
7. Hoffman J, Lindhard A, Jensen H: Appendix mass: Conservative management without interval appendectomy. *Ann J Surg* 1984; 148:379–383.
8. Arnbjornsson E: Management of appendiceal abscess. *Curr Surg* 1984; 41:4–9.
9. Scatarige JC, Fishman EK, Crist DW, et al: Diverticulitis of the right colon: CT observations. *AJR* 1987; 148:737–739.
10. Frick MP, Maile CW, Crass JR, et al: Computed tomography of neutropenic colitis. *AJR* 1984; 143:763–765.
11. Goldberg HI, Gore RM, Margulis AR, et al: Computed tomography in the evaluation of Crohn disease. *AJR* 1983; 140:277–282.
12. Jones B, Fishman EK, Siegelman SS: Computed tomography and appendiceal abscess: Special applicability in the elderly. *J Comput Assist Tomogr* 1983; 7:434–438.
13. Gale ME, Birnbaum S, Gerzof SG, et al: CT appearance of appendicitis and its local complications. *J Comput Assist Tomogr* 1985; 9:34–37.
14. Nunez D Jr, Huber JS, Yrizarry JM, et al: Nonsurgical drainage of appendiceal abscess. *AJR* 1986; 146:587–589.
15. Barakos JA, Jeffrey RB Jr, Federle MP, et al: CT in the management of periappendiceal abscess. *AJR* 1986; 146:1161–1164.
16. Jeffrey RB Jr, Tolentino CS, Federle MP, et al: Percutaneous drainage of periappendiceal abscess: Review of 20 patients. *AJR* 1987; 149:59–62.

CHAPTER 43

Preoperative Assessment of Colorectal Carcinoma

Frederick M. Kelvin, M.D.
Dean D. T. Maglinte, M.D.

Case Presentation

A 63-year-old man had a 4-month history of intermittent rectal bleeding. Physical examination, including digital rectal examination, yielded normal findings; subsequent 30 cm flexible sigmoidoscopy failed to show any cause for the rectal blood loss. What further studies should be performed?

DISCUSSION

Of the numerous causes for rectal bleeding the most common are hemorrhoids, diverticular disease, polyps, and primary carcinoma. Because a 30 cm flexible sigmoidoscopic examination on average reaches only the middle third of the sigmoid colon, negative findings should be followed by a complete evaluation of the colon to exclude a more proximal carcinoma or polyp. This is particularly important in view of the increasing proportion (20% to 25%) of carcinomas that lie in the cecum or ascending colon.[1] Although polyps are much more common than carcinoma, the clinician's main concern is to exclude carcinoma. A colorectal carcinoma is found in approximately 10% of patients older than 40 years of age with recent onset of rectal bleeding.[2] Examination of the entire colon may be accomplished by either barium enema or colonoscopy; the choice remains highly controversial.

A double-contrast barium enema examination demonstrated a large, irregular polypoid mass in the proximal sigmoid colon (Fig 43–1). This appearance is virtually pathognomonic of a primary carci-

noma. Histologic confirmation of the diagnosis by colonoscopic biopsy is therefore unnecessary in this case. Colorectal carcinoma typically produces a large intraluminal mass or annular stricture with abrupt margins (Fig 43–2); both types of lesions usually are irregular.

COLORECTAL EXAMINATION

Barium Enema or Colonoscopy?

Barium enema has a high sensitivity (approximately 95%) for detecting colorectal carcinoma.[3] However, gastroenterologists and general surgeons are increasingly advocating colonoscopy rather than barium enema as the initial method of examining the entire colon when carcinoma is suspected clinically. The main advantage of colonoscopy, other than the ability to perform concurrent polypectomy, is its somewhat greater sensitivity for detecting polyps. It is probably no more sensitive than a well-performed barium enema study for the detection of carcinoma. Colonoscopy costs approximately three to four times as much as barium enema and is asso-

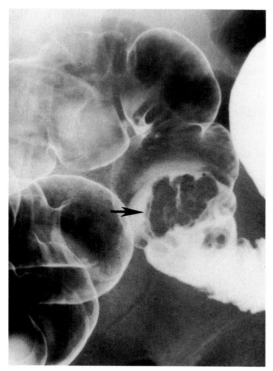

FIG 43–1.
Polypoid carcinoma of the sigmoid colon. A large, irregular, lobulated mass *(arrow)* occupies much of the lumen in the proximal sigmoid colon. Note absence of any retrograde obstruction despite its size.

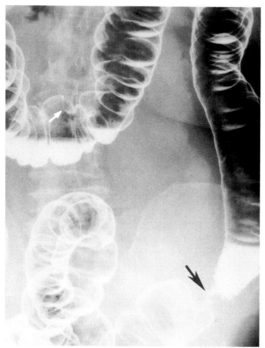

FIG 43–2.
Synchronous carcinomas. An irregular annular carcinoma *(black arrow)* with characteristically abrupt proximal and distal margins is present in the lower descending colon. A smaller, polypoid mass *(white arrow)* is demonstrated in the mid–transverse colon. Colonoscopic biopsy findings showed this more proximal neoplasm to be a second carcinoma.

ciated with approximately tenfold greater risk of perforation. Although expert colonoscopists reach the cecum in 90% to 95% of cases, this is not representative of general standards of practice. For example, a recent national survey of members of the American Society of Gastrointestinal Endoscopy found that colonoscopy was complete in only 65% of cases.[4] Based on these considerations, it seems prudent to retain the traditional role of the barium enema for examining the colon in cases such as the one described.

Barium Enema: Problems in Detection

Although the well-performed barium enema is highly accurate in detecting colorectal carcinoma, it is essential to recognize the problems that may be encountered. When residual stool is present a carcinoma can be excluded only if the fecal mass is shown unequivocally to be mobile. The presence of severe sigmoid diverticulosis may make recognition of a coexistent carcinoma difficult (Fig 43–3). With the single-contrast study vigorous compression is essential for maximal detection of neoplasms; this is

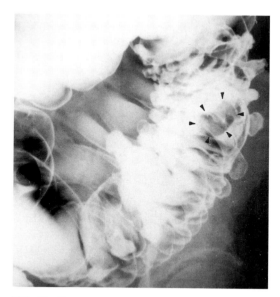

FIG 43–3.
Carcinoma in an area of severe diverticulosis. A polypoid carcinoma produces a filling defect *(arrowheads)* within the barium pool. This was overlooked, probably because the examiner was distracted by the severe diverticulosis. (From Kelvin FM, Maglinte DDT: *Radiology* 1987; 164:1–8. Used by permission.)

rarely performed.[5] The majority of failures to detect carcinoma with a double-contrast study are due to errors of perception.[6] When the tumor lies on the nondependent surface of the bowel, only part of its surface may be coated with barium; under these circumstances the only evidence of the neoplasm may be slightly irregular linear or curvilinear shadow (Fig 43–4). The barium pool also must be examined carefully on double-contrast studies; a filling defect within the pool should suggest a dependent wall lesion or fecal material.

PREOPERATIVE EVALUATION FOR SYNCHRONOUS NEOPLASMS

After detection of a colorectal carcinoma preoperative evaluation should be directed toward two main considerations: examination of the entire large bowel for synchronous neoplasms and a possible search for metastatic disease. In the case described the double-contrast study that detected the carcinoma in the sigmoid colon provided a technically satisfactory examination of the remainder of the colon, which was shown to be entirely normal. However, when a carcinoma is detected by digital rectal examination or sigmoidoscopy, barium enema or colonoscopy is essential to identify additional neoplasms. Approximately 5% of patients harbor multiple (synchronous) carcinomas (see Fig 43–2). Recognition of such lesions is particularly important because synchronous carcinomas are frequently impalpable at laparotomy. Because the large bowel contains at least one adenomatous polyp in more than one third of patients with colorectal carcinoma, careful assessment is essential when a single neoplasm is found. The entire colon should be visualized unless the neoplasm causes obstruction; barium does not become inspissated above a distally located nonobstructing carcinoma.

Preoperative colonoscopy as a means to achieve maximal detection of synchronous neoplasms has been widely recommended. Its value in this setting is predominantly in the detection of additional adenomas[7]; the cost effectiveness of identifying an occasional synchronous carcinoma has been questioned.[8] When a high-quality double-contrast barium enema has unequivocally demonstrated a carcinoma and shows no other lesions, as in the case described, preoperative colonoscopy is probably unjustified. Instead, colonoscopy should be performed 3 to 6 months after surgery to assess the anastomosis and to detect small polyps that can be

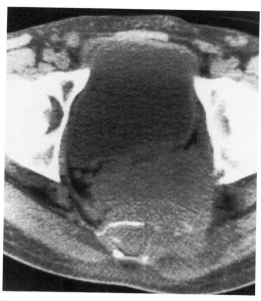

FIG 44–3.
Recurrent rectal carcinoma. This patient had severe pelvic pain. He had undergone an abdominoperineal resection because of rectal cancer 3 years earlier. The CT demonstrates a larger recurrent tumor destroying the sacrum. (From Thompson WM, Halvorsen RA Jr: *Invest Radiol* 1987; 22:96–105. Used by permission.)

(overall accuracy, 26 of 28, or 93%). Moss et al.[6] used their CT staging system and reported a 95% accuracy, with no false negative results and 5% false positive results, in 39 patients with recurrent rectocarcinomas. One false positive result was due to a uterine mass (surgically proved uterine fibroid) that could not be separated from the rectum. The other false positive result was a diagnosis of stage II recurrence; examination of multiple biopsy specimens and surgery revealed only a fibrosis.[6]

Grabbe and Winkler[8] found that CT was a useful means of observing 51 patients after sphincter-saving resection because of rectosigmoid cancer; most recurrences occurred extraluminally, and CT could detect the pericolonic extent of the tumor. They concluded that CT is essential in these patients if repeat resection is contemplated.

Freeny et al.[11] and Thompson et al.[12] reported that CT can identify recurrent colorectal carcinoma. CT correctly detected recurrent tumors in seven of eight patients, missing only one hepatic metastasis.[11] The overall accuracy in 46 patients examined by Thompson et al.[12] for recurrent rectosigmoid carcinoma was 87%, with a sensitivity of 91% and a

specificity of 72%. CT accurately detected local recurrence as well as lymph node metastases. A biopsy was done of all suspect lesions. Aggressive use of percutaneous biopsy and serial CT scans allows detection of early recurrences and differentiation of recurrent tumors from postoperative change. In terms of technique, other than receiving oral contrast medium, patients should fast before a colorectal CT. The entire abdomen through the pelvis, including the ischiorectal fossa, should be scanned.[24] Contiguous 1 cm slices are obtained with the patient supine after ingestion of 3 to 600 ml 1% to 2% meglumine diatrizoate (Gastrografin) or barium solution. To opacify the colon completely this material should be administered 4 to 5 hours before the examination. Dilute rectal contrast medium can be used if the colon is not considered adequately opacified.[24] Use of rectal air insufflation and bowel preparation enhance visualization of the large bowel on CT, as does scanning with the patient prone for evaluation of the rectum and rectosigmoid colon. Intravascular contrast material is used to answer specific questions, to improve detection of liver metastases, and to opacify vessels when evaluating for

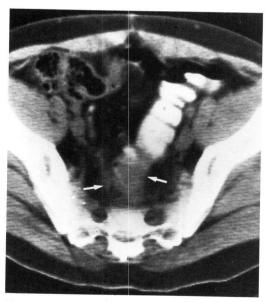

FIG 44–4.
Recurrent sigmoid carcinoma. Computed tomographic scan 18 months after anterior resection of sigmoid carcinoma. Recurrence of disease is demonstrated at the anastomosis *(arrows)*. (From Thompson WM, Halvorsen RA Jr: *Invest Radiol* 1987; 22:96–105. Used by permission.)

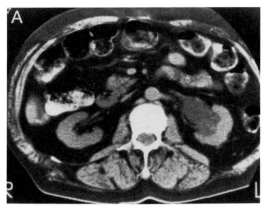

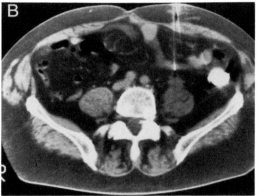

FIG 44–5.
Recurrent sigmoid carcinoma. **A,** computed tomographic (CT) scan through level of kidneys demonstrates hydronephrosis on the left. The patient had microscopic hematuria 2 years after anterior resection of a sigmoid carcinoma. An intravenous pyelogram demonstrated a nonfunctioning left kidney. **B,** CT in the same patient demonstrates a needle placed in a small mass that was obstructing the left ureter. Cytologic evaluation revealed recurrent adenocarcinoma.

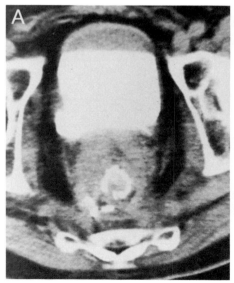

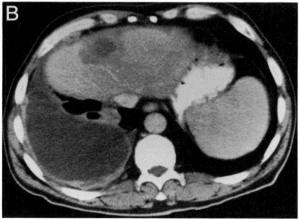

FIG 44–6.
Recurrent rectosigmoid carcinoma. **A,** computed tomographic (CT) scan through the pelvis demonstrates recurrent tumor at the site of a prior anastomosis. **B,** CT of the liver in the same patient demonstrates metastases.

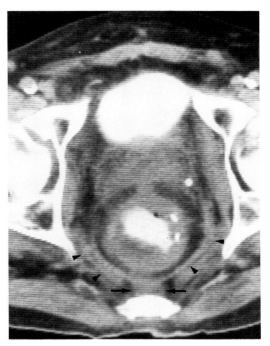

FIG 44-7.
Postradiation change and recurrent rectosigmoid carcinoma. Computed tomographic scan through the pelvis demonstrates recurrent tumor extending posterior to the sacrum *(arrows)* and thickening of the perirectal fascia *(arrowheads)* due to prior radiation therapy.

The criteria used to determine recurrent disease are (1) a mass not present on the first postoperative CT scan (Figs 44-2 to 44-4), (2) a mass invading adjacent organs, (3) enlarged lymph nodes (Fig 44-2), greater than 1.5 cm, (4) hydronephrosis due to an obstructing mass (Fig 44-5), and (5) distant metastases, especially to the liver (Fig 44-6).

The difficulty in distinguishing local recurrent rectosigmoid carcinoma from postradiation fibrosis (Fig 44-7), postoperative change (hematoma, abscess [Fig 44-8], fibrosis, and normal pelvic structures) has been described (Figs 44-9 and 44-10).[12, 24-27] Whereas the CT characteristics of the normal postoperative presacral space have been described and differentiated from recurrent tumor, these features on a single CT examination are not totally definitive. Kelvin et al.[26] reported that although 60% of presacral masses due to postoperative fibrosis diminished in size and became better defined over time, 40% of the abnormalities showed no change (Fig 44-10). Masses due to recurrent tumor enlarge and become less defined on serial stud-

metastatic lymphadenopathy. The bladder should be full or intravenous contrast should be administered during the examination. A tampon in the vagina is helpful in women.[24]

The normal colorectal wall is no more than 3 to 5 mm thick when the lumen is adequately distended. Although detectable by CT, interluminal abnormalities are best demonstrated by barium enema examination or endoscopy. Evaluation of the intraperitoneal and extraperitoneal structures related to the colon and rectum is important. An attempt should be made to identify the primary recurrent tumor and to evaluate its relationship to surrounding structures, especially the genitourinary system.

Lymph nodes follow the major vessels in the pelvis and are located in the internal and external iliac areas, the femoral regions, and in the deep pelvis adjacent to the obturator muscles. Periaortic and mesenteric lymph nodes are evaluated in all patients. Lymph nodes larger than 1.5 cm in diameter are abnormal and consistent with metastatic disease.

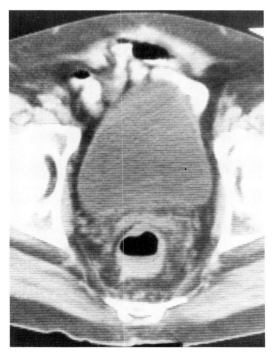

FIG 44-8.
Postoperative abscess. Computed tomographic scan through the pelvis after an abdominoperineal resection demonstrates a pelvic mass containing an air-fluid level. This was a sterile abscess, not a recurrent tumor.

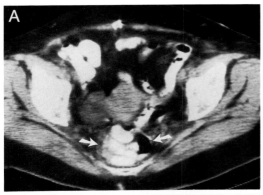

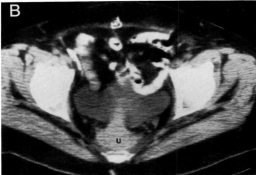

FIG 44—9.
Normal variants. **A,** computed tomographic (CT) scan after abdominoperineal resection demonstrates small bowel in the presacral space *(arrows)*. **B,** CT after abdominoperineal resection demonstrates a presacral mass *(U)*, which is a retroverted uterus.

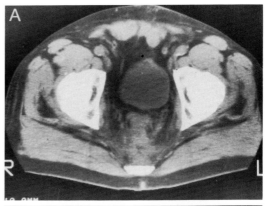

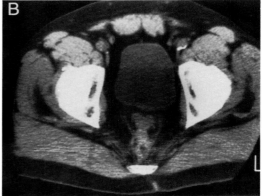

FIG 44—10.
Postoperative changes. **A,** computed tomographic (CT) scan through the pelvis 3 weeks after abdominoperineal resection because of rectal carcinoma. A large irregular mass in the presacral space could be confused with recurrent tumor. **B,** CT 12 months later demonstrates marked resolution in the mass. Note that not only has the mass diminished in size but the margins are much better defined. (From Thompson WM, Halvorsen RA, Foster WL Jr, et al: *AJR* 1986; 146:703–710. Used by permission.)

ies. These results[26] differ from those of Lee et al.,[25] who found no abnormal soft tissue densities in 11 patients without recurrent disease. Reznek et al.[27] reported a prospective series of 10 patients with no recurrence, in which five patients had essentially normal findings on postoperative CT scans and five had presacral soft tissue masses. The masses tended to diminish in size, although some remained unchanged for 28 months. Currently most authors recommend baseline CT scans of the postoperative presacral space 3 to 4 months after surgery. These scans permit identification of postoperative change so that follow-up scans at regular intervals can detect the minor changes that may represent early recurrence. Butch et al.[9] described the CT examination of 28 patients with presacral masses after abdominal perineal resection because of rectosigmoid cancer. The masses were divided into three catego-

ries according to their CT appearance: a solid mass, a mass with a central low-density area, and a mass containing gas (see Fig 44–8). Percutaneous biopsy of all lesions showed that 15 of the 19 (79%) solid masses were recurrent tumor, three of the five lesions with central low density were recurrent carcinomas, and none of the four gas-containing masses contained tumors. One of the four lesions was an abscess; three were sterile fluid collections. These results emphasize the necessity to perform CT-guided percutaneous biopsy of suspect presacral or pelvic masses in patients after surgery for rectosigmoid carcinoma. Biopsy can be avoided only when comparison with baseline CT shows that the mass is diminishing in size.[9, 11, 12, 27]

Laboratory tests, such as carcinoembryonic antigen (CEA), are of uncertain value in detecting recurrent colorectal carcinoma. McCarthy et al.[10] compared CT and CEA for detection of recurrent rectosigmoid carcinoma in 28 patients. Thirteen patients had recurrence of disease, seven without and six with symptoms. CT findings were positive in nine of 10 patients scanned, and CEA was abnormal in only six of 11. The CT scan detected every incidence of local recurrence but was falsely negative in one patient with peritoneal seating. In the nonrecurrence group there were two false positive studies; in each case a mass was identified that was not tumor. Percutaneous biopsy in one case and laparotomy in the other revealed only postoperative fibrosis. These results indicate that serial CT scanning with percutaneous CT-guided biopsy is the most sensitive method for detecting recurrent rectosigmoid carcinoma.[9–13]

The exact role of MRI in patients who have undergone surgery because of rectosigmoid carcinoma is unknown. Gomberg et al.[22] reported that MRI successfully differentiated current tumor from postoperative fibrosis in two patients. These investigators correctly predicted tumor recurrence in one patient and fibrosis in another, based on a high signal on the T_2-weighted sequences in the patient with recurrent tumor and low signal on the T_2-weighted sequences in the second patient. These authors indicated that biopsy confirmation of suspected malignancy is necessary prior to treatment because other pathologic entities can have high signal intensity on T_2-weighted sequences. In a more recent study, Johnson et al.[23] used T_1 and T_2 relaxation times in 30 patients with rectal carcinoma and seven patients with a fibrotic postoperative pelvic mass. Their results demonstrated that the calculated T_1 relaxation value is useful in discriminating between carcinoma and pelvic fibrosis, whereas the calculated T_2 values were not. Universally, the T_1 values were longer than 725 msec in most patients with recurrent tumor; the T_1 values in the fibrosis group were all less than 700 msec, with a mean of 458 msec. These authors believe the factors responsible for this probably were related to greater water content in the tumor and the fact that less water was bound to macromolecules. Considerably more work is needed to verify these two reports.

Currently the majority of patients who undergo resection of a rectosigmoid carcinoma are observed with endoscopy and barium enema examinations. The barium enema is of little value in patients who have had an abdominoperineal resection but is useful in patients who have had an interior resection. In a comparative study using both CT and the barium enema, Chen et al.[14] reported that sensitivity of the barium enema for detecting local recurrence was 88%; for CT it was only 69%. Conversely, the barium enema examination was not useful for detecting remote metastasis shown on CT scans, which disclosed disease at one or more sites in more than 90% of the patients. CT, as would be expected, is best for evaluating recurrences remote from the anastomosis, pelvic recurrence in patients with colostomies, and hepatic metastases. The authors conclude that the barium enema examination and CT are therefore complementary and should be used together, particularly in patients who have had an anterior resection.

Recurrent carcinoma confined to the pelvis occurs in 30% to 50% of patients after resection of rectosigmoid carcinoma.[20] Isolated pelvic recurrence is a major cause of death in these patients, and in one series it was responsible for death in 45% of the patients who died of recurrent disease.[16] More than 80% of recurrent pelvic tumors occur within 2 years.[16, 26] Based on these facts and prior CT reports, the consensus is that all patients who have undergone resection for rectal or sigmoid carcinoma should have a baseline CT 3 to 4 months after surgery and then every 6 months for 2 years.[4, 7, 11–13] CT should then be performed at yearly intervals in conjunction with endoscopy and barium enema examination. A CT-guided biopsy should be done on any new or enlarging presacral mass or enlarged lymph node not present on a previous study. This protocol should permit detection and treatment of early asymptomatic recurrences, an approach that may prolong survival in these patients.

In the patient presented (see Fig 44–1) the differential diagnosis is recurrent tumor and postoperative fibrosis. The size and irregularity of the mass 12 to 18 months after surgery suggest a recurrent tumor. Because no baseline CT study was available for comparison, CT-guided biopsy (Fig 44–11) was performed, which confirmed recurrent rectosigmoid carcinoma. The extension of the mass to the sacrum and pelvic sidewalls precluded resection, and the patient was treated with radiation and chemotherapy.

This case emphasizes the importance of appropriate follow-up in patients with a prior rectosig-

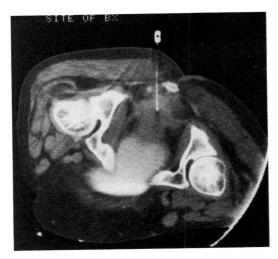

FIG 44–11.
(Same patient as in Fig 44–1) computed tomographic scan obtained during percutaneous needle biopsy confirmed recurrent rectal cancer. (From Thompson WM, Halvorsen RA, Foster WL Jr, et al: *AJR* 1986; 146:703–710. Used by permission.)

moid carcinoma, as well as knowledge of the recurrence patterns, proper CT technique, and proper radiographic evaluation.

REFERENCES

1. *Cancer facts and figures.* New York, American Cancer Society, 1984.
2. Husband JE, Hodson NJ, Parsons CA: The use of computed tomography in recurrent rectal tumor. *Radiology* 1980; 134:677–682.
3. Leer JWH, Scholten ET, Tjho-Heslinga RE, et al: Role of computed tomography in the diagnosis and radiotherapy planning of recurrent and rectal carcinoma. *Diagn Imag* 1980; 149:208–213.
4. Adalsteinsson B, Glimelius B, Graffman S, et al: Computed tomography of recurrent rectal carcinoma. *Acta Radiol* 1981; 22:669–672.
5. Zelas P, Haaga JR, Lavery IC, et al: The diagnosis by percutaneous biopsy with computed tomography of a recurrence of carcinoma of the rectum in the pelvis. *Surg Gynecol Obstet* 1981; 22:669–672.
6. Moss AA, Thoeni RF, Schnyder P, et al: Value of computed tomography in the detection and staging of recurrent rectal carcinomas. *J Comput Assist Tomogr* 1981; 5:870–874.
7. Kelvin FM, Korobkin M, Breiman RS, et al: Recurrent rectal carcinoma in an asymptomatic patient. *J Comput Assist Tomogr* 1982; 6:186–188.
8. Grabbe E, Winkler R: Local recurrence after sphincter-saving resection for rectal and rectosigmoid carcinoma. *Radiology* 1985; 155:305–310.
9. Butch RJ, Wittenberg J, Muller PR, et al: Presacral masses after abdominoperineal resection for colorectal carcinoma: The need for needle biopsy. *AJR* 1985; 144:309–312.
10. McCarthy SM, Barnes D, Deveney K, et al: Detection of recurrent rectosigmoid carcinoma. Prospective evaluation of CT and clinical factors. *AJR* 1985; 144:577–579.
11. Freeny PC, Marks WM, Ryan JA, et al: Colorectal carcinoma evaluation with CT: Preoperative staging and detection of postoperative recurrence. *Radiology* 1986; 158:347–353.
12. Thompson WM, Halvorsen RA, Foster WL Jr, et al: Preoperative and postoperative CT staging of rectosigmoid carcinoma. *AJR* 1986; 146:703–710.
13. Thompson WM: Imaging strategies for tumors of the gastrointestinal system. *CA* 1987; 37:165–185.
14. Chen YM, Ott DJ, Wolfman NT, et al: Recurrent colorectal carcinoma: Evaluation with barium enema examination and CT. *Radiology* 1987; 163:307–310.
15. Gilbertsen VA: Improving the prognosis for patients with intestinal cancer. *Surg Gynecol Obstet* 1967; 124:1253–1259.
16. Welch JP, Donaldson GA: Detection and treatment of recurrent cancer of the colon and rectum. *Am J Surg* 1978; 135:505–511.
17. Olson RM, Perencevich NP, Malcom AW, et al: Patterns of recurrence following curative resection of adenocarcinoma of the colon and rectum. *Cancer* 1980; 45:2969–2974.
18. Nava HR, Pagana TJ: Postoperative surveillance of colorectal carcinoma. *Cancer* 1982; 49:1043–1047.
19. Willett CG, Tepper JE, Cohen AM, et al: Failure patterns following curative resection of colonic carcinoma. *Ann Surg* 1984; 200:685–690.
20. Sugarbaker PH, Gunderson LL, Wittes RE: Colorectal cancer, in DeVita V, Hellman S, Rosenberg S (eds): *Cancer,* ed 2. Philadelphia, JB Lippincott Co, 1985, pp 795–884.
21. Stulc JP, Petrelli NJ, Herrera L, et al: Anastomotic recurrence of adenocarcinoma of the colon. *Arch Surg* 1986; 121:1077–1080.
22. Gomberg JS, Friedman AC, Radecki PD, et al: MRI differentiation of recurrent colorectal carcinoma from postoperative fibrosis. *Gastrointest Radiol* 1986; 11:361–363.
23. Johnson RJ, Jenkins JPR, Ishenwood I, et al:

Quantitive magnetic resonance imaging in rectal carcinoma. *Br J Radiol* 1987; 60:761–764.

24. Thompson WM, Halvorsen RA, Foster WL, et al: Computed tomography of the rectum. *Radiographics* 1987; 7:773–807.

25. Lee JTK, Stanley RJ, Sagel SS, et al: CT appearance of the pelvis after abdominoperineal resection for rectal carcinoma. *Radiology* 1981; 14:737–741.

26. Kelvin FM, Korobkin M, Heaston DK, et al: The pelvis after surgery for rectal carcinoma: Serial CT observations with emphasis on nonneoplastic features. *AJR* 1983; 141:959–964.

27. Reznek RH, White FE, Young JWR, et al: The appearances on computed tomography after abdomino-perineal resection for carcinoma of the rectum: A comparison between the normal appearances and those of recurrence. *Br J Radiol* 1983; 56:237–240.

CHAPTER 45

Segmental Sigmoid Narrowing

C. Daniel Johnson, M.D.

Case Presentation

A 67-year-old man was afebrile with a 3-day history of left lower quadrant pain and leukocytosis. Four years earlier he had had a similar episode, which resolved after oral antibiotic therapy and bed rest. An abdominal computed tomographic (CT) examination (Fig 45–1) was performed. What is the differential diagnosis and what examination should be done to confirm the diagnosis? Is a barium enema examination contraindicated at this time?

DISCUSSION

A CT examination of the pelvis demonstrates bowel wall thickening of the sigmoid colon with associated mesenteric soft tissue stranding (Fig 45–1,A). No pericolonic fluid or gas collection is present. The major differential diagnostic considerations include diverticulitis, primary colonic adenocarcinoma, serosal metastases, inflammatory bowel disease, ischemia, and radiation changes (Table 45–1). Diverticulitis and cancer are statistically the most likely possibilities and should be considered first. A barium enema examination was performed (Fig 45–1,B) in further evaluation: The mid–sigmoid colon is narrowed, colonic folds are thickened, and associated diverticula are deformed and tethered; the underlying colonic mucosa is intact. Findings are those of diverticulitis.

Acute diverticulitis is a common clinical finding, particularly among the elderly.[1] Usually the diagnosis is obvious clinically and treatment is conservative, with antibiotics and bowel rest, without requiring an imaging study. Radiographic evaluation of diverticulitis is helpful when the diagnosis is

uncertain, and barium enema has been the traditional method of imaging these patients. However, recently CT has been used in some centers in the initial screening of these patients.[2–4]

Barium enema study findings of diverticulitis include narrowing of the bowel lumen, localized mass effect, thickened colonic folds, tethered folds, deformed diverticula, an intact mucosa through the affected bowel segment, and localized contrast material extravasation into the pericolonic abscess tract or cavity[5] (Fig 45–2,A). Few patients have all of these findings, but several are usually concurrently present. Contrast material extravasation into the abscess cavity or tract makes the diagnosis straightforward if an intact and normal colonic mucosa can be identified. Indirect evidence of adjacent inflammation usually is manifested radiologically by thickened and tethered folds. Mass effect may or may not be present, depending on the size and location of the pericolonic abscess. In the clinical setting of suspected diverticulitis without an antecedent history of neoplasm, these findings allow the diagnosis to be made with assurance.

CT findings of diverticulitis may be divided

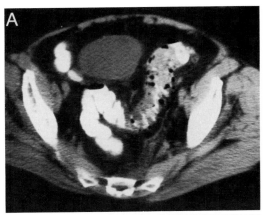

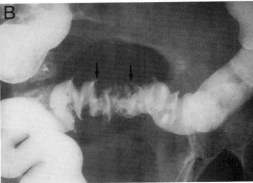

FIG 45–1.
A, computed tomographic scan demonstrates narrowing of the lumen, bowel wall thickening, and soft tissue mesenteric stranding of the sigmoid colon. **B,** barium enema study demonstrates narrowing of the mid–sigmoid colon, thickened folds with deformed and tethered *(arrows)* diverticula. The underlying mucosa is intact. Findings are characteristic of diverticulitis.

TABLE 45–1.

Differential Diagnosis of Segmental Sigmoid Wall Thickening

Neoplasm
  Primary adenocarcinoma
  Metastases
Inflammation
  Diverticulitis
  Inflammatory bowel disease
  Foreign body perforation
  Pseudomembranous colitis
Vascular disease
  Ischemia
  Radiation enteritis

lection, representing the actual diverticular abscess[6] (see Fig 45–2,B and C). A perforated colon cancer can have an identical CT appearance (Fig 45–3,A and B).

The preferred initial imaging study (either barium enema or CT) in suspected diverticulitis is controversial and somewhat dependent on individual preference and patient population. One recent study reported that results of conventional barium enema studies were diagnostic in approximately 80%, indeterminate in 10%, and negative in 10% of patients with diverticulitis.[6] CT scans were diagnostic (abscess identified) in approximately 50%, consistent with but not diagnostic (thickened wall or mesenteric stranding) in 40%, and negative in approximately 10% to 20%.[6] No complications occurred from enemas used during the conventional barium examination or in conjunction with CT in patients with acute diverticulitis. During the CT examination, rectally administered contrast material or air facilitates assessment of bowel wall thickness.

Most authorities would agree that CT is indicated in patients in whom a distant abscess is suspected, those refractory to standard medical therapy, those who are candidates for percutaneous drainage of the diverticular abscess, or in rare patients with large fistulous tracts that prevent filling of the affected sigmoid segment during barium enema studies.

Primary colonic adenocarcinoma is a common radiologic finding among the elderly. The majority of colon cancers do occur in the rectosigmoid, with the cecum being the second most common site. Typical barium enema findings include a polypoid or sessile plaquelike intraluminal growth or annular narrowing with abrupt shouldered edges.[7] Neoplasms presenting as primarily intraluminal growths

into those that are consistent with the diagnosis but nonspecific, and diagnostic findings. Bowel wall thickening and associated mesenteric soft tissue stranding are consistent but nondiagnostic findings of diverticulitis (see Fig 45–1,A). Nearly any cause of segmental colonic narrowing could cause these CT findings; the most important is colon carcinoma. Therefore clinical judgment must be exercised in diagnosing diverticulitis solely on the basis of these radiographic findings. A barium enema examination should be encouraged in these patients to exclude carcinoma by identification of an intact colonic mucosa throughout the diseased bowel segment (see Figs 45–1,B and 45–2,A). Diagnostic CT findings include bowel wall thickening and mesenteric soft tissue stranding plus a pericolonic gas or fluid col-

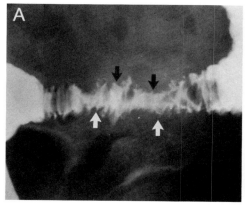 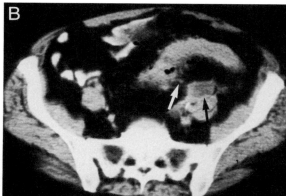 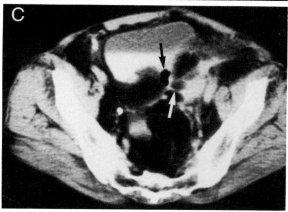

FIG 45–2.
Diverticulitis. **A,** barium enema examination demonstrates narrowing of the mid–sigmoid colon with an intact mucosa, mass effect *(black arrows)*, tethered folds *(white arrows)*, and thickened folds. Contrast extravasation is not seen. Findings are diagnostic of diverticulitis in patients without a prior malignant lesion. Serosal metastases could have similar findings. **B** and **C,** bowel wall thickening is difficult to assess on computed tomographic (CT) scan without intraluminal contrast. Mesenteric soft tissue stranding *(white arrow)* and an extracolonic soft tissue and fluid and gas collection *(black arrow)* representing the localized mesenteric abscess is considered diagnostic of diverticulitis on CT. Diverticulitis was confirmed at surgery.

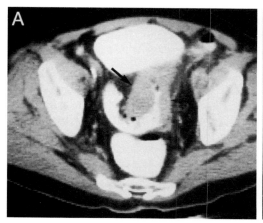 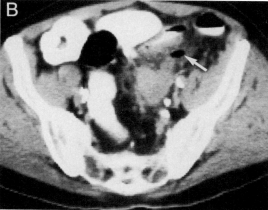

FIG 45–3.
Perforated sigmoid cancer. Computed tomographic (CT) scans demonstrate circumferential bowel wall thickening in the sigmoid *(black arrows, **A**)*, with associated mesenteric soft tissue stranding and extracolonic air *(white arrow, **B**)*. Using strict CT criteria this would have been considered diagnostic of diverticulitis. Barium enema or colonoscopy would be helpful to exclude carcinoma. Perforated adenocarcinoma was found at surgical exploration.

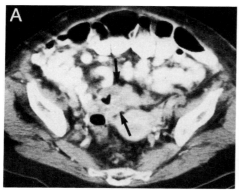
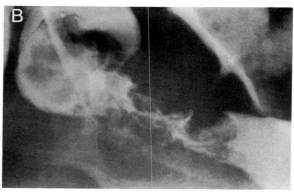

FIG 45–4.

Annular sigmoid carcinoma. **A,** computed tomographic scan demonstrates circumferential thickening of the sigmoid wall, which is nodular *(arrows).* These findings are nonspecific and could be due to many causes of segmental sigmoid wall thickening (see Table 45–1). **B,** barium enema examination of the affected sigmoid colon demonstrates abrupt shouldered margins and nodular mucosa, which is not clearly intact throughout the affected area. Findings are highly suggestive of adenocarcinoma, which was confirmed at surgery.

are rarely confused with diverticulitis. Circumferential tumors occupying a relatively long segment of colon can occasionally create some diagnostic confusion. Findings that favor carcinoma over diverticulitis include a short, abruptly narrowed, ulcerated mucosa with nodular contours. Diverticulitis usually involves a longer colonic segment, tapers gradually, the underlying mucosa is intact, and fistula or sinus tracts may be found.[7] Colonic folds commonly are straight and thickened rather than nodular. Occasionally radiographic distinction between diverticulitis and cancer cannot be made and colonoscopy is necessary for a definitive diagnosis. CT findings of carcinoma are nonspecific and include bowel wall thickening, which may be asymmetric or circumferential, and mesenteric soft tissue stranding (Fig 45–4).

Serosal metastases occasionally mimic diverticulitis. Barium enema findings include mass effect, usually on the superior aspect of the sigmoid colon, with tethered and thickened colonic folds. CT findings include mesenteric soft tissue stranding, bowel wall thickening, or a localized sigmoid mass. In patients with a history of prior malignant disease, radiographic findings of peritoneal implants may be impossible to differentiate from diverticulitis. Multiplicity of lesions most commonly identified in the pouch of Douglas, ileocecal region, and superior sigmoid surface is helpful in suggesting metastases.[8, 9] These regions should be carefully studied in patients with suspected metastases (Fig 45–5).

Other less common causes of sigmoid wall thickening include inflammatory bowel disease, foreign body perforation, pseudomembranous colitis, ischemic colitis, and radiation enteritis.

Crohn's disease may mimic diverticulitis on CT examination, with findings of symmetric wall thickening (with irregular inner and outer wall con-

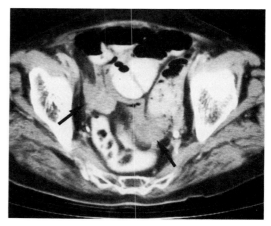

FIG 45–5.

Serosal metastases. Computed tomographic scan of the pelvis demonstrates two large masses *(arrows),* one in the right side of the pelvis adjacent to a dilated loop of ileum, which is partially obstructed by the mass; the second mass abuts the sigmoid colon. The multiplicity of lesions in these particular locations is highly suggestive of serosal metastases, which were confirmed at surgery.

tours), luminal narrowing, ulcerations within the thickened colonic wall, and mesenteric changes (soft tissue stranding, abscess, either local fat hypertrophy or edematous infiltration, fibrosis, and adenopathy).[10] Double-contrast barium enema examinations usually provide specific diagnostic findings of segmental asymmetric bowel disease, which spares the rectum and commonly involves the terminal ileum. Mucosal changes, depending on disease activity and age, include early aphthoid ulcers, inflammatory polyps, deep transmural ulcerations, and cobblestoning. Fistulas, sinus tracts, and disease away from associated diverticula are frequently identified.[11] Barium enema findings of Crohn's disease are seldom confused with those of diverticulitis.

Ulcerative colitis usually presents with nonspecific CT findings: thickened colonic wall, sometimes with smooth outer contours, minimally narrowed lumen, and associated mesenteric soft tissue stranding.[10] A target appearance of the colon in cross section (rings of high and low density, with the middle of three rings being low density) reportedly is highly specific for ulcerative colitis.[12] Usually only bowel wall thickening is seen. Double-contrast barium enema examinations usually can provide a specific diagnosis by indicating rectal involvement, symmetric and continuous granular appearing mucosal ulcerations, inflammatory polyps, backwash ileitis, and absent fistulas or sinus tracts.

Foreign body perforation, commonly due to swallowed bones or toothpicks, presents with findings indistinguishable from diverticulitis on both CT and contrast enema examination.[13]

Pseudomembranous colitis and ischemic colitis present with nonspecific findings of acute colitis on both CT and barium enema studies; regular or irregular bowel wall and fold thickening usually are the major findings on both examinations. Pseudomembranous colitis commonly involves the entire colon, but may be segmental. Ischemic colitis usually is segmental, often involving the distribution of one of the main mesenteric colonic arterial branches.[10, 14]

Radiation enteritis also presents with acute nonspecific CT findings, including wall and fold thickening of the colon and, commonly, adjacent small bowel loops confined within the radiation ports. Mesenteric soft tissue stranding is usually identified. Late changes include stricture and adherence of small bowel loops.[7, 10, 15] These later findings are rarely confused with diverticulitis. Correlation of the clinical history and physical findings with the radiologic changes usually leads to the correct diagnosis (Fig 45–6).

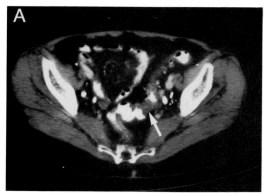

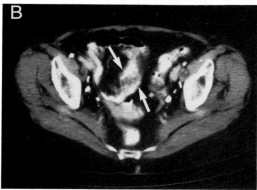

FIG 45–6.
Radiation enteritis. **A** and **B,** computed tomographic scan of the pelvis demonstrates irregular wall thickening of the sigmoid colon and several loops of ileum *(arrows)*. Increased soft tissue stranding of the mesentery is also present. The patient had received radiation therapy for cervical carcinoma.

CONCLUSION

The CT examination in our patient illustrates segmental sigmoid wall thickening and mesenteric stranding that can be seen in a number of different diseases. In this patient the findings are secondary to diverticulitis. The barium enema study is diagnostic of diverticulitis. A CT examination should be considered diagnostic of diverticulitis only when a pericolonic fluid or gas collection is identified. The conventional barium enema remains an excellent examination for initial evaluation of suspected diverticulitis and for exclusion of an underlying carcinoma. In most patients no further imaging studies are required, and CT is reserved for patients with suspected remote abscess, those not responding to standard medical treatment, and those in whom percutaneous drainage of the diverticulitis abscess is considered.

debilitating disease. The cytopathic clostridial toxin causes mucosal destruction. An adherent pseudomembrane composed of fibrin, mucin, white blood cells, and necrotic debris then develops over the necrotic mucosa. Diarrhea is the prominent symptom, and the diagnosis is made by assay of the stool for the *C. difficile* toxin and endoscopic visualization of the characteristic pseudomembrane. Because the diagnosis is usually suspected clinically, and confirmed endoscopically, barium enema examination is seldom indicated, and in fact may exacerbate the condition. If air contrast barium enema examination is performed, rounded, irregular plaquelike areas of pseudomembrane may be seen covering the mucosal surface, causing 2 to 7 mm multiple "filling defects" (Fig 46–3). Frequently, excessive mucus and secretions or confluence of the pseudomembrane obscure visualization of the plaques by barium enema.[13] Later, in more severe cases, the entire mucosa develops a shaggy appearance, and submucosal edema causing thumbprinting may develop.

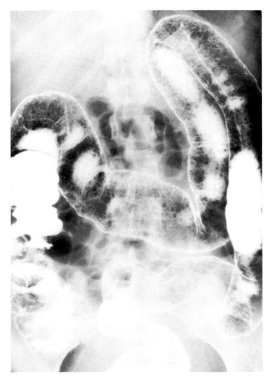

FIG 46–3.
Multiple small, irregular plaques of pseudomembrane are visualized on air contrast barium enema in this patient with antibiotic-related pseudomembranous colitis. (Courtesy Robert N. Berk, M.D., San Diego, Calif.)

Artifacts

Occasionally diagnostic confusion may arise because stool or foreign material in the colon stimulates polypoid lesions on barium enema studies. Careful examination and spot filming can usually differentiate polyps from diverticulae. However, diverticulae containing fecaliths cannot always be differentiated.[14] Stool alone in a poorly cleansed colon may obscure lesions or be confused with polyps (Fig 46–4).

A second barium enema examination after proper preparation of the colon should eliminate any confusion caused by stool or foreign bodies. Poor preparation and faulty technique are major factors contributing to missed carcinomas on barium enema examination.

Inflammatory and Postinflammatory Polyps

Inflammatory polyps, commonly referred to as pseudopolyps, are masses of inflammatory and granulation tissue and residual islands of undermined mucosa surrounded by ulceration. They develop during acute episodes of ulcerative and granu-

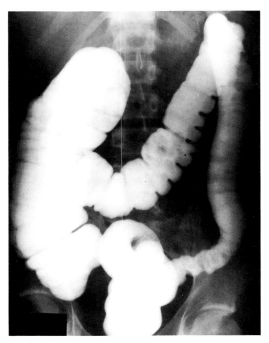

FIG 46–4.
Stool in an inadequately prepared colon may be mistaken for polyps and can be an important factor in the incidence of missed carcinoma on barium enema.

lomatous colitis. After the acute inflammatory episode subsides the polyps may reepithelialize and persist for years. These small postinflammatory polyps often assume a characteristic elongated, branching configuration. They are benign lesions with no malignant potential.[15]

Radiographically, in the acute phase the background of mucosal inflammation reveals the correct diagnosis. If encountered later the multiple postinflammatory polyps appear as multiple filling defects on a background of normal mucosa. They are most commonly 2 to 15 mm in diameter and sessile, elongated, filiform, or branching (Fig 46–5). Bridges of regenerated mucosa may join some of the lesions. This characteristic appearance along with the history of inflammatory bowel disease allows the correct diagnosis. Larger polypoid masses as well as conglomerate masses of postinflammatory polyps may occur, and occasionally even result in colonic obstruction.

Lymphoid Follicular Pattern and Lymphoid Hyperplasia

Lymphoid follicles are widely recognized as a normal feature of the colonic mucosa.[16] They are uniform, less than 2 to 3 mm in diameter, and are seen scattered on a background of normal mucosa on good quality air contrast barium enema examination (Fig 46–6). The follicles are more commonly visualized in children and are frequently umbilicated in this age group. In most instances the lymphoid follicular pattern is a normal variation in both children and adults and is not associated with symptoms or clinical disease. Prominent lymphoid follicles in adults may occur in association with colonic carcinoma.[17] Careful evaluation of the entire colon is necessary when a lymphoid follicular pattern is found in patients older than 60 years.

Hyperplasia and enlargement of lymphoid follicles may occur in response to a variety of conditions, including hypogammaglobulinemia, infections, inflammatory bowel disease, or lymphoma.[18] Visualization of follicles 4 mm or larger should prompt a search for one of these underlying conditions.

Gastrointestinal Polyposis Syndromes

Multiple polyps of the colon are present in all of the gastrointestinal polyposis syndromes listed in Table 46–1. The radiographic appearance of the

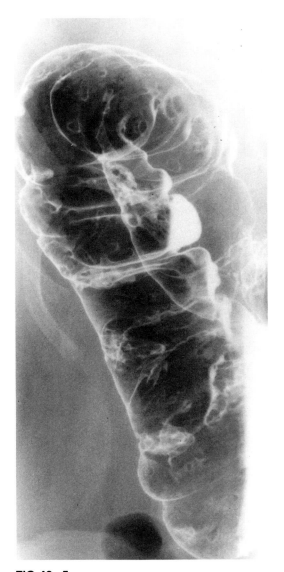

FIG 46–5.
Multiple elongated postinflammatory polyps are present in the right colon in this patient with a past history of ulcerative colitis.

polyps is virtually the same in these diseases, with minor variations. Accurate classification of the syndromes is based on histologic analysis of the polyps.

Familial Polyposis Coli and Gardner's Syndrome.—Differences between familial polyposis coli (FPC) and Gardner's syndrome are becoming less distinct, and many investigators believe they

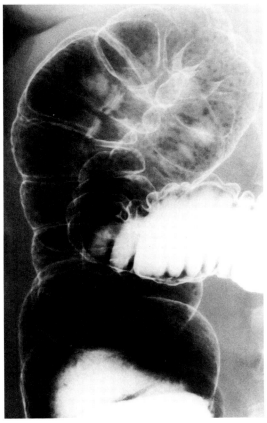

FIG 46–6.
Lymphoid follicular pattern, as illustrated in the hepatic flexure in a 61-year-old woman, may be a normal feature of the colonic mucosa.

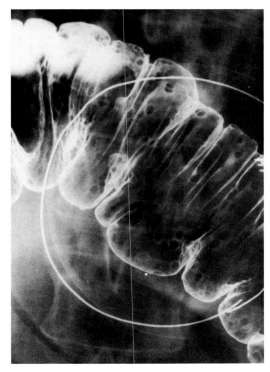

FIG 46–7.
Multiple small colonic adenomas that are typical of familial multiple polyposis are best visualized by air contrast barium enema.

are different expressions of a single genetic defect and should be considered one disease (FPC).[19]

FPC is inherited as an autosomal dominant trait with almost 100% penetrance. The age range at diagnosis is 24 to 35 years. The colonic polyps are tubular adenomas, and adenocarcinoma of the colon may develop in 100% of patients with untreated FPC. Extracolonic neoplasms are not uncommon, and there is a high incidence of gastric, duodenal, and small bowel polyps with variable malignant potential. Ampullary and thyroid carcinomas, mesenteric fibromatosis, and skin and bone lesions all have an increased incidence in patients with FPC.[20]

The radiologist, using meticulous double-contrast technique, has an important role in diagnosing this disease (Fig 46–7). Colonic polyps in FPC number at least 100 and range from 2 to 5 mm in diameter.[21] The majority of polyps are sessile, but larger polyps may be pedunculated. In most cases the polyps are diffusely distributed throughout the colon and rectum. Early in the course of FPC, however, polyps may be sparse and scattered, appearing as tiny nodules with apparently normal intervening colonic mucosa.

Turcot Syndrome.— Turcot syndrome is characterized by a combination of colon adenomas and central nervous system (CNS) tumors.[22] An autosomal recessive mode of inheritance has been suggested, with symptoms commonly present in the second decade. Colon malignancies may develop, but patients more often die of the CNS neoplasms. Multiple café-au-lait spots have been described, and a genetically determined neuroectodermal abnormality may be responsible for the skin and CNS lesions in this syndrome.[23]

The radiographic appearance and distribution of the colonic polyps are similar to those of FPC. In a few reported cases the number of polyps was less than 100.

Peutz-Jeghers Syndrome.—Hamartomatous polyps involving all segments of the gastrointestinal tract, mucocutaneous melanotic pigmentation, extragastrointestinal neoplasms, and autosomal dominant inheritance characterize Peutz-Jeghers syndrome. Hamartomas are found in the small bowel in 90% to 100% of patients, in the colon in 30%, and in the stomach in 25%. Rarely they occur in the esophagus and respiratory and urinary tracts. There is a 2% to 12% incidence of gastrointestinal carcinomas, predominantly in the duodenum and colon.[24] Extraintestinal tumors include carcinoma of the breast and ovarian tumors in women and testicular neoplasms in men.

Radiographically the hamartomatous polyps of the colon usually are not as diffusely distributed and tend to be larger than the adenomas found in FPC.

Multiple Hamartoma Syndrome (Cowden's Disease).—Multiple hamartoma syndrome is an uncommon genodermatosis with an autosomal dominant pattern of inheritance. It is characterized by mucocutaneous lesions, gastrointestinal polyposis, and an increased incidence of thyroid and breast lesions, including thyroid and breast carcinoma.[25] Approximately 30% to 40% of patients have polyps involving all segments of the gastrointestinal tract, most commonly the colon.[26] The reported histopathologic characteristics of the polyps vary and include hamartomatous, juvenile, inflammatory, lymphomatous, and occasionally adenomatous types.[26] At least one colon cancer has been reported.[25]

The radiographic appearance of the colon polyps is not distinctive. In most reported cases the polyps were 5 mm or smaller and distributed in all segments of the colon and rectum.

Cronkhite-Canada Syndrome.—Cronkhite-Canada syndrome is an unusual disease with no familial tendency. Diffuse gastrointestinal polyposis, alopecia, skin hyperpigmentation, onychotrophia, weight loss, diarrhea, and general inanition are characteristic. In most cases the patients have been older than 50 years of age at onset. Histologic analysis shows the polyps to be hamartomas of the juvenile type. At least 14 cases of gastrointestinal malignant disease have been reported, most of them involving the colon.[27]

Radiographically the polyps are distributed uniformly in the colon and rectum and may be superimposed on an edematous mucosa.[27] The clinical signs, symptoms, and age of the patients help to differentiate this disease from other gastrointestinal polyposis syndromes.

Familial Juvenile Polyposis Coli.—Familial juvenile polyposis coli may be transmitted as an autosomal dominant trait. The polyps are hamartomas of the juvenile type and are most common in the colon and rectum but may be found in the stomach and small bowel.[28] There is an increased incidence of colon cancer in these patients and their family members. A subset of nonfamilial juvenile polyposis coli exists, with an increased incidence of congenital abnormalities. The colonic polyps of familial juvenile polyposis coli average 1 to 2 cm in diameter, number 10 or more, and often are pedunculated.[28]

Malignant Lymphoma

The colon is often involved in patients with malignant lymphoma and may be the site of initial clinical findings. The multinodular variety, diffuse colonic involvement with multiple lymphomatous nodules, occurs in 30% to 50% of patients with colonic lymphoma (Fig 46–8). Several characteristic radiographic features of lymphoma are helpful in suggesting the correct diagnosis.[29] The nodules typically are quite variable in size, averaging 7 mm in diameter. They are usually sessile, smooth, and closely spaced. A larger cecal mass is frequently associated. The haustra are often distorted, and barium evacuation is incomplete because of infiltration of the muscularis propria. All segments of the colon and rectum may be involved. Because malignant lymphoma is usually systemic at the time of presentation, splenomegaly and associated involvement of the stomach and small bowel may provide additional clues to the diagnosis. Less commonly, irregular, pedunculated, filiform or umbilicated lymphomatous polyps occur. Biopsy of the nodules is required for confirmation of the diagnosis.

CONCLUSION

In the case presented (see Fig 46–1) the nodules are closely spaced, sessile, smooth, and average 5 mm to 1 cm in diameter; a bulky cecal mass is also present. This combination of features suggests

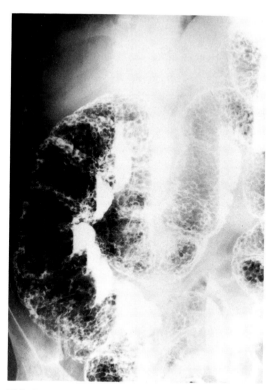

FIG 46—8.
Small closely spaced nodules of lymphoma are present throughout the colon. (From Williams SM, Berk RN, Harned RK: *AJR* 1984; 143:87–91. Used by permission.)

the correct diagnosis of malignant lymphoma. Biopsy of the nodules confirmed non-Hodgkin's lymphoma.

REFERENCES

1. Abrams JS, Reines HD: Increasing incidence of right-sided lesions in colorectal cancer. *Am J Surg* 1979; 137:522–526.
2. Gillespie PE, Chambers TJ, Chan KW, Doronzo F, et al: Colonic adenomas—A colonoscopic survey. *Gut* 1979; 20:240–245.
3. Nebel OT, El Masry NA, Castell DO, et al: Schistosomal disease of the colon: A reversible form of polyposis. *Gastroenterology* 1974; 67:939–943.
4. Cardoso JM, Kimura K, Stoopen M, et al: Radiology of invasive amebiasis of the colon. *AJR* 1977; 128:935–941.
5. Seaman WB, Clements JL: Urticaria of the colon: A nonspecific pattern of submucosal edema. *AJR* 1982; 138:545–547.
6. Rabin MS, Bledin AG, Lewis D: Polypoid leukemic infiltration of the large bowel. *AJR* 1978; 131:723–724.
7. Sacks BA, Joffe N, Antoniolli DA: Metastatic melanoma presenting clinically as multiple colonic polyps. *AJR* 1977; 129:511–513.
8. Wall SD, Ominsky S, Altman DF, et al: Multifocal abnormalities of the gastrointestinal tract in AIDS. *AJR* 1986; 146:1–5.
9. Rose HS, Balthazar EJ, Megibow AJ, et al: Alimentary tract involvement in Kaposi sarcoma: Radiographic and endoscopic findings in 25 homosexual men. *AJR* 1982, 139:661–666.
10. Wayte DM, Helwig EB: Colitis cystica profunda. *Am J Clin Pathol* 1967; 48:159–169.
11. Marshak RH, Linder AE, Maklansky D: Pneumatosis cystoides coli. *Gastrointest Radiol* 1977; 2:85–89.
12. Bartlett JG, Chang TW, Gurwith M, et al: Antibiotic-associated pseudomembranous colitis due to toxin-producing clostridia. *N Engl J Med* 1978; 298:531–534.
13. Stanley RJ, Melson GL, Tedesco FJ: The spectrum of radiographic findings in antibiotic-related pseudomembranous colitis. *Radiology* 1974; 111:519–524.
14. Keller CE, Halpert RD, Feczko PJ, et al: Radiologic recognition of colonic diverticula simulating polyps. *AJR* 1984; 143:93–97.
15. Munyer TP, Montgomery CK, Thoeni RF, et al: Postinflammatory polyposis (PIP) of the colon: The radiologic-pathologic spectrum. *Radiology* 1982; 145:607–614.
16. Kelvin FM, Max RJ, Norton GA, et al: Lymphoid follicular pattern of the colon in adults. *AJR* 1979; 133:821–825.
17. Bronen RA, Glick SN, Teplick SK: Diffuse lymphoid follicles of the colon associated with colonic carcinoma. *AJR* 1984; 142:105–109.
18. Kenney PJ, Koehler RE, Shackelford GD: The clinical significance of large lymphoid follicles of the colon. *Radiology* 1982; 142:41–46.
19. Haggitt RC, Reid BJ: Hereditary gastrointestinal polyposis syndromes. *Am J Surg Pathol* 1986; 10:871.
20. Harned RK: Radiological aspects of the gastrointestinal cancer-associated genodermatoses, in Lynch HT, Fusaro RM (eds): *Cancer Associated Genodermatoses*. New York, Van Nostrand Reinhold Co, 1982.
21. Bartram CI, Thornton A: Colonic polyp patterns in familial polyposis. *AJR* 1984; 142:305.
22. Turcot J, Depres J, St Pierre F: Malignant tumors of the central nervous system associated

with familial polyposis of the colon: Report of two cases. *Dis Colon Rectum* 1959; 2:465.

23. Radin R, Foregan KC, Zee C, et al: Turcot syndrome: A case with spinal cord and colonic neoplasms. *AJR* 1984; 142:475.

24. Reid JD. Intestinal carcinoma in the Peutz-Jeghers Syndrome. *JAMA* 1974; 229:833.

25. Erbe RW, Compton CC: Case records of the Massachusetts General Hospital. *N Engl J Med* 1987; 316:1531.

26. Chen YM, Ott DJ, Wu WC, et al: Cowden's disease: A case report and literature review. *Gastrointest Radiol* 1987; 12:325.

27. Munitz HA: Polyposis syndromes, in Ott DJ, Wu WC (eds): *Polypoid Disease of the Colon.* Baltimore, Urban & Schwarzenberg Inc, 1986.

28. Bussey HJR, Veale AMO, Morson BC: Genetics of gastrointestinal polyposis. *Gastroenterology* 1978; 74:1325.

29. Williams WM, Berk RN, Harned RK: Radiologic features of multinodular lymphoma of the colon. *AJR* 1984; 143:87–91.

CHAPTER 47

Inadequate Colon Preparation

Reed P. Rice, M.D.

Case Presentation

A 75-year-old man had blood in his stool. A single-contrast examination was performed because of limited patient mobility (Fig 47–1). What is the diagnosis, and what further steps should be taken?

DISCUSSION

Most adenocarcinomas of the colon and rectum arise from adenomatous polyps[1, 2]; removal of colonic rectal adenocarcinomas still limited to the wall of the bowel offers the best chance for cure, with 5-year cure rates of 85% or better for Duke class A lesions.[3] Small premalignant or early malignant polyps can be detected by double-contrast barium enema studies or full-column single-contrast examination with effective compression.[4, 5] The controversy regarding the preferred technique for routine examination of the colon is not within the scope of this chapter. Radiologists should be skilled in both techniques and choose that most suitable based on considerations such as age, patient mobility, and coexisting medical problems.

The main deterrent to the radiologic detection of small polypoid lesions of the colon is poor bowel cleansing before the examination. A report indicating that findings are "grossly negative, but small polyps cannot be excluded because of poor preparation" is not acceptable. Patients' lives depend on our ability to find or exclude small polyps.

Methods for preparation of the colon before radiologic examination include strict adherence to a clear liquid diet for several days, mucosal contact irritant cathartics, saline cathartics in combination with forced hydration, mucosal irritant suppositories, large-volume oral balanced electrolyte solutions (Go-lytely), and large-volume enemas. These methods may be used singly or in combination. We prefer a combination of saline cathartics with forced fluid intake starting approximately 20 hours before the examination, a clear liquid evening meal prior to the examination, mucosal irritant type of laxative given orally at approximately 6:00 PM, and a suppository or large-volume tap water enema several hours before the examination. This format generally is effective and does not interfere with adequate sleep in most patients. Other regimens are equally effective. Regardless of the technique, the radiologist must ensure that the colon is suitably prepared. The most important aspect of this responsibility is to see that each patient is screened on arrival in the radiology department. If the adequacy of the overnight preparation is questionable, a large-volume tap water enema should be administered in the radiology department (Figs 47–2 and 47–3). Occasionally more than one large-volume enema is necessary.

Use of the double-contrast technique requires a 1-hour interval between the cleansing enema and the

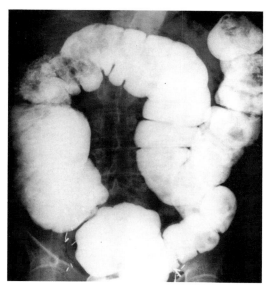

FIG 47–1.
Single-contrast examination demonstrates gross fecal residue in spite of preparation with laxatives and a suppository.

examination. We have found that patients are very receptive to this approach and appreciate our efforts to assure the best possible examination. If patients realize they are "in the system" and the radiology department personnel are communicating with them, they generally do not object to the delay.

In spite of careful screening and administration of cleansing enemas in the radiology department, some patients will not be adequately prepared. If the preparation is not too poor, the decubitus and upright films obtained as part of a double-contrast examination may permit exclusion of polyps. Floating particulate stool tends to drop away from the nondependent surface. However, if the amount of stool or adherence of stool to the nondependent surface of the bowel precludes adequate evaluation, there are at least two options. If the area that cannot be completely evaluated is limited to a single segment of the colon, a supplementary single-contrast enema after the initial evacuation may permit completion of the examination. We have used this technique frequently to complete an otherwise inadequate examination of the right colon. If the amount of fecal residue is so great that the examination is totally in-

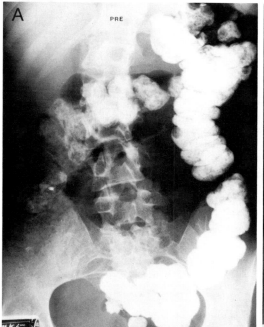
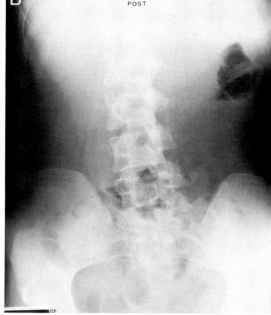

FIG 47–2.
Example of efficacy of single large-volume (2,000 ml) tap water enema in a patient who had had an upper gastrointestinal tract examination the day before these abdominal films. **A,** before cleansing enema. **B,** a satisfactory single-contrast barium enema examination was performed after the cleansing enema.

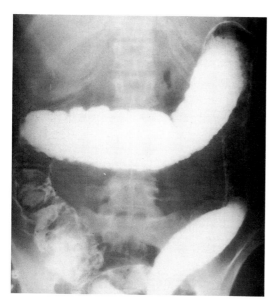

FIG 48–1.
Single film from a barium enema revealing diffuse mucosal irregularity. What is the differential diagnosis? How should it be confirmed?

have characteristic features of both early Crohn's disease and ulcerative colitis.[1–6] The typhloappendiceal form of amebiasis refers specifically to abnormalities that affect only the cecum and appendix. The terminal ileum is normal (Fig 48–2,B). The ameboma is a segmental lesion characterized by marked thickening of the bowel, producing an excrescent mass that narrows the lumen (Fig 48–2,C). These can be solitary or multiple, and in order of decreasing frequency occur on the cecum, ascending colon, rectosigmoid, transverse colon, and descending colon. The barium enema demonstrates a narrow segment of bowel of variable length with irregular mucosa, lack of distensibility, and loss of haustration. The lesions may mimic a primary carcinoma (Fig 48–2,C). The fulminating form of invasive colonic amebiasis follows a rapid acute toxic course and has a mortality rate of 90%. This is the least common form of the disease. Patients can have clinical findings similar to those of toxic megacolon seen in ulcerative or granulomatous colitis. The radiographic findings are indistinguishable from those of ischemic colitis and other edematous or hemorrhagic processes (Fig 48–2,D). There may be diffuse thumbprinting due to marked thickening of the folds, which can be identified on both the plain films and the barium enema study. The barium enema examination

should be performed cautiously because of the risk of perforation in severe cases. Toxic megacolon is an extremely rare complication of amebiasis. The presence of toxic megacolon in amebiasis, as in other entities, is a contraindication to barium enema examination. A high clinical suspicion must be maintained to evaluate the disease appropriately.

Behçet's Syndrome

Behçet's syndrome comprises oral and genital ulceration with ocular lesions. Any segment of the gastrointestinal tract may be involved. The appearance on the barium enema varies from mild proctitis to pancolitis, with multiple discrete ulcers and inflammatory polyposis.[1, 7, 8] Long linear intramural ulcers and deep ulcers have been reported. Aphthoid ulcers (Fig 48–3) and skip lesions are common. The terminal ilium may be involved. Though more often resembling Crohn's disease, occasional cases of Behçet's syndrome cannot be distinguished from idiopathic ulcerative proctocolitis. All three conditions may produce arthritis, thrombophlebitis, and aphthoid stomatitis.

Campylobacter-associated Colitis

Campylobacter has recently been reported as a cause of acute diarrhea in children and adults.[1] It is a common cause of acute infectious colitis. The disease is usually self-limiting, and a barium enema examination is seldom performed. Symptoms vary from abdominal cramps and mild diarrhea to severe febrile illness with fulminant bloody diarrhea.[1] Abdominal pain is prominent and may be severe. Radiographic appearance of *Campylobacter*-associated colitis similar to Crohn's disease in the ileum and transverse colon was described by Lambert et al.[9] A diffuse granular mucosal pattern that is distinguishable from acute ulcerative colitis has also been reported.[10] The diagnosis should be suspected when abdominal pain is disproportionately severe in a patient with apparent acute mild to moderate ulcerative colitis. Transient ischemic colitis in young adults and ischemic colitis related to oral contraceptive use produce a similar radiographic appearance (Fig 48–4). It is also tempting to regard a relapse of ulcerative colitis as possibly an acute attack of *Campylobacter* colitis. When confronted with colitis suspected of being ischemic or related to the contraceptive

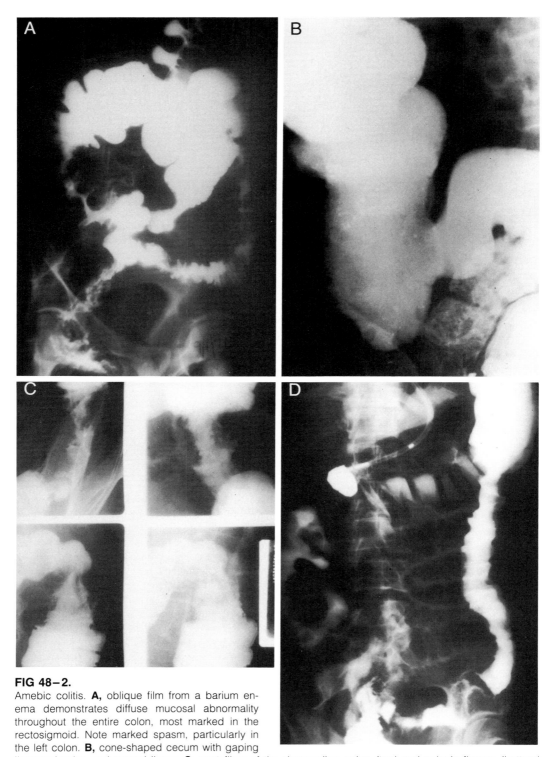

FIG 48–2.
Amebic colitis. **A,** oblique film from a barium enema demonstrates diffuse mucosal abnormality throughout the entire colon, most marked in the rectosigmoid. Note marked spasm, particularly in the left colon. **B,** cone-shaped cecum with gaping ileocecal valve and normal ileum. **C,** spot films of the descending colon *(top)* and splenic flexure *(bottom)* demonstrate circumferential narrowing due to amebomas. Findings are consistent with circumferential adenocarcinoma. **D,** left posterior film from a barium enema demonstrates marked mucosal ulceration, spasm, thumbprinting, and some dilation of the small bowel due to severe amebic dysentery. The patient died 48 hours later.

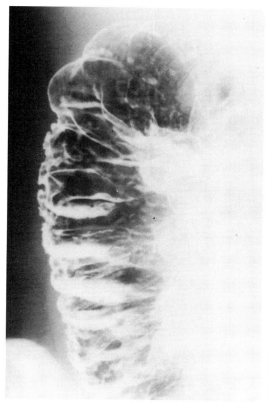

FIG 48–3.
Behçet's syndrome. Spot film from a double-contrast examination. Numerous areas of superficial aphthous ulceration mimic Crohn's disease.

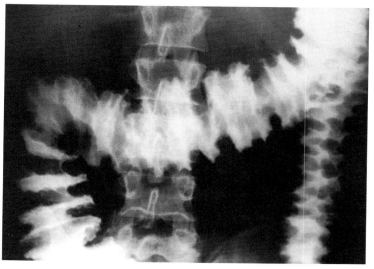

FIG 48–4.
Campylobacter colitis. Radiograph of colon during a barium enema demonstrates diffuse mucosal edema with marked thumbprinting. Diffuse distribution mili- tates against ischemic colitis. *Campylobacter* was cultured from the stool. (Courtesy David Stephenens, M.D., Rochester, Minn.)

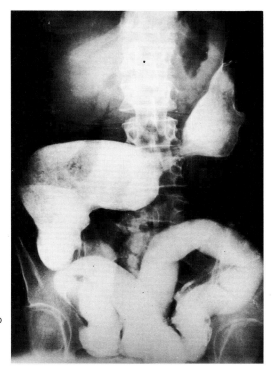

FIG 48–5.
Cathartic colon. Barium enema in a patient known to be a chronic laxative abuser. Note loss of haustration, dilation, and foreshortening of the right colon. (Courtesy R. Meisell, M.D., New York, N.Y.)

pill, stool cultures for *Campylobacter* or *Clostridium difficile,* responsible for pseudomembranous colitis, may help provide the correct diagnosis.[11]

Cathartic Caustic and Soap Enema Colitis

Cleansing of the large bowel is not without some hazard.[12–14] There have been reports of soapsuds enemas causing transitory colitis and of a detergent enema producing severe colitis after self-administration in demented patients.[14] More commonly encountered is cathartic colon, a syndrome that follows prolonged laxative abuse.[12] The radiographic and pathologic appearances superficially mimic ulcerative colitis. Classic full-blown radiographic findings include spasm in the left colon and shortened right colon, with loss of haustrations, patulous ileocecal valve, and dilated terminal ilium (Fig 48–5). The areas of spasm may be confused with true strictures, but change slowly during fluoroscopy. They are associated with hypertrophy of the muscular mucosa,[13, 14] similar to the benign strictures of ulcerative colitis. In advanced cases the diagnosis is not difficult to establish with an appropriate history and biopsy confirmation.

Cytomegalovirus Colitis

Sixty percent to 90% of patients with immunocompromise after renal transplantation with immunosuppressive therapy will have reactivation of latent cytomegalovirus (CMV) infection. Hemorrhage is the most common gastrointestinal complication after renal transplantation, with bleeding from the upper gastrointestinal tract occurring in the vast majority of patients. In some 20% of patients with hemorrhage occurring from the colon the most common cause is cecal ulceration secondary to CMV infection. In this clinical situation barium enema findings of mucosal changes, including thumbprinting, luminal narrowing, and even tumor-like defects due to severe local inflammation, are virtually diagnostic of CMV vasculitis of the cecum or terminal ilium.[1, 13] The condition is associated with high mortality, and surgical resection may be required once the bleeding is localized by angiography or colonoscopy. CMV may also be manifested in the early stages with the demonstration of aphthoid ulcers radiographically indistinguishable from Crohn's disease (Fig 48–6).

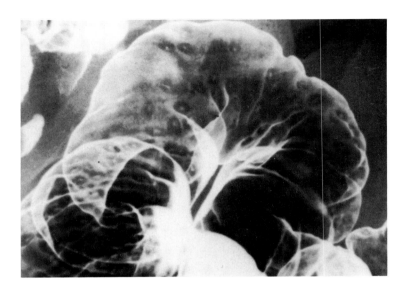

FIG 48−6.
Cytomegalovirus colitis. Spot film of the sigmoid colon from a double-contrast barium enema in a patient with proved cytomegalovirus infection. Note numerous aphthoid ulcers indistinguishable from Crohn's disease. (Courtesy Emil Balthazar, M.D., New York.)

Ischemic Colitis

Ischemic colitis characteristically develops in elderly patients with diminished flow, specifically with decreased cardiac output,[1, 14, 15] and in patients with colonic ischemia from thrombosis of the mesenteric vessels. The range of the disease is extreme in both severity and in acuteness of presentation. Diagnosis should be considered in the elderly patient with sudden onset of abdominal pain and bloody diarrhea. Depending on the clinical presentation and the time of radiographic evaluation, there is a broad spectrum of radiographic abnormalities, varying from an almost normal appearing colon to haustral thickening with thumbprinting (Fig 48−7,A) to severe ulcerating colitis that can at times mimic idiopathic ulcerative colitis or Crohn's disease.[1] In the vast majority of patients with radiographic abnormalities demonstrated by barium enema the colon will return to normal in 2 to 3 weeks (Fig 48−7,B).[14] Very rarely patients will have severe pain and bloody diarrhea and an abdominal radiograph will show evidence of intramural colonic gas and portal venous gas. These patients have gangrene of the colon. Less severely affected patients with a subacute course have bloody diarrhea and mild abdominal pain. The barium enema confirms intramural edema with thumbprinting in the affected area. The most common areas involved are the splenic flexure and sigmoid colon. Recovery is usually complete (Fig 48−7,A and B) except for occasional loss of haustration and distensibility. Rarely, in fewer than 5% of patients, healing will progress to a stricture, which may require resection because of obstruction (Fig 48−7,C).[14] Occasionally the disease may have so insidious a course that it is not evaluated until late and a stricture is the first manifestation of ischemia (Fig 48−7,C). There have been reports of ischemic colitis developing proximal to an obstructing lesion, particularly a carcinoma.[1, 16] Inasmuch as the colitis usually presents the more dramatic radiographic findings, the tumor may be overlooked unless a careful barium enema is performed. In patients with apparent clinical ischemic colitis with thumbprinting and ulceration in the proximal colon, the distal colon must be examined and even reexamined for a possible cause of neoplastic obstruction, even though this occurs in a small percentage of patients.

The radiologist should participate in the evaluation of suspected ischemic colitis. In the absence of any peritoneal signs it is safe to perform a barium enema, and once the classic radiographic changes are identified, the radiologist should recommend a follow-up examination in 2 to 3 weeks to confirm that the colon has returned to normal and no neoplasm is present.

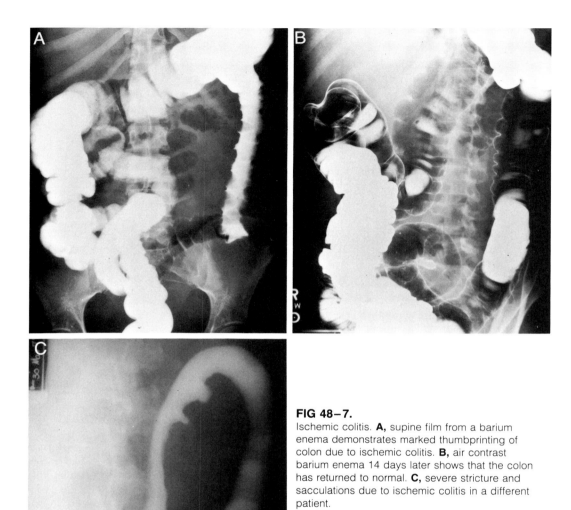

FIG 48–7.
Ischemic colitis. **A,** supine film from a barium enema demonstrates marked thumbprinting of colon due to ischemic colitis. **B,** air contrast barium enema 14 days later shows that the colon has returned to normal. **C,** severe stricture and sacculations due to ischemic colitis in a different patient.

Pseudomembranous Colitis

Pseudomembranous colitis usually, but not always, follows antibiotic administration and is caused by a mucosal toxin produced by overgrowth of *C. difficile*.[17, 18] The diagnosis can be established by observing pseudomembranous plaques on the rectal and colonic mucosa endoscopically and by culturing the organism from the stool. Prompt treatment with vancomycin eliminates the organism from the stool within 5 days.[18] Severe cases may require colonic resection. Characteristically the co-

lonic mucosa is erythematous and studded with elevated cream-colored mucosal plaques. Early on there may be only mild granular proctitis or discrete ulcers. The plaques, too, may be more prominent proximally in the colon and not seen in the rectum. Classically the plain abdominal radiograph will show mild colonic dilation with marked thickening of haustrations and even thumbprinting (Fig 48–8,A).[19] Occasionally the small flat-topped plaques can be identified on the edematous mucosa. In a patient with acute diarrhea these radiographic

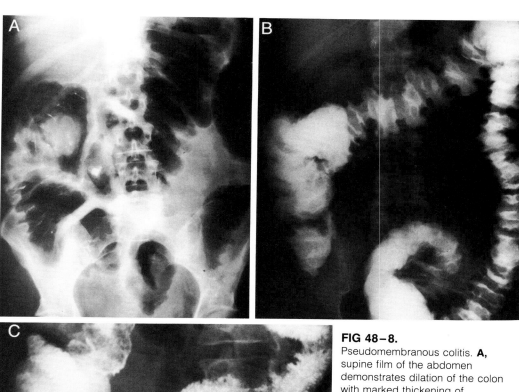

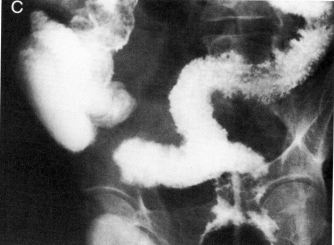

FIG 48–8.
Pseudomembranous colitis. **A,** supine film of the abdomen demonstrates dilation of the colon with marked thickening of haustrations in a patient who was taking clindamycin. Findings are those of pseudomembranous colitis. **B,** barium enema in a patient taking antibiotics exhibits diffuse mucosal edema and marked thickening of haustrations. **C,** right posterior oblique view from a barium enema demonstrates marked mucosal irregularity, with barium localized between the diffuse plaque formation, in a patient with pseudomembranous enterocolitis.

findings are strongly suggestive of pseudomembranous colitis, especially if the patient gives a history of taking antibiotics, specifically clindamycin or ampicillin. A barium enema is contraindicated in patients with severe pseudomembranous colitis because it can exacerbate the clinical condition and even lead to perforation of the colon.[19] Barium enemas have been performed in patients with mild to moderate disease. The findings vary from focal disease to severe colitis (Fig 48–8,B and C).[20] Mucosal irregularity may be marked because of barium filling areas between mucosal plaques (Fig 48–8,C).[21] Occasionally the findings can be misleading, and recognizing the differences on proctosigmoidoscopy and knowing the history are therefore of paramount importance.

Strongyloides-associated Colitis

Strongyloidiasis is a parasitic infection with worldwide distribution. The reported incidence is high in endemic areas in Africa, Asia, and South America, and infection with *Strongyloides stercoralis* is also being recognized with greater frequency in metropolitan areas of the United States.[21, 22] Many of the infections are trivial or asymptomatic and remain undiagnosed for years. Changes in the host-parasite relationship, especially in older patients, can change from chronic asymptomatic infestation to debilitating and even lethal infection. In the upper gastrointestinal tract mild mucosal edema may progress to eventual effacement of the mucosa in the duodenum and jejunum. The motility of the duodenum is decreased and may be associated with dilation. Narrowing of the small bowel, resulting in a "pipestem" appearance, with hypomotility may ensue. Colitis may develop in these patients, resembling both the radiographic and endoscopic features of ulcerative or amebic colitis (Fig 48–9).[22] In chronic disease the colon can lose its normal haustral pattern entirely and become narrow and tubular, indistinguishable from that in chronic ulcerative colitis. Acute disease can produce severe findings radiographically indistinguishable from those of acute ulcerative colitis.

Tuberculous Colitis

The ileum and cecum are involved in 80% of all patients with gastrointestinal tuberculosis. Clinical symptoms, often vague and ill-defined, include diarrhea, constipation, abdominal cramps, fever, weight loss, and at times a palpable mass. Radiographically gastrointestinal tuberculosis most commonly mimics Crohn's disease (Fig 48–10).[6, 23, 24] On barium enema a conical shrunken and contracted cecum is often associated with a narrow ulcerated terminal ileum. The cecal changes usually result from spasm early in the disease and from transmural infiltration with fibrosis in later phases. In advanced cases, similar to Crohn's disease, ileal narrowing may result from stricture, with ulceration and thickening of the bowel wall. It is probable that many conditions diagnosed as gastrointestinal tuberculosis in the past were in fact Crohn's disease, and difficulty in differentiating the two diseases persists. Tuberculosis should be considered when radiographic

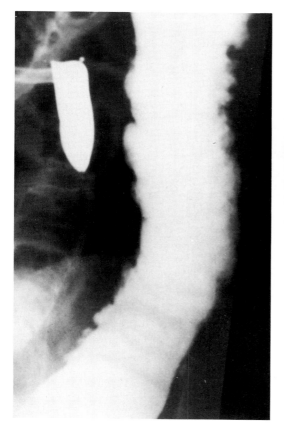

FIG 48–9.
Strongyloides colitis. Spot film of the descending colon from a barium enema in a patient with strongyloidiasis shows diffuse ulceration. (Courtesy Arthur Clemett, M.D., New York.)

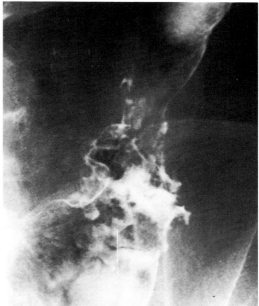

FIG 48–10.
Tuberculous colitis. Coned down view of the sigmoid colon from a barium enema in a patient with tuberculous colitis. There is irregularity, narrowing, and ulceration.

CHAPTER 49

Cholelithiasis

William M. Thompson, M.D.

Case Presentation

A 42-year-old woman had vague right upper quadrant abdominal pain, especially after meals. Physical examination and laboratory workup yielded normal findings. Ultrasonography of the gallbladder was ordered (Fig 49–1). What are the findings? What is the differential diagnosis? How confident are you of your diagnosis? How would you confirm the diagnosis?

DISCUSSION

Until the 1970s the oral cholecystogram was the major radiographic procedure of choice for evaluation of gallstones. During the past 10 to 12 years real-time ultrasound has become the major screening method for the detection of gallstones.[1] Ultrasound has been shown to be highly accurate for diagnosing cholelithiasis and for examining patients with suspected acute cholecystitis, empyema of the gallbladder, pericholecystic abscess, and gallbladder neoplasm.[1-4] Sonography has become the primary radiographic procedure for evaluating the gallbladder, but plain films,[5-7] oral cholecystography,[6-8] radionuclide scanning,[1, 9, 10] and computed tomography (CT)[11] have been used in the evaluation of gallbladder disease, and there may even be a role for magnetic resonance imaging (MRI).[12]

Techniques for Examining the Gallbladder

The plain film of the abdomen is the simplest and least expensive method for examining a patient with suspected cholelithiasis.[5-7] Although most gallstones are composed of cholesterol, calcium bilirubinate may account for all or part of these entities. However, only 10% to 15% of gallstones have enough calcium to be detected on plain abdominal radiographs (Fig 49–2,A).[5] There are other causes of calcification in the gallbladder as well as in the right upper quadrant (see Chapter 1). Rarely, noncalcified fissuring gallstones are demonstrated due to a lucent stellate appearance resembling the insignia of a Mercedes-Benz automobile (Fig 49–2,C). This appearance is thought to be caused by nitrogen within clefts in predominantly cholesterol-laden gallstones.[13] Two findings occur on plain films in patients with acute cholecystitis: a right upper quadrant mass in a hydropic gallbladder and air within the wall or lumen due to emphysematous cholecystitis (Fig 49–2,D).

The advantages of real-time sonography include lack of dependence on absorption of a contrast medium from the bowel, no dependence on liver and gallbladder function, and lack of exposure to ionizing irradiation.[1-4] Also, the examination can be performed at the bedside. In addition cholecystosonography usually can be performed in 15 to 20 minutes, with a greater than 95% success rate. Ultrasonography and oral cholecystography are equally accurate in detecting cholelithiasis.[1-4] Reports that sonography can detect stones missed by oral cholecystography (see Fig 49–2,A and B) suggest that the false negative rate for oral cholecystog-

403

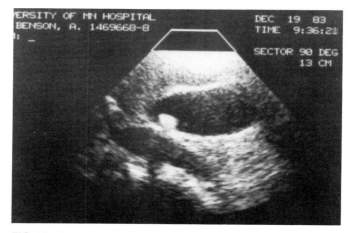

FIG 49–1.
Sonogram demonstrates the gallbladder. What is the finding? What is
the differential diagnosis? How would you confirm the diagnosis?

raphy is higher than previously believed, perhaps as high as 8% to 10%. Certainly stones overlooked on sonography are detected by oral cholecystography, and occasionally false positive results of sonography are encountered, primarily due to polyps and folds in the gallbladder. Overall, the sensitivity, specificity, and accuracy of cholecystosonography are equal to, if not superior to, oral cholecystography. Also, the frequency of indeterminate studies is lower with sonography than with oral cholecystography.

In spite of these problems the oral cholecystogram remains an accurate and specific study for the detection of gallstones.[6–8] The two most common agents for oral cholecystography are iopanoic acid (Telepaque) and tyropanoate sodium (Bilopaque). Each requires different patient preparation.[8] Fat, which produces gallbladder contraction, should be given in the diet at the same time that iopanoic acid is administered. The active enterohepatic recirculation of bile salts plays a major role in facilitating both the intestinal absorption and hepatic excretion of this agent.[5] If fat is not administered in the diet with iopanoic acid, adequate opacification of the gallbladder will not be achieved as reliably as when fat is given. This agent and the evening meal should be ingested 16 to 18 hours before the study. Tyropanoate sodium is not affected by dietary fat; in fact, because fat promotes gallbladder emptying, fat in the patient's evening meal may interfere with gallbladder opacification. When this agent is used the patient should be given a fat-free diet and the contrast administered 10 to 12 hours before the study. The usual dosage of either agent is 3 gm

given orally the evening before the study. If there is poor opacification or no visualization, a second dose of 3 gm should be administered and the patient examined the following day. A second dose is necessary in approximately 25% of patients and improves visualization in approximately half. Some workers advocate giving the 6 gm over 2 days and examining the patient on the third day.[8] This method has the advantage of higher accuracy and more efficiency; the disadvantage is that approximately 75% of the patients receive a second dose of oral cholecystopaque unnecessarily. Failure of the gallbladder to take up the contrast agent implies cystic duct obstruction due to gallstones; additional causes of faint or no visualization of the gallbladder are given in Table 49–1. Some of these causes are difficult to exclude clinically, but as a result of the wide availability of ultrasound, nonvisualization of the gallbladder usually is not a major issue. The use of a fatty meal during the examination causes gallbladder contraction, which may aid in evaluation of gallbladder wall function and detection of small stones, adenomyomatosis (Fig 49–3), cholesterolosis, and polyps; contraction also changes the position of the gallbladder, freeing it from overlying bowel gas.

Real-time sonography has become the procedure of choice in the evaluation of the gallbladder and detection of gallstones.[1–4] The only prerequisite is that the patient fast for at least 6 hours before the study to allow the gallbladder to fill with bile, thus enhancing the acoustic visibility of gallstones. In emergency situations the gallbladder can be ex-

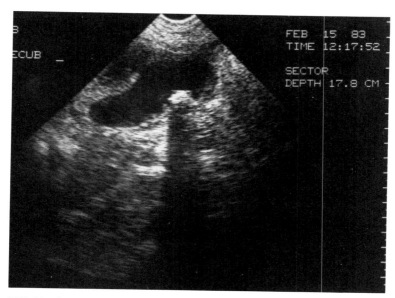

FIG 49–8.
Sonogram in a patient with cholelithiasis pattern 1. The sonogram demonstrates an echogenic shadowing focus, which moved with change in position.

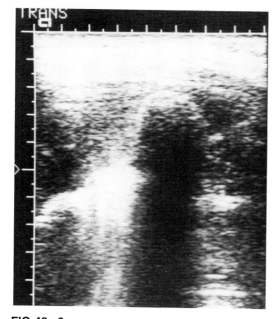

FIG 49–9.
Sonogram in a patient with cholelithiasis pattern 2. Real-time sonogram through region of the gallbladder fossa demonstrates an echogenic focus with a clean posterior acoustic shadow.

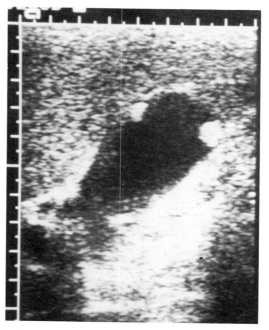

FIG 49–10.
Sonogram in a patient with cholelithiasis pattern 3. Real-time sonogram of the gallbladder demonstrates two echogenic foci that do not shadow and did not move. The lack of dependency and motion suggests that these lesions are not stones. They were found to be caused by candidiasis.

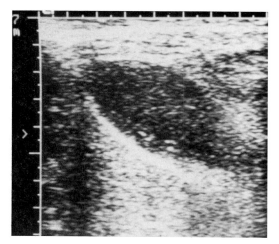

FIG 49–11.
Sludge. Sonogram in a patient who had received a bone marrow transplant demonstrates low-level echoes within the gallbladder that do not shadow.

Complications of Cholelithiasis

A significant complication of cholelithiasis is acute cholecystitis, usually resulting from a gallstone obstructing the cystic duct.[8] The gallbladder becomes distended with bile and inflammatory exudate; in severe cases gross pus is found (empyema). Acalculous cholecystitis is an infrequent, severe variant that usually occurs in debilitated, bedridden older patients. It has a high incidence of gangrenous necrosis, with air in the gallbladder wall. This combination of findings is called emphysematous cholecystitis.

When acute cholecystitis is suspected, both real-time ultrasonography and cholescintigraphy are highly accurate.[21–26] Although first choice of method varies among institutions, 60% to 70% of radiologists prefer sonography as the initial imaging technique, over cholescintigraphy.[8] Each technique has advantages and disadvantages.

The two most specific sonographic findings in acute cholecystitis are the detection of gallstones and a positive Murphy's sign.[25] Gallstones do not in themselves suggest a diagnosis of acute cholecystitis; however, acute cholecystitis without gallstones is extraordinarily rare. Thus gallstones almost always are present in patients who eventually are shown to have acute cholecystitis. When the ultrasonographer or patient can place the transducer over the gallbladder and elicit maximum tenderness, a positive sonographic Murphy's sign has been elicited and is specific for acute cholecystitis. Another sign that may prove useful is thickening of the gall-

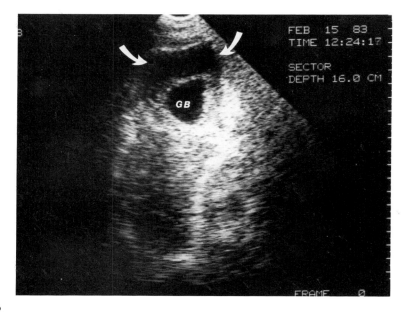

FIG 49–12.
Sonogram demonstrates a fluid collection *(arrows)* over the dorsal surface of the gallbladder *(GB)*. There is slight thickening of the gallbladder wall. Surgery revealed acute cholecystitis with a pericholecystic abscess.

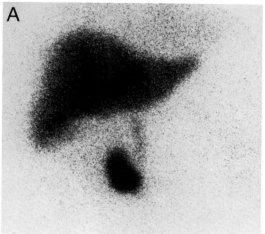

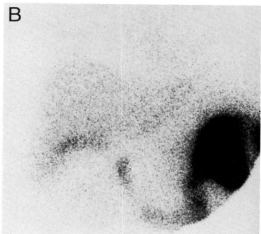

FIG 49–13.
Cholescintigram in a patient with acute cholecystitis. **A,** image obtained at 30 minutes demonstrates normal liver and a normal common duct. The area of tracer adjacent to the distal common duct is in the duodenum, not the gallbladder. **B,** delayed image at 90 minutes shows that the radionuclide has virtually cleared the liver and passed into the bowel. There is an area of increased tracer in the gallbladder fossa, highly suggestive of acute cholecystitis.

bladder wall.[27–29] When the gallbladder is distended the normal thickness of the gallbladder wall is 2 to 3 mm; thickening of the wall to more than 4 to 5 mm is common in both acute and chronic cholecystitis. (For a discussion of gallbladder wall thickening see Chapter 50.) The clinician must rule out other causes of gallbladder wall thickening. A lucent fluidlike rim surrounding the gallbladder is believed to represent inflammatory edema and is a sensitive indicator of complicated cholecystitis (Fig 49–12).[30] Again, just thickening of the gallbladder wall is not specific for acute cholecystitis, because it may occur in ascites or hepatitis. Finally, a complex mass surrounding or adjacent to a stone-filled gallbladder usually represents a pericholecystic abscess.[30] Such an abscess or air in the gallbladder wall is specific for complicated acute cholecystitis. These findings may indicate the need for immediate operative intervention. Air is much more easily detected within the gallbladder wall on plain films or CT scans (see Fig 49–2,D). One advantage of real-time sonography compared with the radionuclide scan is that the right upper quadrant and remainder of the abdomen can be evaluated. This is important because only one half to two thirds of patients with right upper quadrant pain have acute or chronic cholecystitis.[24] Other advantages of sonography have been mentioned.

Acute cholecystitis may be diagnosed by cholescintigraphy when the gallbladder is not visualized with passage of the radionuclide from the liver into the small bowel.[9, 10, 21–23] Failure to fill the gallbladder implies cystic duct obstruction, the hallmark of acute cholecystitis. Delayed views often are needed and should be obtained at 2 and 4 hours and even 24 hours when the gallbladder cannot be visualized on the images obtained within the first hour. Increased radionuclide uptake in the region of the gallbladder fossa due to hyperemia from gallbladder inflammation has been reported (Fig 49–13).[31] This finding coupled with nonvisualization of the gallbladder is specific for acute cholecystitis. Cholescintigraphy demonstrates other hepatobiliary disorders such as liver abscesses, dilated bile ducts, and masses in the porta or pancreas. Because cystic duct rarely occurs when the gallbladder is normal, nonfilling of the gallbladder at 24 hours generally indicates acute cholecystitis. Another advantage of the examination is that normal findings (i.e., filling of the gallbladder) effectively exclude acute cholecystitis.[9, 10] The only real disadvantage of cholescintigraphy is the relatively high percentage of false positive results due to bile stasis. This is common in patients with prolonged fasting, as seen in pancreatitis, alcoholism, long-term parenteral nutrition, and cirrhosis. False positive results

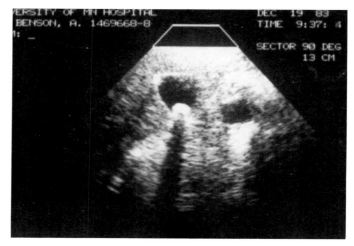

FIG 49–14.
Sonogram from the same examination as in Figure 49–1 demonstrates that the echogenic focus does shadow. This is virtually diagnostic of cholelithiasis.

are particularly troublesome in gravely ill patients, in whom the possibility of acute cholecystitis is often high. Thus some surgeons will not operate on the basis of positive radionuclide findings and require sonography or a CT study for more complete evaluation.

A number of filling defects within the gallbladder that may be demonstrated by ultrasonography and oral cholecystography are not gallstones (see Fig 49–7). Usually these are fixed filling defects that do not change position even after ingestion of a fatty meal (see Fig 49–7). The most common filling defects occur in patients with adenomyosis and cholesterolosis.[32] Adenomatous polyps also can occur within the gallbladder. Rarely a primary malignant neoplasm in the gallbladder is demonstrated as an intraluminal mass. Metastatic disease to the gallbladder is extraordinarily uncommon; melanoma occurs most frequently.

CONCLUSION

In the case presented, the sonogram demonstrated an intrinsic filling defect within the gallbladder, which does not produce a definite shadow in Figure 49–1. Further sonographic evaluation confirmed that the echogenic focus not only moved but also produced shadowing, thereby confirming the diagnosis of cholelithiasis (Fig 49–14).

REFERENCES

1. Berk RN, Ferrucci JT Jr, Fordtran JS, et al: Radiological diagnosis of gallbladder disease: An imaging symposium. *Radiology* 1981; 141:49–56.
2. Cooperberg P, Burhenne H: Real-time ultrasonography. Diagnostic technique of choice in calculous gallbladder disease. *N Engl J Med* 1980; 302:1277–1280.
3. Hessler PC, Hill DS, Detorie FM, et al: High accuracy sonographic recognition of gallstones. *AJR* 1981; 136:517–520.
4. Krook PM, Allen FH, Bush WH Jr: Comparison of real-time cholecystosonography and oral cholecystography. *Radiology* 1980; 135:145–148.
5. Berk RN: The plain abdominal radiograph, in Berk RN, Ferrucci JT Jr, Leopold GR (eds): *Radiology of the Gallbladder and Bile Ducts: Diagnosis and Intervention.* Philadelphia, WB Saunders Co, 1983, pp 1–29.
6. Simeone JF: The gallbladder: Anatomy and examination technique, in Tavaras W, Ferrucci JT Jr (eds): *Radiology: Diagnosis, Imaging, Intervention.* New York, JB Lippincott Co, 1987, pp 1–9.
7. Simeone JF: The gallbladder: Pathology, in Tavaras W, Ferrucci JT Jr (eds): *Radiology: Diagnosis, Imaging, Intervention.* New York, JB Lippincott Co, 1987, pp 1–14.
8. Berk R: Oral cholestography, in Berk RN, Ferrucci JT Jr, Leopold GR (eds): *Radiology of the Gallbladder and Bile Ducts: Diagnosis*

and Intervention. Philadelphia, WB Saunders Co, 1983, pp 83–162.

9. Weissmann HS, Badia J, Sugarman LA, et al: Spectrum of 99m-Tc IDA cholescintigraphic patterns in acute cholecystitis. *Radiology* 1981; 138:167–175.

10. Weissman HS: Cholescintigraphy, in Berk RN, Ferrucci JT Jr, Leopold GR (eds): *Radiology of the Gallbladder and Bile Ducts. Diagnosis and Intervention*. Philadelphia, WB Saunders Co, 1983, pp 261–313.

11. Barakos JA, Ralls PW, Lapin SA, et al: Cholelithiasis: Evaluation with CT. *Radiology* 1987; 162:415–418.

12. Hricak H, Filley RA, Margulis AR: MRI, NMR imaging of the gallbladder. *Radiology* 1983; 147:481–484.

13. Meyers MA, O'Donohue N: The Mercedes-Benz sign: Insight into the dynamics of formation and disappearance of gallstones. *AJR* 1973; 119:63–70.

14. Sommer FG, Taylor KJW: Differentiation of acoustic shadowing due to calculi and gas collections. *Radiology* 1980; 135:399–403.

15. Callen PW, Filly RA: Ultrasonographic localization of the gallbladder. *Radiology* 1979; 133:687–691.

16. Shuman WP, Gibbs P, Rudd TG, et al: PIP-IDA scintigraphy for cholecystitis: False positives in alcoholism and total parenteral nutrition. *AJR* 1982; 138:1–5.

17. Conrad MR, Leonard J, Landay MJ: Left lateral decubitus sonography of gallstones in contracted gallbladder. *AJR* 1980; 134:141–144.

18. Simeone JF, Mueller PR, Ferrucci JT Jr, et al: Significance of nonshadowing focal opacities at cholecystosonography. *Radiology* 1980; 137:181–185.

19. Filly R, Allen B, Minton M, et al: In vitro investigation of the origin of echoes within biliary sludge. *J Clin Ultrasound* 1980; 8:193–196.

20. Filly R, Moss AA, Way LW: In vitro investigation of gallstone shadowing with ultrasound tomography. *J Clin Ultrasound* 1979; 7:255–262.

21. Shuman WP, Mack LA, Rudd TG, et al: Evaluation of acute right upper quadrant pain. Sonography and 99m Tc–PIPIDA cholescintigraphy. *AJR* 1982; 139:61–64.

22. Samuels BI, Freitas JE, Bree RL, et al: Comparison of radionuclide hepatobiliary imaging and real-time ultrasound for the detection of acute cholecystitis. *Radiology* 1983; 147:207–210.

23. Caldwell JH: Ultrasound vs radionuclide scan in evaluation of acute right upper quadrant abdominal pain: Clinicians' comments. *J Clin Ultrasound* 1983; 11:201–202.

24. Laing FC, Federle MP, Jeffrey RB, et al: Ultrasonic evaluation of patients with acute right upper quadrant pain. *Radiology* 1981; 140:449–455.

25. Ralls PW, Halls J, Lapin SA, et al: Prospective evaluation of the sonographic Murphy sign in suspected acute cholecystitis. *J Clin Ultrasound* 1982; 10:113–115.

26. Parulekar SG: Sonographic findings in acute emphysematous cholecystitis. *Radiology* 1982; 145:117–119.

27. Marchall GJF, Casaer M, Baert AL, et al: Gallbladder wall sonolucency in acute cholecystitis. *Radiology* 1979; 133:429–433.

28. Engel JM, Daitch BA, Sikkema W: Gallbladder wall thickness. Sonographic accuracy and relation to disease. *AJR* 1980; 134:907–909.

29. Ralls PP, Quinn MF, Juttner H-U, et al: Gallbladder wall thickening. Patients without intrinsic gallbladder disease. *AJR* 1981; 137:65–68.

30. Bergman AB, Neiman HL, Kraut B: Ultrasonographic evaluation of pericholecystic abscesses. *AJR* 1979; 132:201–203.

31. Smith R, Rosen JM, Gallo LN, et al: Pericholecystic hepatic activity in cholescintigraphy. *Radiology* 1985; 156:797–800.

32. Berk RN, van der Vegt JH, Lichtenstein JE: Hyperplastic cholecystoses, cholesterolosis and adenomyomatosis. *Radiology* 1983; 146:593–601.

CHAPTER 50

Gallbladder Wall Thickening

Christopher C. Kuni, M.D.

Case Presentation

A 35-year-old man was hospitalized because of renal colic. Earlier in the day he had exercised vigorously for a long time in very warm weather and became dehydrated. During the 10 hours after admission he received 30 mg morphine sulfate and 10 L fluid intravenously. A ureteric stone was passed spontaneously, and the patient was discharged. The next day right upper quadrant pain different from the renal colic developed and the patient returned to the hospital, where an ultrasonogram (Fig 50–1,A) was obtained and he was discharged without further treatment. The pain subsided, and follow-up ultrasonography (Fig 50–1,B) was performed 1 week after the first study.

What is the thickness of the normal gallbladder wall? Did the initial ultrasonographic examination reliably exclude acute cholecystitis? What is the differential diagnosis of gallbladder wall thickening?

DISCUSSION

The positive finding in Figure 50–1,A is gallbladder wall thickening (GBWT); the thickness is about 1 cm. The wall appears as three concentric bands. The inner and outer bands are relatively echodense and are separated by a relatively echolucent region. The gallbladder wall appears normal in Figure 50–1,B.

Several ultrasonographic studies have shown that the thickness of the normal gallbladder wall is 3 mm or less.[1-6] Nonpathologic factors that affect the apparent thickness are beam angle and the state of gallbladder filling.[2,7] Ascites may accentuate the effect of inappropriate beam angle but probably does not affect the wall thickness measurement if the beam angle is appropriate. Whether ascites is present or not, the ultrasound beam should be perpendicular to the gallbladder wall for accurate measurement (Fig 50–2). The wall thickness of a normal but contracted gallbladder may be more than 3 mm.

In the case presented there are no stones in the gallbladder. Because ultrasonography detects gallstones in at least 83% of patients with acute cholecystitis,[8] this diagnosis is unlikely. However, the patient has two findings that support the diagnosis of acute cholecystitis: GBWT and point tenderness over the sonographically located gallbladder. Therefore acute acalculous cholecystitis, although unlikely, was possible at the time of the initial study. In one series of patients[9] careful attention was directed to the pattern of wall thickening; relatively few (8%) of those with our patient's three-layer pat-

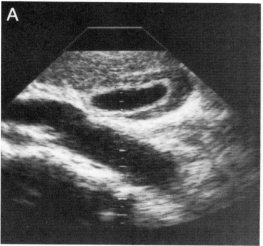
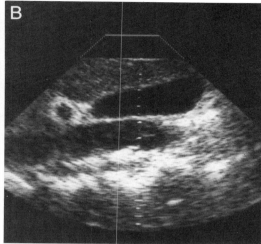

FIG 50–1.
A, initial ultrasonographic study shows gallbladder wall thickness of more than 1 cm. **B,** follow-up study 1 week later shows wall thickness of 2 to 3 mm. (Courtesy M.L. Daves, M.D., Denver.)

tern, consisting of a single lucent zone between two echodense layers, had acute cholecystitis. A striated pattern consisting of alternating irregular discontinuous lucent and echodense bands (Fig 50–3) was seen in 62% of patients with acute cholecystitis.[9] Thus the simple three-layer pattern seen in Figure 50–1,A militates against acute cholecystitis; although this diagnosis remains possible, other causes of GBWT must be considered, including chronic inflammation, tumor infiltration, increased oncotic pressure, and increased portal venous pressure.

In the limited number of published studies that correlate gallbladder wall thickness with pathologic findings in which chronic and acute inflammation are differentiated, 62% to 73% of patients with GBWT have chronic cholecystitis.[1, 3] Ultrasonographic examination of patients with chronic cholecystitis and GBWT but no acute inflammation usually reveals a relatively uniformly echodense band surrounding the gallbladder lumen, rather than either continuous or interrupted lucencies in the gallbladder wall (Fig 50–4). The high likelihood of chronic cholecystitis in a patient with GBWT presents the radiologist with a difficult dilemma in the setting of clinically suspected acute cholecystitis, GBWT, and cholelithiasis. Additional information

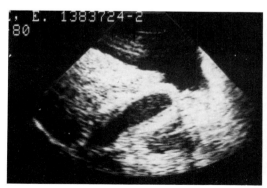
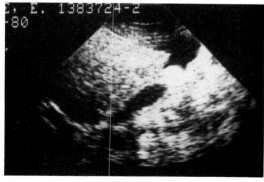

FIG 50–2.
Importance of ultrasound beam angle in a patient with ascites. Incorrect beam angle in the sonogram on the *right* causes the wall of the fundus to appear thicker than in that on the *left,* in which the beam is closer to perpendicular to wall.

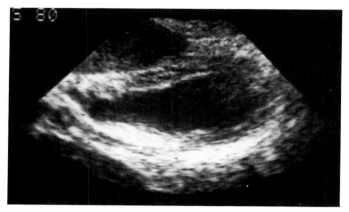

FIG 50–3.
Acalculous acute cholecystitis. Thickened wall contains discontinuous lucent bands.

must be relied on to distinguish acute from chronic cholecystitis. The presence and pattern of gallbladder lucencies are helpful. Point tenderness over the gallbladder localized by ultrasound is important; the combination of such tenderness, cholelithiasis, and GBWT is highly specific for acute cholecystitis.[8] However, evaluation of point tenderness over the gallbladder requires that the patient be lucid and cooperative. Another finding suggestive of acute rather than chronic cholecystitis is fluid around the gallbladder, but this finding is not often present. The question of whether cholecystitis is acute or chronic often can be answered with radionuclide hepatobiliary imaging.[10]

The same factors that cause ascites, namely, increased intravascular oncotic pressure and increased portal venous pressure, also tend to cause GBWT. Thus when ascites is present GBWT frequently is also present; causes of ascites not associated with GBWT include peritoneal tumor implants[11] and peritoneal dialysis.[12] Ascites may increase the need for accurate transducer alignment but otherwise does not cause the appearance of thickening of the normal gallbladder wall.[7] Al-

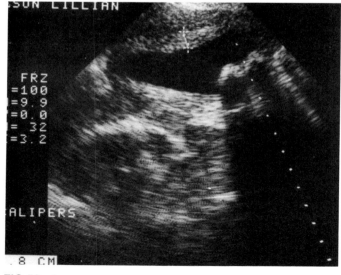

FIG 50–4.
Chronic cholecystitis. Thickened wall is homogeneously echodense.

though several studies have stressed the relationship between hypoproteinemia and GBWT, a series of patients without liver disease but with hypoproteinemia secondary to renal disease did not have GBWT.[4-6, 12] Some controversy surrounds the relationship between hypoproteinemia and wall thickening, yet the preponderance of evidence suggests a causal relationship. In a retrospective evaluation of a patient group containing a large number of alcoholics, 95% of those with GBWT had hypoproteinemia, compared with only 25% of patients with normal gallbladder wall thickness. Because GBWT in patients with hypoproteinemia or increased portal venous pressure is the result of edema, ultrasonography typically shows the three-layer pattern, in which the middle edematous layer is relatively echolucent.

Right-sided congestive heart failure presumably causes GBWT by increasing portal venous pressure, resulting in edema in the gallbladder, with venous drainage via the portal system. This cause of GBWT is relatively uncommon: In two series of a total of 34 patients with GBWT without intrinsic gallbladder disease only three had heart failure.[5, 6] The degree of failure must be severe or other predisposing factors must be present for GBWT to result. This condition may be associated with right upper quadrant pain and gallbladder tenderness. Therefore careful consideration must be given to the possibility of congestive failure when right upper quadrant processes amenable to surgery are being considered. Ultrasonographic hints that congestive failure is the cause of GBWT include enlarged hepatic veins, an enlarged portal vein, and the three-layer pattern with echolucent middle layer (Fig 50–5).

Two benign hyperplastic conditions, cholesterolosis and Rokitansky-Aschoff sinus formation (sometimes called adenomyomatosis), are common, one or the other being found in approximately 25% of gallbladders removed at surgery.[13] Although the precise relationship between these conditions and right upper quadrant pain is uncertain, the conditions probably are usually asymptomatic. Neither predisposes to cancer. Cholesterolosis is characterized by the abnormal accumulation of fatty deposits in macrophages in the gallbladder mucosa and wall, frequently leading to the formation of luminal polyps. Associated mucosal hyperemia may result in diffuse wall thickening. The radiologic hallmark of cholesterolosis is one or more fixed luminal nodules on oral cholecystography or ultrasonography. The nodules do not form acoustic shadows. Rokitansky-Aschoff sinuses are hyperplastic mucosal outpouchings through the muscularis. The sinuses frequently communicate with the lumen and are seen on oral cholecystography as small collections of contrast medium peripheral to the lumen. Ultrasonography reveals an irregularly thickened wall containing small echo-free spaces representing the bile-filled sinuses (Fig 50–6).

On ultrasonography, carcinoma of the gallbladder usually manifests as a mass that fills or replaces the gallbladder; this finding is observed in about 42% of patients. In 23% of patients a mass protrudes into the lumen, and in only 15% is the gallbladder wall diffusely thickened[14] (Fig 50–7). Computed tomography (CT) offers the possibility of differentiating cholecystitis complicated by pericholecystic fluid, gallbladder necrosis, perforation,

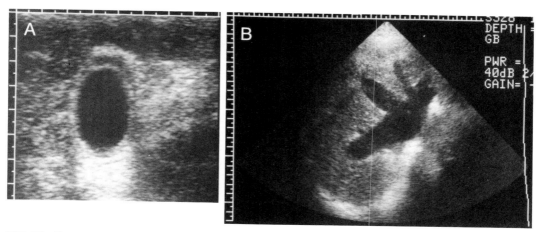

FIG 50–5.
Congestive heart failure. The gallbladder wall is thickened **(A)** and the hepatic veins are enlarged **(B)**.

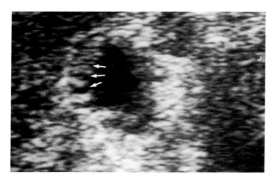

FIG 50–6.
Rokitansky-Aschoff sinuses. The gallbladder wall is 1 cm thick and contains lucent bile-filled sinuses *(arrows).*

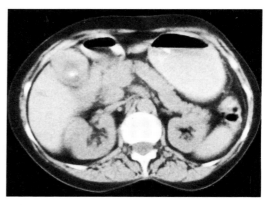

FIG 50–7.
Carcinoma of the gallbladder. This gallbladder with diffusely thickened wall contains a stone.

or cholecystocolonic fistula from gallbladder carcinoma; a low-attenuation curvilinear halo surrounding the gallbladder wall suggests complicated cholecystitis rather than carcinoma.[15] The finding of common bile duct obstruction at the level of the porta hepatis suggests tumor rather than cholecystitis, whereas obstruction at the papilla of Vater suggests obstruction from a gallstone associated with cholecystitis. Ascertaining the level of obstruction may be easier with CT, or possibly with magnetic resonance imaging (MRI), than with ultrasonography. A patient with gallbladder carcinoma imaged with MRI reportedly had a large gallstone surrounded by GBWT and a contiguous mass extending into the liver.[16] The signal strength of the mass relative to that of the liver was low on spin-echo 500/28 images and high on spin-echo 2,000/28 images.

Hepatitis was reported as the apparent cause of GBWT in 14% of one series of patients without intrinsic gallbladder disease and in 50% of similar patients in another series; the cause of hepatitis was unspecified in these series[5, 6] (Fig 50–8). In patients with acute viral hepatitis gallbladder wall thickness correlates with the severity of hepatitis, ranging from 2.5 to 4.5 mm in patients with aspartate and alanine aminotransferase (AST, ALT) values above 500 IU and between 2.0 and 3.5 mm in patients with transaminase values below 500 IU.[17] The mechanism of GBWT in these patients is unclear and appears to be independent of hypoproteinemia.

Unusual conditions associated with GBWT include gallbladder varices in patients with portal hypertension, multiple myeloma, and lymphatic ob-

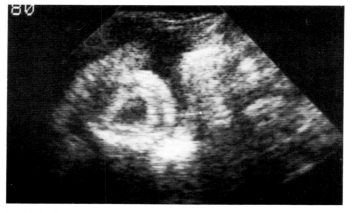

FIG 50–8.
Hepatitis. Gallbladder wall is more than 1 cm thick and shows the three-layer pattern.

struction.[6, 18, 19] In a single reported case the thickening in gallbladder varices was focal and was seen on ultrasound, CT, and oral cholecystography; the diagnosis was established with pulsed Doppler examination of the thickened region and by comparison of CT scans done with and without intravenous contrast medium. A patient with lymphoma and GBWT with gallbladder fossa adenopathy, both seen on ultrasonography, had histopathologic changes indicative of gallbladder wall lymphedema secondary to lymphatic obstruction. The mechanism for GBWT reported in a patient with myeloma is unknown.

CONCLUSION

For several years since the sonogram in Figure 50–1 was obtained the patient has remained healthy and free of right upper quadrant pain; therefore most of the diagnoses discussed are unlikely. There have been several cases of rapidly resolving GBWT associated with right upper quadrant pain, morphine administration, and vigorous hydration but no gallbladder disease (Daves, personal communication, 1988). The importance of morphine remains to be elucidated, but intravenous fluid administration probably is important in the pathogenesis of GBWT. This patient illustrates the caveat that GBWT may result in right upper quadrant pain even when the gallbladder is intrinsically normal; watchful waiting is in order when a process extrinsic to the gallbladder is likely to be the cause of GBWT in a patient with right upper quadrant pain.

REFERENCES

1. Finberg JH, Birnholz JC: Ultrasound evaluation of the gallbladder wall. *Radiology* 1979; 133:693–698.
2. Handler SJ: Ultrasound of gallbladder wall thickening and its relation to cholecystitis. *AJR* 1979; 132:581–585.
3. Engel JM, Deitch EA, Sikkema W: Gallbladder wall thickness: Sonographic accuracy and relation to disease. *AJR* 1980; 134:907–909.
4. Fiske CE, Laing FC, Brown TW: Ultrasonographic evidence of gallbladder wall thickening in association with hypoalbuminemia. *Radiology* 1980; 135:713–716.
5. Ralls PW, Quinn MF, Juttner HU, et al: Gallbladder wall thickening: Patients without intrinsic gallbladder disease. *AJR* 1981; 137:65–68.
6. Shlaer WJ, Leopold GR, Scheible FW: Sonography of the thickened gallbladder wall: A nonspecific finding. *AJR* 1981; 136:337–339.
7. Lewandowski BJ, Winsberg F: Gallbladder wall thickness distortion by ascites. *AJR* 1981; 137:519–521.
8. Laing FC, Federle MP, Jeffrey RB, et al: Ultrasonic evaluation of patients with right upper quadrant pain. *Radiology* 1981; 140:449–455.
9. Cohan RH, Mahony BS, Bowie JD, et al: Striated intramural gallbladder lucencies on US studies: Predictors of acute cholecystitis. *Radiology* 1987; 164:31–35.
10. Kuni CC, Klingensmith WC: *Atlas of Radionuclide Hepatobiliary Imaging.* Boston, GK Hall Publishing Co, 1983, pp 121–145.
11. Tsujimoto F, Miyamoto Y, Tada S: Differentiation of benign from malignant ascites by sonographic evaluation of gallbladder wall. *Radiology* 1985; 157:503–504.
12. Kaftori JK, Pery M, Green J, et al: Thickness of the gallbladder wall in patients with hypoalbuminemia: A sonographic study of patients on peritoneal dialysis. *AJR* 1987; 148:1117–1118.
13. Berk RN, van der Vegt JH, Lichtenstein JE: The hyperplastic cholecystoses: Cholesterolosis and adenomyomatosis. *Radiology* 1983; 146:593–601.
14. Weiner SN, Koenigsberg M, Morehouse H, et al: Sonography and computed tomography in the diagnosis of carcinoma of the gallbladder. *AJR* 1984; 142:735–739.
15. Smathers RL, Lee JK, Heiken JP: Differentiation of complicated cholecystitis from gallbladder carcinoma by computed tomography. *AJR* 1984; 143:255–259.
16. Rossmann MD, Friedman AC, Radecki PD, et al: Case Report: MR imaging of gallbladder carcinoma. *AJR* 1987; 148:143–144.
17. Juttner HU, Ralls PW, Quinn MF, et al: Thickening of the gallbladder wall in acute hepatitis: Ultrasound demonstration. *Radiology* 1982; 142:465–466.
18. Saigh J, Williams S, Cawley K, et al: Varices: A cause of focal gallbladder wall thickening. *J Ultrasound Med* 1985; 4:372–373.
19. Carroll BA: Gallbladder wall thickening secondary to focal lymphatic obstruction. *J Ultrasound Med* 1983; 2:89–91.

CHAPTER 51

Filling Defect in the Gallbladder

Joel E. Lichtenstein, M.D.

Case Presentation

A 56-year-old woman had vague right upper quadrant pain after meals, suggestive of gallbladder disease. A gallbladder sonographic study shows several nodular filling defects apparently attached to the gallbladder wall and projecting into the lumen (Fig 51–1, A and B). No ultrasonic shadowing is demonstrated and no free intraluminal stones are visible. The wall is not thickened and there is no pericholecystic fluid. Oral cholecystography was performed to confirm and further delineate the findings and to investigate gallbladder function. The gallbladder is well visualized after a single dose of oral contrast medium, but the lesions are not clearly demonstrated (Fig 51–2). Upright compression spot films (Fig 51–3) obtained after partial gallbladder contraction stimulated by intravenous injection of a synthetic analog of cholecystokinin confirm the presence of several small irregularly shaped fixed filling defects attached to the upper body of the organ. Given the data from these studies, what is an appropriate differential diagnosis? Is any further radiologic workup indicated?

DISCUSSION

Gallbladder disease, the most common indication for abdominal surgery in the United States, leads to about 500,000 cholecystectomies per year. Gallstones constitute approximately 95% of cases of gallbladder disease and occur in about 20% of the adult population of the United States. Thus it is not surprising that most diagnostic efforts related to the gallbladder are directed toward demonstration of calculi.[1–3] Because only about 15% to 20% of gallstones are calcified sufficiently to be visible on plain abdominal radiographs, other techniques that permit visualization of the gallbladder and filling defects within it generally are required.

GALLBLADDER IMAGING

For many years oral cholecystography was the unchallenged procedure of choice for the diagnosis of gallbladder disease.[4] However, the recent revolution in new imaging methods, particularly ultrasound and radioisotope cholescintigraphy, have called into question the preeminent role of this traditional technique.[5, 6] Computed tomography (CT) is less useful in the diagnosis of stones, although it may be helpful in the diagnosis of related complications or other disease.[7–9] The role of magnetic resonance imaging (MRI) has not been fully explored, but at present it does not appear to be cost effective in study of the gallbladder.[10, 11]

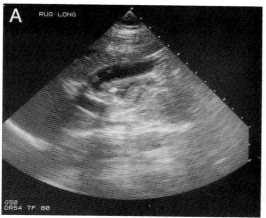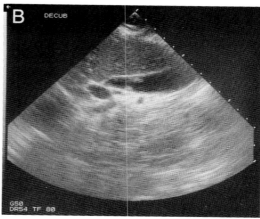

FIG 51–1.

Longitudinal supine **(A)** and decubitus **(B)** right upper quadrant real-time ultrasound study. Several small filling defects in the upper body of the gallbladder appear to be fixed to the wall and do not produce significant acoustic shadowing. The gallbladder wall is otherwise normal, and there is no pericholecystic fluid.

Oral Cholecystography

Oral cholecystography, introduced by Graham and Cole in 1924, was long considered one of the safest and most accurate of radiographic studies. Visualization of the gallbladder with this technique, however, depends on ingestion and retention of an oral cholecystographic contrast agent, which must be absorbed from the bowel, bound to albumin, transported to the liver, extracted by the hepatocytes, conjugated to a glucuronide, and then excreted into the biliary tree. Then it must have access through a patent cystic duct to the gallbladder, where normally it is concentrated to make it visible. Nonvisualization of the gallbladder is evidence of gallbladder disease in more than 97% of patients.

FIG 51–2.

Oral cholecystogram. An upright compression spot film shows dense opacification of the gallbladder. Filling defects in the upper body were suspected but were not clearly seen on the original films.

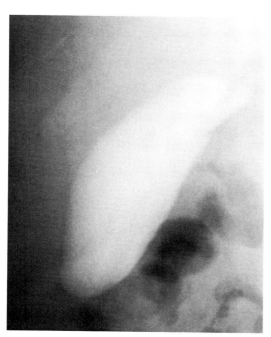

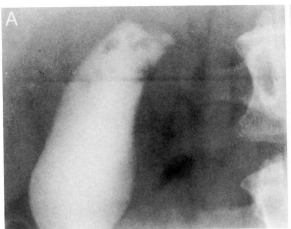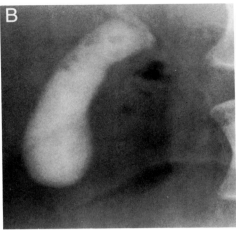

FIG 51–3.
Oral cholecystograms. Spot films before **(A)** and after **(B)** cholecystokinin stimulation. The gallbladder has partially emptied, making the contrast-filled lumen less opaque and better filling the neck and part of the cystic duct. The small irregular fixed filling defects are now well seen.

This high degree of reliability, however, is predicated on the ability to exclude any abnormality in the above steps that might lead to nonvisualization. If the gallbladder is opacified, false positive findings are rare. On the other hand, false negative results were not accurately assessed prior to the advent of diagnostic ultrasound. A gallbladder that opacified without the demonstration of stones was assumed to be normal, and generally no further studies were performed. Stones found on subsequent examination were assumed to have formed in the interval. Recent studies suggest, however, that the false negative rate with oral cholecystography may be as high as 6% to 8%, with small calculi often overlooked in the opacified bile.[12] Indeed, although a common problem is obtaining adequate visualization of the gallbladder, early concern that the oral contrast agents would be so dense as to hide small calculi appears to have been well founded.

Gallstones generally are mobile within the lumen of the gallbladder. They tend to settle in a dependent position or to float at a level determined by their specific gravity relative to the enhanced bile. Thus horizontal beam films and compression are useful for the detection of small lucent stones (Fig 51–4). Nevertheless, application of these techniques failed to demonstrate mobile, or layering, filling defects in the case presented.

Stimulating contraction of the gallbladder with a fatty meal or intravenous cholecystokinin may be useful in demonstrating small stones or other findings in equivocal cases. Tomography may be help-ful in otherwise inconclusive oral studies, and in the case of a nonvisualized gallbladder CT may demonstrate cystic duct obstruction by showing an opacified common duct or an otherwise undetected stone.[13]

Ultrasonography

With current refinements, ultrasonography essentially has supplanted oral cholecystography as the primary diagnostic method in gallbladder disease. Well over 95% of intraluminal calculi are identified routinely. They typically present as echogenic foci that can be demonstrated to move and have posterior ultrasonic shadows because of their intensely reflective properties. The demonstration of typical findings is diagnostic in more than 95% of cases. False positive findings are very rare, and although false negative results are somewhat more of a problem, they too are rare. Ultrasonography also permits examination of the gallbladder wall and the surrounding organs. It is excellent for the diagnosis of stones but does not give direct information about gallbladder function, nor does it provide an accurate determination of the number and size of stones. Oral cholecystography remains valuable as a second method for demonstrating gallbladder morphology and especially for indicating gallbladder function. The need to demonstrate gallbladder function and to determine the size and number of stones prior to treatment with chemolytic agents or extra-

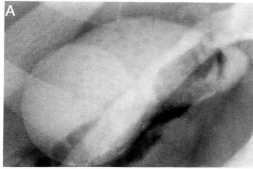

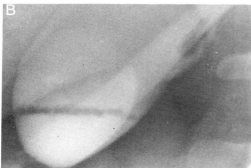

FIG 51–4.
Layering gallstones on oral cholecystography. **A,** closely collimated supine spot film of the gallbladder suggests a faintly mottled pattern, but definitive diagnosis of stones is difficult. **B,** upright compression spot film clearly reveals horizontal layer of lucent calculi.

corporeal shock wave lithotripsy presages a renewed interest in oral cholecystography.

NONCALCULOUS GALLBLADDER DISEASE

Although stones account for the vast majority of gallbladder problems, approximately one in 20 patients with gallbladder disease has non-stone-related disease. The case presented is an example. The filling defects appear adherent to the wall, do not demonstrate pronounced posterior shadowing, and are less reflective than typical stones. Despite some debate, the consensus is that gallstones rarely adhere to the gallbladder wall. It would be unlikely for all of several calculi to be adherent, with none found free within the lumen. Thus the sonogram demonstrates abnormal gallbladder findings suggestive of polypoid excrescences arising from the epithelial surface.

The oral cholecystogram confirms the presence of the wall abnormalities and demonstrates that the gallbladder is functional. It also fails to demonstrate any calculi, although it is less definitive than sonography in this regard.

An acalculous inflammatory process is unlikely because the gallbladder functions well. Sonographically, acalculous cholecystitis more typically presents with a diffusely thickened wall, pericholecystic fluid, and sometimes with gas within the gallbladder wall, but usually not with discrete excrescences.

Carcinoma of the gallbladder is an important lesion to consider clinically. However, it generally occurs in elderly patients with chronic cholecystitis and is therefore almost never seen in association with a functioning gallbladder on oral cholecystography.[14, 15] In addition, gallstones are associated with carcinoma in 80% to 90% of cases. A 4:1 female-to-male predominance reflects the higher incidence of stones in women. Most tumors are found late, when symptoms relate to metastases or to local extension obstructing the biliary tree, and the prognosis is very poor. Carcinoma ordinarily should not be considered in a case such as the one presented, with the gallbladder visualized on oral cholecystography and small excrescences seen on an otherwise normal wall on both oral cholecystography and ultrasonography.

Other filling defects generally are fixed to the wall and are smaller than 1 or 2 cm. Cholesterol polyps are by far the most common of these.[16] They are quite small, irregular, and usually multiple. They are best thought of as a localized form of cholesterolosis and may be associated with the simultaneous presence of the more generalized form. No relationship to stones has been established, and the significance of cholesterol polyps is questionable.

In cholesterolosis the subepithelial tissue of the gallbladder becomes filled with foamy, cholesterol-laden cells (Fig 51–5). The cause and alleged hyperplastic nature of this process have not been established.[17, 18] The more common, relatively flat diffuse form gives rise to the pathologic curiosity called strawberry gallbladder but has little radiographic manifestation. The increased surface area of the gallbladder may result in enhanced concentration of oral cholecystographic contrast medium and more intense than usual visualization of the gallbladder. In spite of the enhanced visualization, the irregularity of the edge may cause it to be somewhat fuzzy, suggesting the diagnosis. Cholesterolosis is

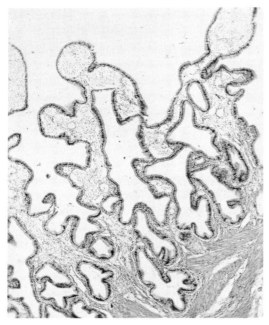

FIG 51–5.
Photomicrograph in a patient with cholesterolosis shows proliferation of foamy appearing lipid-laden cells beneath the redundant epithelial layer of the gallbladder lumen. (Hematoxylin and eosin; original magnification ×50.) (Armed Forces Institute of Pathology Neg. #58-5224.)

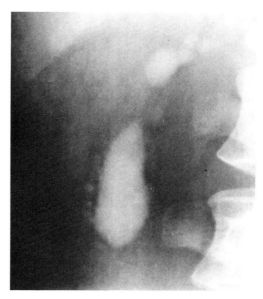

FIG 51–6.
Adenomyomatosis. Multiple tiny diverticula-like out-pouchings of the lumen fill with contrast material. These are enlarged Rokitansky-Aschoff sinuses and are actually confined within a thickened, hyperplastic muscular wall.

one of the two main forms of the hyperplastic cholecystosis described by Jutras et al.[19] in 1960.

The other major form of hyperplastic cholecystosis is adenomyomatosis, or hyperplastic Rokitansky-Aschoff sinuses.[17, 20, 21] Usually these sinuses appear as tiny diverticula-like outpouchings from the lumen; they fill with contrast on oral cholecystography and thicken the wall but do not significantly protrude into the lumen on ultrasonography (Fig 51–6). A variation of this condition, sometimes called an adenomyoma, usually is seen as a small sessile defect in the fundus of the gallbladder (Fig 51–7). Adenomyoma does not have the configuration or distribution seen in the case presented and thus is an unlikely diagnosis.

Benign neoplastic adenomas do occur in the gallbladder but are uncommon.[16] Their relationship to invasive carcinoma is questionable. Adenomas arise through metaplasia of the normal absorptive surface of the gallbladder epithelium and may be sessile or pedunculated, papillary or smooth. They generally are benign and are believed to remain be-

nign. However, occasionally papillary carcinoma of the gallbladder may have similar appearing tissue in its periphery, raising the possibility of an adenoma-carcinoma sequence in rare cases. Gallbladder carcinoma usually is an infiltrative and polypoid combination with no obvious adenoma present. It is generally believed to be a new lesion. Adenomas usually are solitary and are much less common than cholesterol polyps. Thus multiple adenoma is a much less likely diagnosis in the case presented.

The term "papilloma" commonly is applied to excrescences from the gallbladder wall. However, it is an ill-defined term and is not included in the World Health Organization nomenclature for gallbladder disease. In other contexts papilloma usually refers to a papillary tumor of squamous cell origin; this is inappropriate in the gallbladder, which is lined with a columnar absorptive cell epithelium. As used in the gallbladder, papilloma generally refers to a papillary adenoma, which is far less likely than cholesterol polyps in the case presented. In general, papilloma should be abandoned as a radiographic diagnosis in the gallbladder.

Other rare causes of fixed filling defects in the gallbladder include inflammatory fibroid polyps and inflammatory polyps related to parasite eggs, partic-

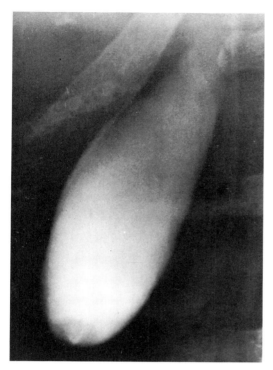

FIG 51–7.
Localized fundal adenomyomatosis or "adenomy-oma." Pathologically these lesions are similar to the more diffuse form of adenomyomatosis, but they tend to occur as a sessile mass at the apex of the fundus. They have a characteristic appearance that depends on whether they are everted and whether the Rokitan-sky-Aschoff sinuses fill.

ularly those of *Ascaris*. Rarely a hamartomatous ec-topia involving pancreatic tissue causes a tumor in the gallbladder, but such lesions usually are sessile, solitary, and larger than the nodules seen in the case presented.

Metastases, particularly melanoma, may pre-sent as multiple wall defects; generally the clinical history is helpful in that regard.

CONCLUSION

Multiple fixed filling defects in the gallbladder are overwhelmingly likely to represent cholesterol polyps. This is especially true if on oral chole-cystography the gallbladder can be demonstrated to function and no typical gallbladder calculi are demonstrated. Ordinarily no further radiologic workup is needed. Cholesterol polyps usually are

not associated with symptoms and generally are not an indication for surgery.

REFERENCES

1. Berk RN, Ferrucci JT, Fordtran JS, et al: The radiological diagnosis of gallbladder disease. *Radiology* 1981; 141:49–56.
2. Berk RN, Ferrucci JT, Leopold GR: *Radiology of the Gallbladder and Bile Ducts.* Philadel-phia, WB Saunders Co, 1983.
3. Cooperberg PL, Gibney RG: Imaging of the gallbladder, 1987. *Radiology* 1987; 163:605–613.
4. Shehadi WH: Radiologic examination of the biliary tract, plain film of the abdomen; oral cholecystography. *Radiol Clin North Am* 1966; 4:463–482.
5. Simeone FJ, Ferrucci J: New trends in gall-bladder imaging. *JAMA* 1981; 246:24–31.
6. Cooperberg PL, Burhenne HJ: Real-time ultra-sonography. Diagnostic technique of choice in calculous gallbladder disease. *N Engl J Med* 1980; 302:1277–1279.
7. Barakos JA, Ralls PW, Lapin SA, et al: Cholelithiasis: Evaluation with CT. *Radiology* 1987; 162:415–418.
8. Smathers RL, Lee JKT, Heiken JP: Differenti-ation of complicated cholecystitis from gall-bladder carcinoma by computed tomography. *AJR* 1984; 143:255–259.
9. Toombs BD, Sandler CM, Conoley PM: Com-puted tomography of the nonvisualizing gall-bladder. *J Comput Assist Tomogr* 1981; 5:164–168.
10. Demas BE, Hricak H, Moseley M, et al: Gall-bladder bile: An experimental study in dogs using MR imaging and proton MR spectros-copy. *Radiology* 1985; 157:453–455.
11. McCarthy S, Hricak H, Cohen M, et al: Cholecystitis: Detection with MR imaging. *Radiology* 1986; 158:333–336.
12. Crade M, Taylor KJW, Rosengield AT, et al: Surgical and pathologic correlation of chole-cystography. *AJR* 1979; 131:227–229.
13. Stephens DH, Gisvold JJ, Carlson HC: To-mography of the gallbladder in oral cholecys-tography. *Gastrointest Radiol* 1976; 1:93–98.
14. Arnaud JP, Graf P, Gramfori JL, et al: Pri-mary carcinoma of the gallbladder. *Am J Surg* 1979; 138:403–406.
15. Melson GL, Reiter F, Evans RG: Tumorous conditions of the gallbladder. *Semin Roent-genol* 1976; 11:269–282.
16. Christensen AH, Ishak KG: Benign tumors and pseudotumors of the gallbladder. Report of 180 cases. *Arch Pathol* 1970; 90:423–432.

17. Berk RN, Van der Vegt JH, Lichtenstein JE: The hyperplastic cholecystoses: Cholesterolosis and adenomyomatosis. *Radiology* 1983; 146:593–601.
18. Salmenkivi K: Cholesterolosis of the gallbladder: A clinical study based on 269 cholecystectomies. *Acta Chir Scand* [Suppl] 1964; 324:1–93.
19. Jutras JA, Longtin JM, Levesque MD: Hyperplastic cholecystoses (Hickey Lecture). *AJR* 1960; 83:795–826.
20. Aguirre JR, Boher RO, Guraieb S: Hyperplastic cholecystoses: A new contribution to the unitarian theory. *AJR* 1969; 107:1–13.
21. Fotopoulos JP, Crampton AR: Adenomyomatosis of the gallbladder. *Med Clin North Am* 1964; 48:9–36.

tastases in lymph nodes or the liver. Primary liver tumors can also obstruct the common hepatic duct. Direct invasion of the common hepatic duct is most commonly caused by carcinoma of the gallbladder. These lesions tend to obstruct the proximal periportal biliary system. US and CT (Fig 52–5,A) will show intrahepatic bile duct dilation with a mass in the porta hepatis and a normal sized common bile duct. PTC or ERCP is often needed to determine the exact site and cause of obstruction (Fig 52–5,B). The smooth extrinsic compression due to metastases can usually be differentiated from the irregular narrowing of cholangiocarcinoma. In many patients metastases to the periportal region are managed palliatively with either percutaneous drainage, internal stenting, or nasobiliary drainage. Thus defining the exact site of obstruction is extremely important. Even when the cholangiographic pattern is nonspe-

cific for metastatic periportal disease the diagnosis is rarely difficult, because the cholangiogram will show proximal obstruction and there is usually a clinical history of a primary neoplasm.

Gallbladder Carcinoma

In patients with gallbladder carcinoma bile duct obstruction usually is due to direct invasion of the common bile duct from the primary tumor. In approximately 50% of patients with gallbladder carcinoma US and CT show evidence of biliary dilation with a mass in the gallbladder fossa (Fig 52–6). A cholangiogram will usually reveal obstruction of the extrahepatic bile ducts near the junction of the cystic duct and the extrahepatic duct.

Pancreatic Carcinoma

Complete or subtotal obstruction of the middle or distal common duct is most commonly due to carcinoma in the head of the pancreas. Both US and

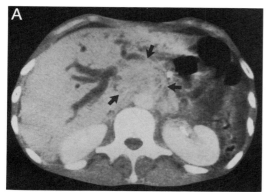

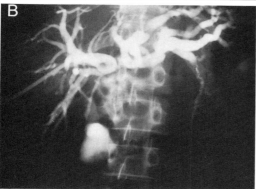

FIG 52–5.
Metastatic disease. **A,** CT scan through the level of the porta hepatis shows a large mass *(arrows)* obstructing the proximal common hepatic duct. **B,** percutaneous cholangiogram in the same patient confirms the proximal obstruction. The patient had undergone palliative resection of a gastric carcinoma 12 months earlier.

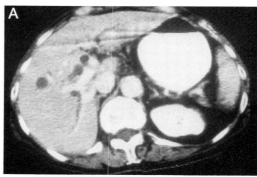

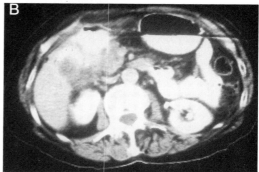

FIG 52–6.
Gallbladder carcinoma. **A,** CT scan through the liver demonstrates intrahepatic bile duct dilation. **B,** CT scan in the same patient demonstrates a large mass in the gallbladder fossa invading the liver and the region of the common hepatic and bile ducts.

CT will reveal extrahepatic bile duct dilation, and in many patients a mass can be detected in the head of the pancreas (Fig 52–7). Other signs of pancreatic cancer include enlargement of the pancreatic duct, atrophy of the body and tail of the pancreas, enlarged peripancreatic, periportal, or celiac lymph nodes, splenic vein occlusion and varices, and extension of the mass into the fat surrounding the celiac and superior mesenteric arteries. Venous or arterial encasement indicates that the tumor is unresectable. The classic finding on PTC is a "rattail" configuration of the contrast-filled duct at the site of obstruction (Fig 52–8). Because most of these tumors are unresectable, treatment of the biliary obstruction is often palliative, using percutaneous or endoscopic biliary drainage.

Ampullary Carcinoma

The classic US and CT appearance of ampullary carcinoma is a distal obstruction of the common bile duct without evidence of a pancreatic mass or stone in the bile duct (Fig 52–9,A and B). Rarely the tumor has been identified on CT as a mass projecting into the duodenal lumen or distal bile duct, mimicking an uncalcified common duct stone. The classic cholangiographic appearance is that of distal obstruction of the common bile duct (Fig 52–9,C). A polypoid mass growing within the distal duct may be identified. These tumors may also produce lesions difficult to differentiate from pancreatic and duodenal cancer or even benign ampullary stenosis.

Common Duct Stones

Choledocholithiasis is a relatively straightforward cholangiographic diagnosis. The demonstration of one or more rounded, faceted, or squared intraluminal filling defects makes the diagnosis in most cases. With complete obstruction from an impacted stone only a meniscus may be demonstrated (Fig 52–10,A). Also, with complete obstruction in-

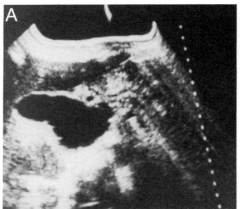
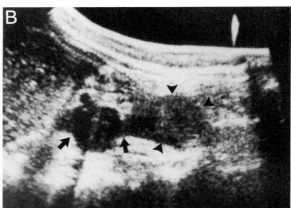
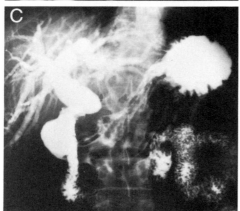

FIG 52–7.
Pancreatic cancer. **A,** sonogram demonstrates massive enlargement of the common duct at the level of the porta hepatis. **B,** longitudinal sonogram in the same patient shows a dilated distal common bile duct *(arrows)* ending in a large pancreatic head mass *(arrowheads).* **C,** percutaneous cholangiogram demonstrates extrahepatic bile duct obstruction. The patient was given barium to opacify the duodenum.

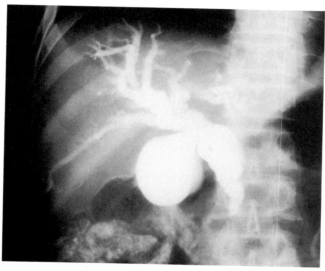

FIG 52−8.
Pancreatic carcinoma. Transhepatic cholangiogram demonstrates classic "rattail" configuration of the common bile duct related to pancreatic carcinoma.

fection of the bile occurs in approximately 80% of patients, and care must be taken not to overfill the ducts, to avoid producing septicemia. Most patients with complete obstruction require immediate percutaneous, nasobiliary, or surgical drainage.

Both US and CT can be used to diagnose common duct stones. With US common bile duct stones appear as echogenic foci within the lumen of the bile duct that shadow (Fig 52−10,B). Most authors report a 25% to 50% detection rate of common duct stones with US. By modifying the US technique one group reports demonstrating common duct stones in 75% of patients.[17] With CT the demonstration of a calcification within a dilated common bile duct is diagnostic of choledocholithiasis (Fig 52−10,C). Other CT findings suggestive of the diagnosis include abrupt termination of a dilated bile duct without an apparent mass, a circular line of high density within the bile duct, and a vague high-density focus within the bile duct. All three of these findings also can be caused by other entities.[17]

If a definite diagnosis of a common duct stone is made by US or CT the patient should undergo a definitive therapeutic procedure without ERCP or PTC just for diagnostic purposes. However, in a number of patients with common duct stones CT or US findings will be indeterminate and either PTC or ERCP is needed for diagnosis.

Benign Stricture

Most benign strictures of the common bile duct not secondary to pancreatitis are posttraumatic, following cholecystectomy. Any mid−common duct stricture in a patient who has had a previous cholecystectomy is a benign iatrogenic stricture until proved otherwise. With an intact gallbladder and no evidence of acute or chronic pancreatitis the stricture should be considered a malignant lesion. Dilation of the intrahepatic and common hepatic ducts will be detected by US and CT without any evidence of an apparent cause. On cholangiography the strictures usually appear as a short focal area of narrowing near the cystic duct; occasionally a long stricture may be demonstrated.

Chronic Pancreatitis

Chronic relapsing pancreatitis may produce severe narrowing of the intrapancreatic portion of the common bile duct due to periductal inflammation. Chronic biliary obstruction may lead to serious problems, such as suppurative cholangitis and biliary cirrhosis. Typically the extrahepatic common duct shows a smooth elongated stricture involving the intrapancreatic common bile duct (Fig 52−11). Although complete obstruction is not common with strictures due to pancreatitis, there can be significant

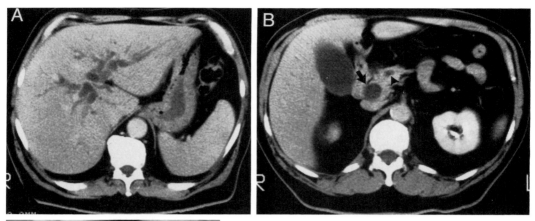

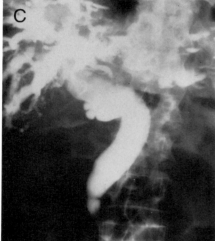

FIG 52–9.
Ampullary carcinoma. **A,** CT scan demonstrates intrahepatic bile duct dilation. **B,** CT scan shows dilated distal common bile duct *(arrow)* and pancreatic duct *(arrowhead).* **C,** transhepatic cholangiogram demonstrates a common bile duct dilated down to the level of the duodenum.

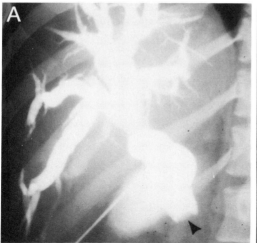

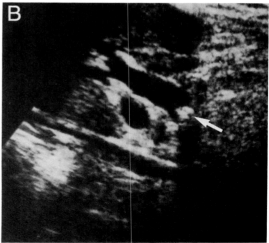

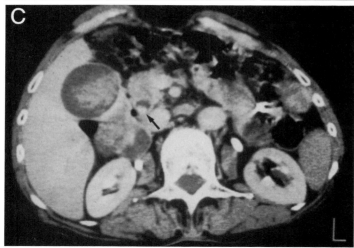

FIG 52–10.
Common duct stones. **A,** percutaneous cholangiogram demonstrates an impacted common duct stone *(arrow).* **B,** sonogram through common hepatic duct shows an echogenic shadowing focus *(arrow).* **C,** a small high-density focus is seen in the distal common duct *(arrow).* Multiple common duct stones were obstructing the bile ducts. The high-density material in the gallbladder was due to hemorrhage from a small gallbladder carcinoma.

dilation of the proximal biliary system. US and CT will demonstrate the bile duct dilation, and both may also show findings of chronic pancreatitis. These findings, especially pancreatic calcifications, are more easily seen on CT. Most patients with strictures due to pancreatitis have a long history of pancreatitis.

Sclerosing Cholangitis

Sclerosing cholangitis is a diffuse periductal inflammatory process that usually affects the extrahepatic bile ducts but may also involve the intrahepatic biliary system. US and CT may not demonstrate any abnormalities or may show subtle segmental areas of intrahepatic bile duct dilation and significant thickening of the extrahepatic ducts. Typical cholangiographic features of sclerosing cholangitis include irregular multisegmental areas of narrowing of both the intrahepatic and extrahepatic

ducts. The intrahepatic ducts may show various degrees of narrowing and distal segmental obstruction (Fig 52–12). There is an increased incidence of bile duct carcinoma in patients with sclerosing cholangitis. Thus any new focal stricture in a patient with known sclerosing cholangitis should raise the consideration of a malignant lesion. A significant percentage of patients with sclerosing cholangitis have chronic ulcerative colitis, although the exact frequency is not well established.

CONCLUSION

The sonogram in Figure 52–1 clearly shows a dilated biliary system, and in the dilated common bile duct there is an echogenic shadowing focus diagnostic of a common duct stone. According to Figure 52–2, CT or direct cholangiography (ERCP or PTC) should be performed. It might also be suggested that the patient be taken straight to surgery

FIG 52–11.
Chronic pancreatitis. Transhepatic cholangiogram demonstrates a long distal common bile duct stricture. Note numerous pancreatic head calcifications.

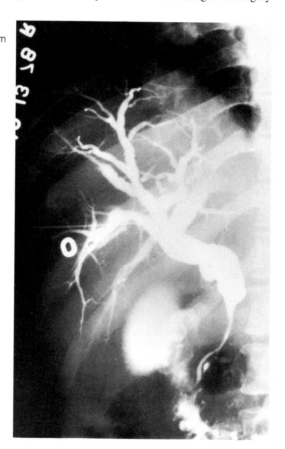

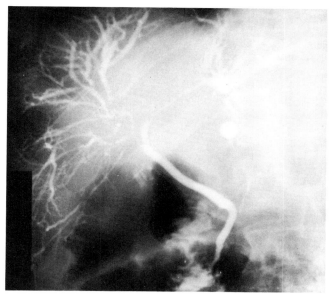

FIG 52–12.
Sclerosing cholangitis. Multiple areas of stenosis of the intrahepatic ducts. Common bile duct is normal.

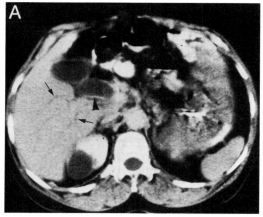

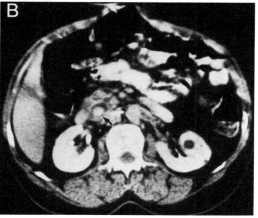

FIG 52–13.
Case presentation. **A,** CT scan shows minimally dilated intrahepatic ducts *(arrows)* and marked dilation of the common bile duct *(arrowhead)*. **B,** CT scan in the same patient demonstrates a high-density distal common bile duct stone *(arrow)*.

for endoscopic sphincterotomy. A CT scan in this patient (Fig 52–13) confirmed the diagnosis and, as important, ruled out other possible causes of obstruction, such as pancreatic cancer. A common duct stone was successfully removed at operation.

REFERENCES

1. Berk RN, Cooperberg PL, Gold RP, et al: Radiology of the bile ducts: A symposium on the use of new modalities for diagnosis and treatment. *Radiology* 1982; 145:1–9.
2. Cooperberg PL, Goling RH: Advances in ultrasonography of the gallbladder and biliary tree. *Radiol Clin North Am* 1982; 20:611–633.
3. Ferrucci JT Jr, Adson MA, Mueller PR, et al: Advances in the radiology of jaundice: A symposium and review. *AJR* 1983; 141:1–20.
4. Berk RN, Ferrucci JT Jr, Leopold GR: *Radiology of the Gallbladder and Bile Ducts: Diagnosis and Intervention*. Philadelphia, WB Saunders Co, 1983.
5. Simeone JF: The biliary ducts: Anatomy and examination techniques, in Taveras J, Ferrucci JT Jr (eds): *Radiology: Diagnosis, Imaging, Intervention*. Philadelphia, JB Lippincott Co, 1987, pp 1–13.
6. Mueller PR: Imaging in obstructive jaundice, in Taveras J, Ferrucci JT Jr (eds): *Radiology: Diagnosis, Imaging, Intervention*. Philadelphia, JB Lippincott Co, 1987, pp 1–13.
7. Mueller PR, Harbin WP, Ferrucci JT Jr, et al: Fine-needle transhepatic cholangiography: Reflections after 450 cases. *AJR* 1981; 136:85–90.
8. Freeny PC, Lawson TL: *Radiology of the Pancreas*. New York, Springer-Verlag, 1982, pp 111–119.
9. Sample WF, Sarti DA, Goldshein LI, et al: Gray-scale ultrasonography of the jaundiced patient. *Radiology* 1978; 128:719–725.
10. Quinn MF, Ralls PW, Boswell WD, et al: Predicting the cause of common bile duct obstruction with sonographic data analysis of binary variables. *Invest Radiol* 1982; 17:316–323.
11. Honickman SP, Mueller PR, Wittenberg J, et al: Ultrasound in obstructive jaundice: Prospective evaluation of site and cause. *Radiology* 1983; 147:511–515.
12. Goldstein CI, Sample WF, Kaddell BM, et al: Gray-scale ultrasonography and thin-needle cholangiography: Evaluation of the jaundiced patient. *JAMA* 1977; 238:221–223.
13. Zeman RK, Dorfman GS, Burrell MI, et al: Disparate dilatation of the intrahepatic and extrahepatic bile ducts in surgical jaundice. *Radiology* 1981; 138:129–136.
14. Shawker TH, Jones BL, Girton ME: Distal common bile duct obstruction: An experimental study in monkeys. *J Clin Ultrasound* 1981; 9:77–82.
15. Pedrosa CS, Casanova R, Rodriquez R: Computed tomography in obstructive jaundice. Part I. The level of obstruction. *Radiology* 1981; 133:627–634.
16. Pedrosa CS, Casanova R, Jezana AH, et al: Computed tomography in obstructive jaundices. Part II. The cause of obstruction. *Radiology* 1981; 133:635–645.
17. Baron RL, Stanley RJ, Lee JTK, et al: A prospective comparison of the evaluation of biliary obstruction using computed tomography and ultrasonography. *Radiology* 1982; 145:991–998.
18. Matzen P, Hauberk A, Holst-Christensen J, et al: Accuracy of direct cholangiography by endoscopic or transhepatic route in jaundice: A prospective study. *Gastroenterology* 1981; 81:237–241.

CHAPTER 53

Abnormal Operative Cholangiogram

Mary Ann Turner, M.D.

Case Presentation

A 54-year-old woman had a 1-year history of intermittent right upper quadrant pain and progressive jaundice over 3 weeks. Ultrasonography revealed gallstones and dilated bile ducts. She underwent a cholecystectomy, and a cholangiogram was performed in the operating room (Fig 53–1). What is the interpretation? What should be done next?

DISCUSSION

Operative cholangiography, first described by Mirizzi[1] in 1932, has become a widely used adjunct to biliary tract surgery. It is well recognized that the procedure can detect unsuspected stones, decrease instances of retained stones, and illustrate bile duct anatomy.[2, 3] Unsuspected disease such as tumor, stricture, or sclerosing cholangitis may be identified as well.

The primary role of operative cholangiography is the detection of unsuspected or overlooked calculi; despite the widespread use of this procedure, however, retained stones occur in 3% to 10% of patients.[4, 5] The most common cause of retained stones is related to unsatisfactory operative cholangiography[5]; errors in diagnosis may result from suboptimal technique or incorrect interpretation.

The diagnostic accuracy of operative cholangiography depends on meticulous attention to technique and rigid criteria for interpretation of the films. The technical considerations in operative cholangiography have been well described.[3, 6–9] Most common technical errors that result in misin-terpretation are listed in Table 53–1.[10] Stones may be obscured by inadequate penetration of the contrast material, grid lines, the overlying spine, and superimposition of tubes or instruments. Significant disease may be overlooked if the films are poorly exposed, the intrahepatic ducts are incompletely filled, or the distal end of the common duct is not visualized.

After completion of a technically satisfactory examination careful, systematic evaluation of the operative cholangiogram is necessary for accurate interpretation. The typical cholangiographic appearance of common biliary tract disorders such as stone, tumor, or stricture usually is easily recognized. However, a number of interpretive pitfalls are inherent in the procedure (Table 53–2).[3, 6–9, 11] The most common problems in interpretation of operative cholangiograms are failure of contrast material to enter the duodenum, inadequate evaluation of the intrahepatic ducts (usually secondary to incomplete filling), and differentiation of air bubbles from stones.[6, 9]

The operative cholangiogram in our patient (see Fig 53–1) shows dilated ducts, a filling defect

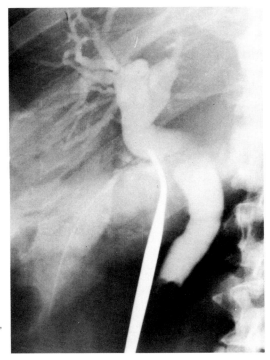

FIG 53–1.
Operative cholangiogram shows a dilated bile duct, a distal common duct defect, and absence of contrast material in the duodenum.

in the distal common duct, and no contrast material entering the duodenum. The upper margin of the defect is meniscoid and slightly irregular; the lower margin is not defined. The intrahepatic ducts are filled, and no intrahepatic ductal defects are seen. There is slight underfilling of the oblique segment of the common hepatic duct just proximal to the cystic duct.

This case demonstrates failure of contrast material to enter the duodenum, one of the more commonly observed difficulties in operative cholangiography. This finding may be related to an impacted stone, tumor, stricture, or spasm. The

characteristic defects produced by these lesions usually are easily recognized (Fig 53–2): an impacted stone typically presents as a smooth meniscoid defect; tumors may demonstrate a smooth or irregular margin; strictures typically are smoothly tapered and unchanging; spasm produces a short segment gradual smooth narrowing of the distal duct.[6] The appearance may be confusing when irregular or multiple stones present an irregular

TABLE 53–2.

Common Interpretive Problems in Operative Cholangiography

Failure of contrast material to enter the duodenum
  Spasm
  Stone
  Tumor
  Stricture
Inadequate evaluation of intrahepatic ducts
  Incomplete filling of intrahepatic ducts
  Failure to account for all major bile ducts
  Superimposition of intrahepatic ducts
Differentiation of air bubbles from stones
Difficulty in evaluating the sphincter segment
Problems related to the cystic duct remnant
Failure to identify surgically significant congenital
  ductal anomalies

TABLE 53–1.

Common Technical Problems in Operative Cholangiography

No preliminary film obtained
No collimation to the right upper quadrant
Films poorly centered or poorly exposed
Common duct projected over the spine
Inadequate penetration of contrast medium
  (especially in dilated ducts)
Grid lines or grid cutoff from improper alignment of
  grid and x-ray beam
Incomplete filling of intrahepatic radicles
Failure of contrast material to enter the duodenum

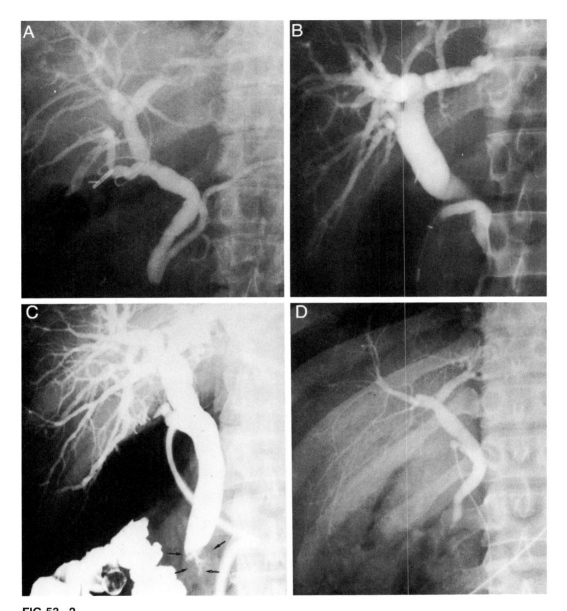

FIG 53–2.
Operative cholangiograms demonstrate failure of contrast material to enter the duodenum secondary to an impacted stone **A** (note also an accessory right hepatic duct inserting into the cystic duct), stricture **B** (chronic pancreatitis), tumor **C,** (bile duct carcinoma), and spasm **(D).** (**A** from Reid SH, Cho SR, Shaw CI, et al: *Am J Roentgenol* 1986; 147:1181–1182. Used by permission.)

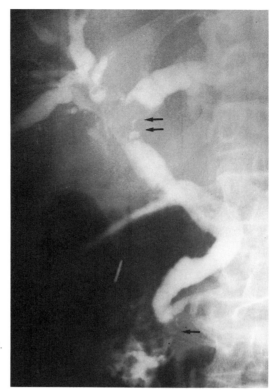

FIG 53–3.
Irregular intraluminal filling defect at bifurcation
(double arrows) that has the appearance of a tumor.
Exploration revealed multiple adherent stones in a
bile plug. Note presence of an additional stone in
the distal duct *(single arrow).*

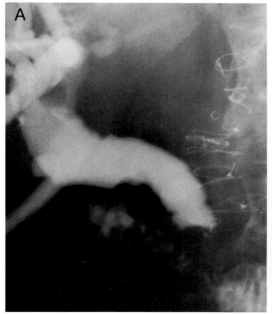

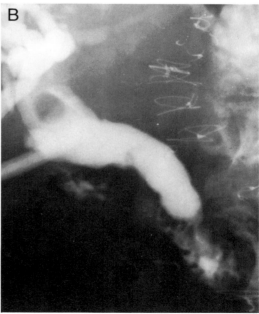

FIG 53–4.
A, pseudocalculus defect at distal end of duct from
sphincteric contraction. **B,** note change in appearance with relaxation. A retained stone in the common
hepatic duct is seen on both films. (From Turner MA,
Cho SR, Messmer JM: *Radiographics* 1987;
7:1067–1105. Used by permission.)

contour mimicking a tumor or when polypoid tumors mimic stones.[12] Calculi mixed with an amorphous bile plug or soft mudlike calculi may have an irregular border or adhere to the wall of the duct, simulating a fixed mural mass (Fig 53–3). Intraductal polypoid tumors may mimic common duct stones, especially if the complete borders of the lesion are not well defined.

Spasm may result in failure of contrast material to enter the duodenum and can be confused with a stricture or an impacted stone. It is a frequent finding on operative cholangiograms, occurring in as many as 25% of patients after common duct exploration.[13] Spasm may be related to rapid or forceful injection of cold or irritating contrast material or to surgical manipulation of the sphincter of Oddi. Anesthetic agents such as morphine sulfate and fentanyl citrate produce spasm.[13]

Contraction of the sphincter of Boyden, the circular muscle fibers of the distal common duct

proximal to the sphincter of Oddi, can produce absence of flow into the duodenum and an obstruction with the radiographic features of an impacted stone. This "pseudocalculus defect"[14, 15] has a meniscoid or flat appearance, is smooth, and seems to fill the lumen without enlarging it (Fig 53–4). The pseudocalculus defect differs from stone by its transient nature and because the inferior border cannot be outlined.

When spasm or the pseudocalculus defect occurs during operative cholangiography additional maneuvers may be necessary to exclude a true obstructing lesion (Fig 53–5). The injection of additional contrast material may be all that is necessary to cause the spasm to disappear. If persistent, spasm may be relaxed by the intravenous administration of glucagon.[16] If this fails, manual compression of the common duct proximal to the injection site before repeating the injection may result in relaxation of the area.[17]

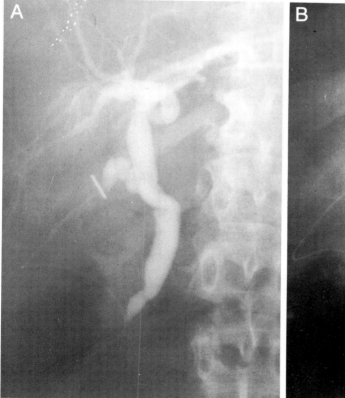 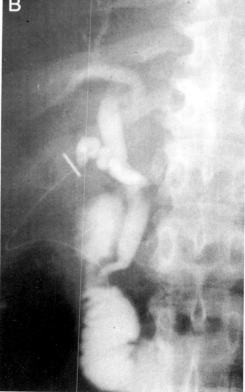

FIG 53–5.
A, operative cholangiogram showing well-filled ducts and distal "obstruction" in a patient with spasm. **B,** note relaxation of spasm after administration of glucagon.

Another common area of difficulty is incomplete evaluation of the intrahepatic ductal system. This may result from failure to account for all major ducts and bifurcations, from incomplete filling of the intrahepatic ducts, especially the left hepatic duct, or from superimposition of intrahepatic branches. Intrahepatic ducts must be demonstrated completely to evaluate for intrahepatic calculi, which occur in 17% to 23% of patients with common duct stones,[6] and to detect the presence of primary intrahepatic ductal diseases such as sclerosing cholangitis or tumor.

An appreciation of normal anatomy is essential to the adequate evaluation of the intrahepatic ductal system; it is impossible to determine if the cholangiogram is complete otherwise. Every major branch must be accounted for. Normally the right and left hepatic ducts converge to form the common hepatic duct. The two major branches of the right hepatic duct are a dorsocaudal branch and a ventrocranial branch. The central portion of the dorsocaudal branch has a characteristic hooklike configuration prior to coursing peripherally.[9, 18] The bifurcation area is the most common site of anatomic variation in the biliary tract, with the dorsocaudal branch of the right hepatic duct draining into the left hepatic duct in 12% of patients and the dorsocaudal branch joining the right and left hepatic ducts to form a trifurcation in 11%.[18]

Superimposition of the major intrahepatic branches is common and is more pronounced in patients with markedly dilated ducts. The bifurcation of the dorsal and ventral branches of the right hepatic duct frequently is superimposed, and thus a stenosing lesion or small stone at the bifurcation may be missed (Fig 53–6). Conversely, overlapping intrahepatic ducts can create the erroneous impression of an intrahepatic calculus. Rotating the patient to an oblique position will separate the ducts so that hidden lesions may be detected.

One of the most common errors in cholangiographic interpretation is overlooking absence of filling of the left hepatic duct. Because of its anterior position, the left hepatic duct is notoriously difficult to fill in the supine patient during operative cholangiography (Fig 53–7). This problem is compounded by the common practice of tilting the patient to the right to avoid ductal overlap from the spine. The common hepatic duct also may be difficult to fill completely in the supine patient, because of its oblique anterior uphill course as it passes caudally to join the cystic duct. Inadequate opacification or "streaming" of contrast material in this area may obscure stones.[11]

Failure to fill the intrahepatic ducts warrants additional examination to exclude obstructing stone or tumor. If a major branch is absent or terminates abruptly, an obstructing calculus must be suspected (Fig 53–8). Use of the left posterior oblique or Trendelenburg position, increased injection pressure, and occlusion of the distal ducts temporarily

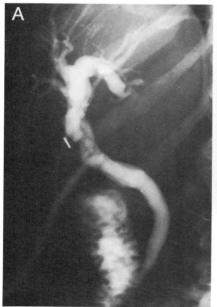
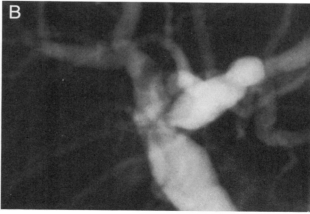

FIG 53–6.
A, overlapping intrahepatic ducts on apparently normal operative cholangiogram obscured a right hepatic duct stone. **B,** Stone was visible after turning the patient to the left oblique position.

tained common duct stones. *Am J Surg* 1973; 125:51–54.

5. Burhenne HJ: Nonoperative extraction of stones from the bile ducts. *Semin Roentgenol* 1976; 11:213–217.

6. Sachs MD: Routine cholangiography, operative and post-operative. *Radiol Clin North Am* 1966; 4:547–569.

7. Goldberg HI: Operative and post-operative cholecystocholangiography. *Semin Roentgenol* 1976; 11:203–211.

8. Clemett AR: Operative and post-operative cholangiography, in Berk RN, Clemett AR (eds): *Radiology of the Gallbladder and Bile Ducts.* Philadelphia, WB Saunders Co, 1977.

9. Thompson WM: The optimal radiographic technique for operative and T-tube cholangiography. *Crit Rev Diagn Imag* 1986; 26:107–176.

10. Burhenne HJ: Problem areas in the biliary tract. *Curr Prob Radiol* 1975; 5:28–40.

11. Monford DC, Clone JN: Source of error in operative cholangiography. *Arch Surg* 1970; 100:664–667.

12. Turner MA, Cho SR, Messmer JM: Pitfalls in cholangiographic interpretation. *Radiographics* 1987; 7:1067–1105.

13. Chessick KC, Black S, Hoye SJ: Spasm and operative cholangiography. *Arch Surg* 1975; 110:53–57.

14. Beneventano TC, Shein CJ: The pseudocalculus sign in cholangiography. *Arch Surg* 1969; 98:731.

15. Mujahed Z, Evans JA: Pseudocalculus defect in cholangiography. *Am J Roentgenol* 1972; 116:337–341.

16. Ferrucci JT Jr, Wittenberg J, Stone LB, et al: Hypotonic cholangiography with glucagon. *Radiology* 1976; 118:446–467.

17. Schwartz SA: A technique for operative cholangiography to evaluate failure of passage of contrast material. *Surg Gynecol Obstet* 1984; 158:589–590.

18. Puente SG, Bannura GC: Radiological anatomy of the biliary tract: Variations and congenital anomalies. *World J Surg* 1983; 7:271–276.

19. Reid SH, Cho SR, Shaw CI, et al: Anomalous hepatic duct inserting into the cystic duct. *Am J Roentgenol* 1986; 147:1181–1182.

20. Baer JW, Abiri M: Right hepatic artery as a cause of pseudocalculus in the biliary tree. *Gastrointest Radiol* 1982; 7:269–273.

21. Ring EJ, Ferrucci JT Jr, Eaton SB, et al: Villous adenomas of the duodenum. *Radiology* 1972; 104:45–48.

22. Miller JH, Gisvold JT, Weiland LH, et al: Upper gastrointestinal tract: Villous tumors. *Am J Roentgenol* 1980; 134:933–936.

CHAPTER 54

Filling Defect in the Common Bile Duct on T Tube Cholangiogram

William M. Thompson, M.D.

Case Presentation

A 52-year-old man had undergone a cholecystectomy and common duct exploration because of cholelithiasis and choledocholithiasis 6 weeks earlier. A follow-up
T tube cholangiogram was obtained (Fig 54–1). What are the findings? What is
the recommended technique for T tube cholangiography? How should this problem be treated?

DISCUSSION

Multiple filling defects within the common bile
duct represent retained common duct stones, a frequent finding in patients undergoing cholecystectomy. In most patients the stones are removed successfully during the initial operation. The routine
use of intraoperative cholangiography and chole-
dochoscopy has aided in their detection and has reduced the incidence of retained common duct
stones. However, retained common duct stones still
occur in 1% to 3% of patients after cholecystectomy.

Before the common duct stones are removed
they must be detected by direct cholangiography.
This chapter describes the technique for T tube
cholangiography and discusses the various methods
for the removal of common duct stones.

The standard technique for T tube cholangiography uses low kilovoltage (70 to 75 kVp) and a dilute contrast agent (10% to 15% iodine solution).
Long exposure times (2 to 4 seconds) are required

for low kVp use, and these long exposure times
may produce significant motion distortion. Compared with high kVp, there is also an increased
amount of radiation to the patient and to medical
personnel. For T tube cholangiography low kVp can
be used effectively because modern fluoroscopic
equipment has very high milliamperage (ma) (800
to 1,200 ma). One disadvantage of the dilute contrast agent and low kVp technique is that there may
be a lack of penetration of the contrast agent–filled
duct and thus failure to detect bile duct calculi.

Thompson et al.[1] reported a technique using a
high kVp–high contrast agent concentration (110
kVp and 38% iodine) for direct cholangiography.
Phantom and clinical results indicated that this technique produced results that were as good as or better
than the standard low kVp–low contrast agent concentration method (70 kVp and 15% iodine; Fig
54–2). The advantages of the high kVp–high contrast agent concentration technique are greater exposure latitude; shorter exposure time and therefore
less motion distortion; less radiation to the patient

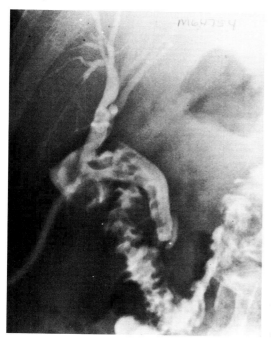

FIG 54–1.
T tube cholangiogram demonstrates multiple filling defects after surgery for cholecystolithiasis and choledocholithiasis. What are the defects?

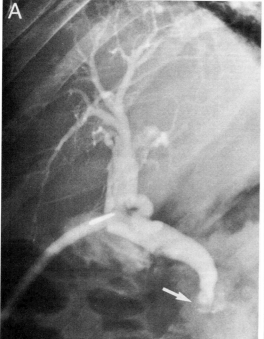 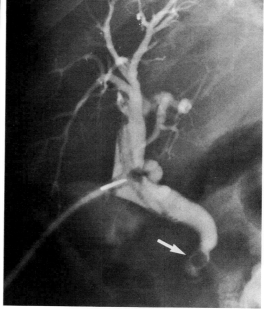

FIG 54–2.
T tube cholangiography. **A,** this film, exposed at 75 kVp, 40 Ma after a 15% iodine solution was injected into the biliary system, is an example of the low kVp–low iodine concentration technique. Note the poor demonstration of the retained stone *(arrow)* and the T tube. **B,** this film, exposed at 110 kVp, 8 Ma after a 38% iodine solution was injected into the biliary system, is an example of the high kVp–high iodine solution technique. Note the distal common duct stone *(arrow)* and the excellent demonstration of the T tube.

and operating room personnel; and most important, adequate penetration of the bile ducts.

Based on these results Thompson et al.[1] recommend using a high kVp (100 to 110 kVp) and high contrast agent concentration (30% to 38% iodine) technique for T tube cholangiography. These same principles apply to operative cholangiography.

ANATOMY

Figure 54–3 shows the anatomy of the intrahepatic bile ducts.[2] The left hepatic ducts are ventral and cross over the spine into the epigastrium and left upper quadrant. These ducts fill well with the patient prone, but poorly with the patient supine. Therefore, to ensure filling of the left hepatic ducts

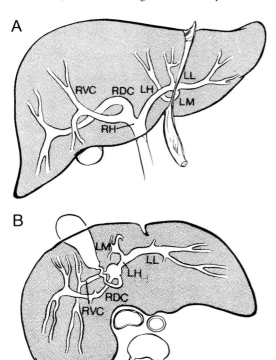

FIG 54–3.
Anatomy of bile ducts, anterior **(A)** and transverse **(B)** views. *RH* = right hepatic duct; *RVC* = right ventrocranial segmental duct; *RDC* = right dorsocaudal segmental duct; *LH* = left hepatic duct; *LM* = left medial segmental duct; *LL* = left lateral segmental duct. (From Thompson WM: *Contemp Diagn Radiol* 1984; 7:1–6. Used by permission.)

patients should be turned from supine to left side down or prone during operative and T tube cholangiography. The right hepatic ducts are dorsal and fill well with the patient supine. Thus, to ensure that the entire right ductal system is completely filled with contrast during endoscopic retrograde cholangiopancreatography (ERCP) the patient must be rotated from the prone to the supine position. Without complete filling of the biliary system abnormalities such as retained duct stones, particularly in the left hepatic ducts, may not be detected in some patients.

REMOVAL OF RETAINED COMMON DUCT STONES

Percutaneous stone removal has become the preferred procedure in most cases, obviating the need for a second operation.[3–7] The procedure initially reported in the early 1970s subsequently was popularized by Burhenne.[3] The technique utilizes a steerable catheter and baskets of different caliber. The procedure can be performed in both inpatients and outpatients.

PATIENT PREPARATION

After common duct exploration surgeons routinely request a T tube cholangiogram prior to withdrawal of the tube. This study is needed to detect retained stones, because most patients with retained stones rarely have symptoms in the immediate postoperative period. For the radiographic technique to be safe and successful the T tube sinus tract must mature. The normal waiting period is 5 to 6 weeks after the operation. Although stones may be extracted earlier than 4 weeks after surgery, frequently this is technically more difficult because the sinus tract is not as well healed and may be harder to cannulate. The longer the T tube is left in place the better the tract will be formed. Similarly, larger T tube tracts (14 F catheter or larger) facilitate the removal of stones. Occasionally the os at the T tube–skin site is inflamed, and manipulation in these instances may be painful to the patient. Very rarely local anesthesia is needed; analgesics and sedatives seldom are necessary during the procedure. Meperidine (Demerol) and diazepam (Valium) can be given intravenously as needed. Routinely we give all patients antibiotic therapy. The agent of choice is cefamandole (Mandol), 1 mg intravenously, administered the evening before and the morning of the procedure. The antibiotic is omitted on the day after the procedure if the patient has no fever; it is continued if fever occurs. Fever, which is the most common complication, occurs after particularly difficult extractions and is presumably from bacterial cholangitis. Because we administer antibiotic therapy routinely, our patients rarely have fever or sepsis.

METHOD

We use polyethylene catheters that can be steered by a control handle (Medi-Tech, Watertown, Mass.) and baskets for the extraction. The equipment is reusable. The baskets come in three sizes, ranging from 9 to 25 mm. The size of the basket and catheter used is determined by the sinus tract and the size of the duct as demonstrated on the T tube cholangiogram. To permit more flexibility in choosing the basket, the largest caliber catheter that

the sinus tract and duct will accept is used. Initially the largest basket that will fit in the duct is tried, because it is effective for both large and small stones. Occasionally a smaller basket proves more successful, particularly with smaller stones.

A second T tube cholangiogram on the day of the procedure is usually necessary, because patients referred for stone removal on the basis of a previous T tube study may have passed the stone or stones. In these cases the T tube is removed and the patient discharged. The initial injection at the time of the stone removal should be performed slowly to ensure that the stone or stones do not become impacted in the distal duct and that the ducts do not become overdistended, thereby risking the development of cholangitis.

After the presence of the stone or stones is confirmed, the T tube is removed and the patient's abdomen is prepared and draped for the insertion of the steerable catheter under sterile conditions (Fig

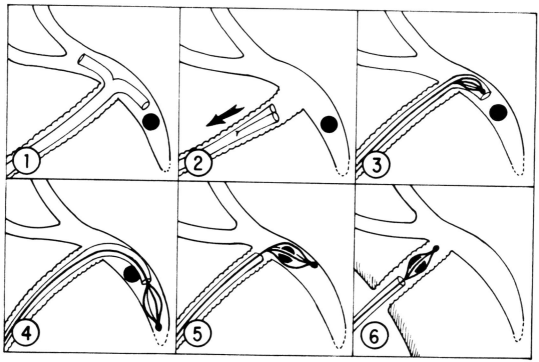

FIG 54–4.
Schematic of the procedure for nonoperative removal of retained common duct stones: *(1)* Obtain a T tube cholangiogram to identify the retained stone. *(2)* Remove the T tube at least 5 to 6 weeks after surgery. *(3)* Advance the steerable catheter into the bile duct via the T tube sinus tract and pass the sheath containing the stone basket through the catheter. *(4)* Open the basket after it has passed the stone. *(5)* Entrap the stone with the basket. *(6)* Remove the stone through the sinus tract. (Adapted from Burhenne HJ: *Am J Roentgenol* 1980; 134:888–898.)

54–4, 1 and 2). After the catheter has been inserted, contrast medium usually is needed to localize the stones.

In most cases guidewires are not necessary. However, if catheter manipulation is difficult, a guidewire (0.035 or 0.038 mm J) may be inserted through the T tube tract and directed toward the stones. Guidewires may be needed in some patients with T tube tracts with multiple angles or in patients in whom the procedure is being performed before the 6-week waiting time has elapsed. The wire is inserted through the T tube into the bile duct; then the tube is removed. A second guidewire is placed through the sinus tract to provide a guide for the catheter, ensuring secure passage back into the biliary system.

After the catheter is introduced into the bile duct the tip is positioned past the stone (Fig 54–4, 3 and 4). The basket is then coaxially introduced through the catheter, advanced past the stone, and opened. This should be done so that the basket does not point into the wall and potentially injure the bile duct. The open basket is moved adjacent to the stone and jiggled, twirled, or moved slightly to and fro until the stone is engaged (Figs 54–4, 5).

After the stone is engaged, fragmentation is

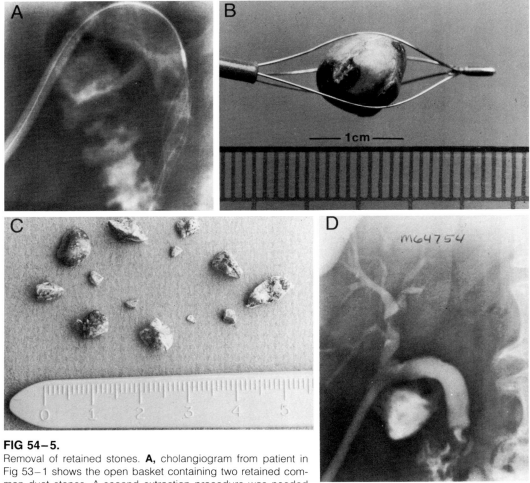

FIG 54–5.
Removal of retained stones. **A,** cholangiogram from patient in Fig 53–1 shows the open basket containing two retained common duct stones. A second extraction procedure was needed to remove all of the stones. **B,** this enlarged photograph shows a stone in the basket after being extracted. **C,** photomicrograph of multiple stones and fragments removed from the common duct. **D,** T tube cholangiogram taken the day after removal of the last stones indicates no evidence of any other retained stones.

avoided by withdrawing the basket only slightly in the catheter and removing the entire system as a unit with a smooth, uninterrupted motion (Figs 54–4, 6). If the stone is large, removal through the tract may be uncomfortable for the patient; withdrawing a stone through the musculature of the abdominal wall may prove difficult. Usually, however, steady gentle pressure allows removal of the stone. Occasionally fragmentation cannot be avoided when a large stone is being withdrawn through a small sinus tract. If the stone fragments or if there are multiple stones the sequence can be repeated (Fig 54–5). A second injection of contrast material is necessary to demonstrate remaining stones and to provide a visual path back into the biliary system.

After completion of the procedure a straight red rubber catheter (10 to 16 F) is inserted into the common bile duct and taped to the skin. This catheter provides easy access for repeat cholangiography and, if necessary, repeated manipulation of the bile duct on subsequent days.

After all of the stones have been extracted another cholangiogram is obtained, usually the next day, to confirm a normal ductal system (Fig 54–5, D). Occasionally tiny (1 to 3 mm) fragments remain. If these cannot be engaged easily they are left in place and will pass spontaneously.

RESULTS AND COMPLICATIONS

Table 54–1 shows the results from five series.[3–7] The overall success rate in more than 1,000 cases reported is 90% to 95%. Failures are related to the inability to catheterize the biliary system via the sinus tract; inability to recatheterize the system after initial stones have been removed; and the presence of stones in cystic duct remnants, in hepatic ducts, and in the distal common bile duct.

In patients with midline sinus tract openings the tracts are tortuous and may be difficult to instrument. These midline tracts may require the radiologist's hands to be directly under the radiation beam, although this usually can be avoided by turning the patient on his or her side. Because midline sinus tracts make manipulation quite difficult, surgeons should be instructed to place the T tube sinus tract opening in the lateral aspect of the abdominal wall as close to the common bile duct as possible.

Our complications[7] and those reported by Burhenne[3] are listed in Table 54–2. Fever and sepsis are the most common complications, but usually can be avoided by administering antibiotics.

OTHER METHODS USING THE T TUBE TRACT

The basket technique is the most popular method of removing retained common duct stones, but other procedures also use the T tube tract. Stones can be pushed through the ampulla of Vater with a straight catheter.[3] Malleable forceps have been used with great success in both the United States and South America.[4] Ultrasound has been used to fragment stones,[8, 9] and mono-octanoate, an investigational dissolving solution, has been used to help diminish the size of large stones, which then can be extracted.[10] Sinus tracts have been dilated up to 20 F to allow passage of a choledochoscope for stone removal under direct vision.[11] Nevertheless,

TABLE 54–1.
Results of Common Bile Duct Stone Removal

Author	Number	%
Burhenne[3]	628/661	95
Mazzariello[4]	204/222	92
Garrow[5]	99/105	94
Bean et al.[6]	33/44	75
Thompson[7]	54/60	90
Total	1018/1092	92

TABLE 54–2.
Complications of Stone Removal

Complication*	Thompson[7] n	%	Burhenne[3] n	%
Sinus tract leak	0		7	
Peritoneal spill	1		2	
Bile collections	0		2	
Fever†	3		11	
Sepsis	1		2	
Pancreatitis	0		2	
Vasovagal reaction	0		1	
Total	5/60	8.3	27/661	4.1

*Only one reported death in more than 1,000 cases in the literature.
†Most common.

the basket technique is the preferred method for removing most retained common duct stones.

OTHER METHODS OF REMOVING COMMON DUCT STONES

Stones have been removed from the common duct after percutaneous cholangiography and placement of a percutaneous biliary drainage catheter[12] (Fig 54–6). Stones have been pushed into the duodenum with a biliary drainage guidewire and standard angioplasty balloons, and peroral endoscopic sphincterotomy has been used successfully for common duct stone removal.[13] Most of these patients have had distal common bile duct stones. In the majority of cases the stones pass spontaneously after sphincterot-

omy. A long basket passed through the endoscope can be used to extract the retained stones that do not pass.

Extracorporeal lithotripsy was developed for urinary stones and gallstones and has been used to treat common duct stones.[14] Although the exact role of lithotripsy in treating biliary stones has not been determined, it is likely to be an adjunctive procedure for common duct stones.

SUMMARY

Basket removal of retained common duct stones is simple and extremely safe. It can be performed in any radiology department with fluoroscopic equipment and saves the patient a second operation.

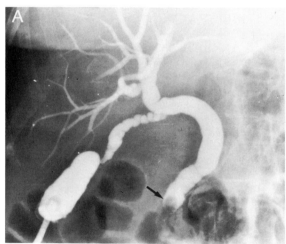

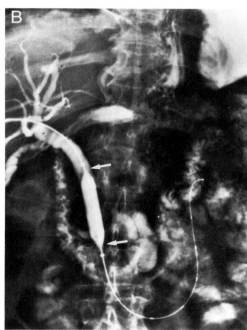

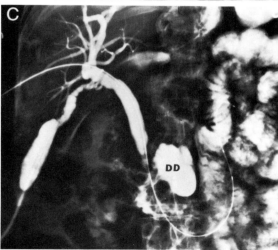

FIG 54–6.
Percutaneous removal of common duct stone. **A,** cholangiogram performed through cholecystectomy tube demonstrates a distal common duct stone *(arrow)* obstructing the bile duct. **B,** radiograph demonstrates contrast agent–filled angioplasty balloon *(arrows)* used to push common duct stone into the duodenum. **C,** follow-up cholangiogram shows normal common bile duct. *DD* = duodenal diverticulum.

REFERENCES

1. Thompson WM, Halvorsen RA, Gedquadas RK: High kVp vs low kVp for T tube and operative cholangiography. *Radiology* 1983; 146:635–642.
2. Wiechel K-L: Surgical anatomy of the bile ducts, in Berci G, Hamlin JA (eds): *Operative Biliary Radiology*. Baltimore, Williams & Wilkins Co, 1981, pp 37–50.
3. Burhenne HJ: Percutaneous extraction of retained biliary tract stones: 661 patients. *Am J Roentgenol* 1980; 134:888–898.
4. Mazzariello R: Review of 220 cases of residual biliary tract calculi treated without reoperation: An eight-year study. *Surgery* 1973; 73:299–306.
5. Garrow DG: The removal of retained biliary tract stones. *Br J Radiol* 1977; 50:777–782.
6. Bean WJ, Smith SL, Calonje MA: Percutaneous removal of residual biliary tract stones. *Radiology* 1974; 113:1–9.
7. Thompson WM: Removal of retained common duct stones. *Contemp Diag Radiol* 1984; 7:1–6.
8. Martin EC, Wolff M, Neff RA: Use of the electrohydraulic lithotriptor in the biliary tree in dogs. *Radiology* 1981; 139:215–217.
9. Bean WJ, Daughtry JP, Rodan BA, et al: Ultrasonic lithotripsy of retained common bile duct stone. *AJR* 1985; 144:1275–1276.
10. Thistle JL, Carlson GL, Hofmann A: Monooctanoate, a dissolution agent for retained cholesterol bile duct stones. *Gastroenterology* 1980; 78:1016–1022.
11. Whelan JG Jr, Moss JP: Biliary tract exploration via T tube tract: Improved technique. *Am J Roentgenol* 1979; 133:837–842.
12. Perez MR, Oleaga JA: Removal of a distal common bile duct stone through percutaneous transhepatic catheterization. *Arch Surg* 1979; 104:107–109.
13. Siegel JH: Endoscopic papillotomy in the treatment of biliary tract disease: 258 procedures and results. *Dig Dis Sci* 1981; 26:1057–1064.
14. Gelfand E, McCullough DL, Myers RT, et al: Choledocholithiasis: Successful treatment with extracorporal lithotripsy. *AJR* 148:1114–1116.

CHAPTER 55

Cholangiography of Biliary Strictures

Robert L. MacCarty, M.D.

Case Presentation

A transhepatic cholangiogram (Fig 55–1) was obtained in a 30-year-old man with a 9-year history of recurrent right upper quadrant pain, epigastric pain, fever, and jaundice. His past history is significant for the presence of intermittent diarrhea since age 14 years. A cholecystectomy was performed at age 25 years. What is the diagnosis? What are the differential diagnostic considerations? What forms of treatment might be considered?

DISCUSSION

The dominant radiographic finding on the cholangiogram is the long stricture involving the common hepatic and common bile ducts. Biliary strictures may be benign or malignant (Table 55–1) and may result from diseases arising primarily in the bile ducts or outside the ducts and affecting them secondarily. The correct diagnosis usually can be made by analyzing the morphologic features of the stricture, its location, the degree of obstruction, and whether there are multiple strictures and by correlating key historical, clinical, and laboratory information.

MALIGNANT BILIARY STRICTURES

Solitary strictures that occur spontaneously (i.e., in the absence of surgical injury or other obvious cause) are overwhelmingly likely to be malignant,[1–4] particularly when they result in high-grade obstruction as evidenced by marked dilation above the stricture (Fig 55–2). Malignant strictures typically are at least 1 cm long and from 0.5 cm to several centimeters in diameter. The location of a malignant stricture is helpful in predicting the histologic findings (Table 55–2). A lesion obstructing an intrahepatic duct (Fig 55–3) is likely to be a metastasis, a cholangiocarcinoma, or a hepatoma. From the hilum of the liver to mid–common duct, malignant biliary strictures are usually the result of cholangiocarcinoma or malignant lymphadenopathy. Lymph nodes in the porta hepatis and hepatoduodenal ligament may be involved by metastasis or lymphoma (Fig 55–2). As they enlarge and coalesce they characteristically encroach on and ultimately obstruct the adjacent bile ducts. Direct invasion of the mid- or upper portions of the common duct is also typical of carcinoma of the gallbladder (Fig 55–4).

In most cases malignant strictures of the lower common duct form as the result of encasement by adenocarcinoma of the head of the pancreas (Fig 55–5). These relatively common tumors also may obstruct the common duct more superiorly as a re-

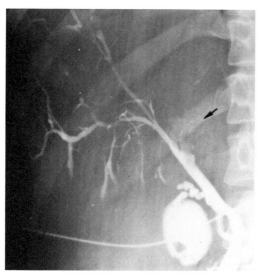

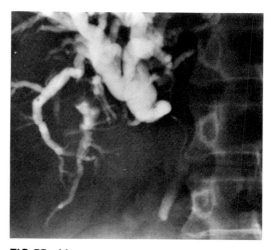

FIG 55–11.
Mirizzi's syndrome. Stricture of the mid–common duct with high-grade obstruction. At surgery, inflammatory reaction from cholelithiasis was found.

FIG 55–9.
Multiple intrahepatic duct strictures due to diffuse cholangiocarcinoma. Note polypoid component obstructing the lumen of the left hepatic duct *(arrow)*.

onset of biliary disease preceded the cholecystectomy by 4 years. These facts effectively rule out surgical injury and primary gallbladder disease as causes of the biliary stricture.

A rare cause of iatrogenic stricture, recently

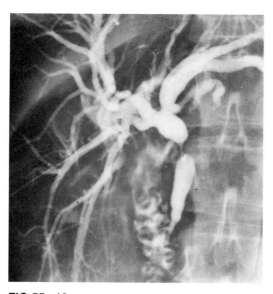

FIG 55–10.
Annular stricture of the mid–common duct after cholecystectomy. Note surgical clip at the inferior margin of the stricture.

recognized, is injury resulting from hepatic artery infusion of chemotherapeutic agents for the treatment of liver metastasis[6] (Fig 55–12). A history of recent infusion chemotherapy in a patient with a new common duct stricture is sufficient to make the diagnosis, but is not a consideration in the case under discussion.

Benign strictures of the lower common duct include those due to papillary stenosis and those due to involvement of the common duct by pancreatitis. Papillary stenosis is often overdiagnosed in patients with unexplained right upper quadrant pain. A proper diagnosis should be made in the setting of focal narrowing in the region of the ampulla of Vater (Fig 55–13) and in a patient with definite evidence of cholestasis (e.g., abnormal results of liver function studies or manometry or failure of the common duct to decrease in size in response to a fatty meal). By the same token, there is grave danger in misdiagnosing papillary stenosis in a patient with periampullary carcinoma. The diagnosis of papillary stenosis therefore is in part a diagnosis of exclusion and should be made only after the papillary region has been visualized directly (at endoscopy or surgery) and adequate biopsy studies have proved the lesion to be benign. The cholangiographer can only suggest the diagnosis, because it is usually impossible to rule out carcinoma solely on the basis of cholangiographic appearances.

Chronic pancreatitis obstructing the common duct also may be difficult or impossible to distin-

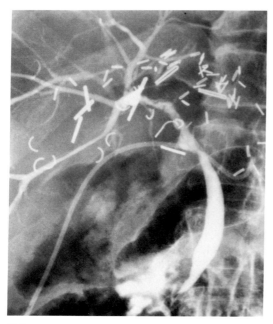

FIG 55–12.
Common hepatic duct stricture secondary to hepatic arterial infusion chemotherapy.

guish from its malignant counterpart. In general, the degree of obstruction from pancreatitis is less than with pancreatic carcinoma, the stricture is longer, and the strictured segment in some cases assumes a more smoothly undulating appearance (Fig 55–14). The presence of calcification in the head of the pancreas strongly favors pancreatitis, and typical changes in the pancreatic ducts on retrograde pancreatography also support the diagnosis of pancreatitis. Even when the diagnosis of pancreatitis is firm, the clinical picture may be confounded by the occasional case in which pancreatic carcinoma arises in a setting of chronic pancreatitis.

Chronic pancreatitis and papillary stenosis are excluded in the case presented because of the length of the stricture, which extends all the way up to the hilum, and because the intrahepatic ducts, although incompletely filled, are on close inspection also abnormal (see Fig 55–1). Note several areas of slight stricture at the origin of the left hepatic duct and along the proximal portion of the inferior segmental branch, and the slight fusiform dilation of a peripheral segment of the superior branch of the left hepatic duct. These findings indicate the presence of a disease process involving the biliary tree diffusely.

The most likely diagnosis in this case is some

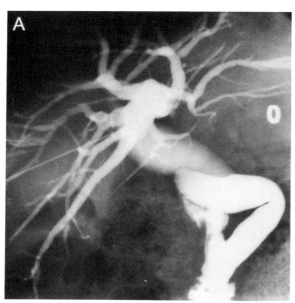
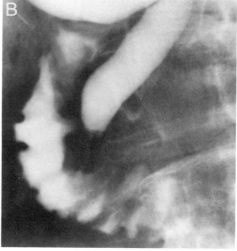

FIG 55–13.
A, dilated intrahepatic and extrahepatic bile ducts on transhepatic cholangiography. **B,** localized view of the lower common duct shows a short stricture of the periampullary portion of the duct. Endoscopy with bi- opsy showed no evidence of malignancy. Clinical follow-up confirmed the diagnosis of benign papillary stenosis.

gives a multilobulated configuration to the surface of the cirrhotic appearing liver.

In this case, because of the importance of distinguishing a benign regenerative nodule from a potentially resectable hepatocellular carcinoma, percutaneous biopsy was performed at the initial CT examination (see Fig 56–1,D). Histologic analysis showed the tumor to be a grade 2 hepatocellular carcinoma. Subsequently a well-defined tumor, 5 cm in diameter, was removed by wedge resection. The cause of cirrhosis was eventually attributed to chronic active liver disease resulting from non-A, non-B viral hepatitis. One potentially helpful diagnostic laboratory test that was not performed prior to biopsy in this case is determination of the serum α-fetoprotein level. This substance is markedly increased in a majority of patients with sizable hepatocellular carcinomas.

A solitary mass is only one of the forms that hepatocellular carcinoma may have at presentation.[21] These tumors may be classified according to gross morphologic features as solitary, multinodular, or diffuse. Multinodular forms occur either as a large dominant mass with one or more smaller satellite lesions nearby or as multiple nodules of similar size. A tumor also may be classified according to its relationship to the adjacent parenchyma. There are well-defined expanding tumors and poorly defined spreading tumors. The masses illustrated in Figures 56–1, 56–3, and 56–7 are of the expanding type. These tumors tend to be relatively slow growing and well differentiated, and the pressure they exert on surrounding parenchyma may cause a reactive fibrous capsule to form at the periphery of the mass. Internally the tumors often contain foci of necrosis (Fig 56–7). The spreading types of hepatocellular carcinomas tend to be higher grade malignancies that infiltrate or invade rather than compress adjacent parenchyma (Fig 56–8).

A distinct histologic subtype of hepatocellular carcinoma that merits separate consideration is fibrolamellar hepatocellular carcinoma. Unlike the ordinary type of hepatocellular carcinoma, this variety typically occurs in adolescents and young adults, is not associated with cirrhosis or hepatitis, and seldom causes elevation of serum α-fetoprotein levels.

Fibrolamellar hepatocellular carcinoma is more likely to be resectable than is the more common form of the tumor, and has a better prognosis. Fibrolamellar hepatocellular carcinomas are typically large, sharply circumscribed expanding masses, often encapsulated by reactive fibrous tissue. Internally they are usually of mixed composition, with hypervascular tumor tissue, necrotic foci, and fi-

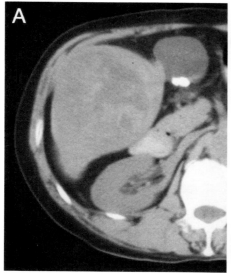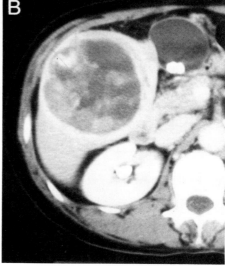

FIG 56–7.
Hepatocellular carcinoma. **A,** unenhanced computed tomographic scan shows well-defined mass of heterogeneous hypodensity. **B,** with contrast enhancement the peripheral rim and well-vascularized internal components of the tumor become hyperdense, whereas major parts, representing ischemic, necrotic, and fibrotic components, remain unenhanced.

brotic scars. Occasionally a central fibrotic scar has a stellate configuration similar to the scar sometimes seen in focal nodular hyperplasia. Internal calcification is also common in fibrolamellar tumors.[22] Although the presence of calcification or a stellate scar in a hepatocellular carcinoma should suggest fibrolamellar disease, these features are not unknown in nonfibrolamellar hepatomas (see Fig 56−4).

Sectional imaging by US, CT, and MRI can display many of the architectural features of hepatocellular carcinomas, and it is worthwhile to make note of these characteristics, because they may have bearing on the prognosis and treatment.

Imaging examinations also can reveal significant secondary effects of hepatocellular carcinoma, the presence or absence of which may be influential in determining the most appropriate method of treatment. It is important to search for evidence of extension of tumor into the portal venous system and to look for invasion of a major hepatic vein or bile duct (see Fig 56−8). Extrahepatic metastases, which occur in a variety of locations, should also be sought. Evaluation for these manifestations, together with a precise assessment of the extent of neoplasm within the liver, is of particular importance in determining the potential resectability of a tumor.

Even tumors that cannot be removed from the liver by resection may be amenable to interventional therapy. Among innovative forms of treatment currently in various stages of development is radiologically directed local ablation of tumors by alcohol injection, cryosurgery, or laser. Complete replacement of the liver with a transplanted organ is also being performed.

COMMENT

Among the many benefits of contemporary abdominal imaging as it applies to the workup in a patient with a mass in the liver is the vast amount of information that it can contribute beyond the identification and evaluation of the mass itself. In the case presented, for example, the discovery of cirrhosis established the likelihood of hepatocellular carcinoma. Incidentally, it is not at all rare for cirrhosis that has not been diagnosed clinically to come to attention first on an imaging examination of the liver. Negative information, such as the absence of metastasis or major vascular involvement, which would have rendered the tumor unresectable, was equally important. In this case conventional real-time US and contrast-enhanced CT were all that was needed to determine patency of the vessels and to exclude gross metastatic disease with reasonable certainty. Had they been needed, Doppler sonogra-

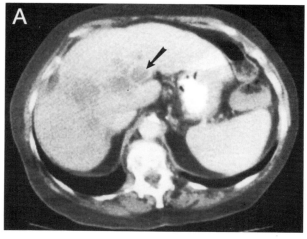 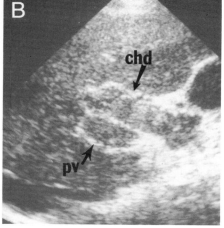

FIG 56−8.
Invasive hepatocellular carcinoma. **A,** computed tomographic scan shows a rather poorly defined multifocal intrahepatic mass, mostly lying across the border between the left and right lobes. The lumen of the portal vein *(arrow)* is not opacified with contrast ma- terial, indicating thrombotic involvement. **B,** sonogram shows the portal vein *(pv)* and dilated common hepatic duct *(chd)* to be filled with echogenic material representing tumor thrombus.

phy, MRI, or angiography also would have been available.

When nonoperative tissue characterization is desired a percutaneous biopsy with precise placement of the needle under US or CT guidance is almost always possible. Without the guidance of imaging, safe or accurate percutaneous biopsy of the mass in Figure 56–1 would not have been feasible. The standard precautions should be observed in the performance of percutaneous biopsy. Especially in cases of impaired liver function, this would include an evaluation of clotting ability. In the case of a potentially resectable mass, it is also worthwhile to know the surgeon's opinion before proceeding with a biopsy; some surgeons object to this preoperative intervention.

REFERENCES

1. Clain JE, Stephens DH, Charboneau JW: Ultrasonography and computed tomography in focal fatty liver. *Gastroenterology* 1984; 87:948–952.
2. Stanley J, Vujic I, Schabel SI, et al: Evaluation of biliary cystadenoma and cystadenocarcinoma. *Gastrointest Radiol* 1983; 8:245–248.
3. Pandolfo I, Blandino G, Scribano E, et al: CT findings in hepatic involvement by *Echinococcus granulosus*. *J Comput Assist Tomogr* 1984; 8:839–845.
4. Didier D, Weiler S, Rohmer P, et al: Hepatic alveolar echinococcus: Correlative US and CT study. *Radiology* 1985; 154:179–186.
5. Thompson WM, Chisholm DP, Tank R: Plain film roentgenographic findings in alveolar hydatid disease—*Echinococcus multilocularis*. *AJR* 1972; 116:345–358.
6. Ralls PW, Colletti PM, Quinn MF, et al: Sonographic findings in hepatic amebic abscess. *Radiology* 1982; 145:123–196.
7. Taboury J, Porcel A, Tubiana J-M: Cavernous hemangiomas of the liver studied by ultrasound: Enhancement posterior to a hyperechoic mass as a sign of hypervascularity. *Radiology* 1983; 149:781–785.
8. Scheible W, Gosink BB, Leopold GR: Grayscale echographic patterns of hepatic metastatic disease. *AJR* 1977; 129:983–987.
9. Stephens DH: The liver, in Haaga JR, Alfidi RJ (eds): *Computed Tomography of the Whole Body*, ed 2. St Louis, CV Mosby Co, 1988, pp 792–853.
10. Scatarige JC, Kenny JM, Fishman EK: CT of giant hemangiomas. *AJR* 1987; 149:83–85.
11. Rabinowitz SA, McKusick KA, Strauss HW: ^{99m}Tc red blood cell scintigraphy in evaluating focal liver lesions. *AJR* 1984; 143:63–68.
12. Brodsky RI, Friedman AC, Maurer AH, et al: Hepatic cavernous hemangioma: Diagnosis with ^{99m}Tc-labeled red cells and single photon emission CT. *AJR* 1987; 148:125–129.
13. Glazer GM, Aisen AM, Francis IR, et al: Hepatic cavernous hemangioma: Magnetic resonance imaging. *Radiology* 1985; 155:417–420.
14. Ros P, Lubbers PR, Olmsted WW, et al: Hemangioma of the liver: Heterogeneous appearance on T2-weighted images. *AJR* 1987; 149:1167–1170.
15. Solbiati L, Livraghi T, DePra L, et al: Fine-needle biopsy of hepatic hemangioma with sonographic guidance. *AJR* 1985; 144:471–474.
16. Welch TJ, Sheedy PF II, Johnson CM, et al: Focal nodular hyperplasia and hepatic adenoma: Comparison of angiography, CT, US, and scintigraphy. *Radiology* 1985; 156:593–595.
17. Mattison GR, Glazer GM, Quint LE, et al: MR imaging of hepatic focal nodular hyperplasia: Characterization and distinction from primary malignant hepatic tumors. *AJR* 1987; 148:711–715.
18. Wilbur AC, Gyi B: Hepatocellular carcinoma: MR appearance mimicking focal nodular hyperplasia. *AJR* 1987; 149:721–722.
19. Lubbers PR, Ros PR, Goodman ZA, et al: Accumulation of technetium-99m sulfur colloid by hepatocellular adenoma: Scintigraphic-pathologic correlation. *AJR* 1987; 148:1105–1108.
20. Alpern MB, Lawson TL, Foley WD, et al: Focal hepatic masses and fatty infiltration detected by enhanced dynamic CT. *Radiology* 1986; 158:45–49.
21. Teefey SA, Stephens DH, James EM, et al: Computed tomography and ultrasonography of hepatoma. *Clin Radiol* 1986; 37:339–345.
22. Freidman AC, Lichtenstein JE, Goodman Z, et al: Fibrolamellar hepatocellular carcinoma. *Radiology* 1985; 157:538–587.

CHAPTER 57

Fever, Increased White Blood Cell Count: Abnormal Liver

Robert A. Halvorsen Jr., M.D.

Case Presentation

A 59-year-old woman with a history of aplastic anemia came to the emergency room complaining of right upper quadrant pain. The patient had fever, and a computed tomographic (CT) scan was obtained to rule out liver abscess (Fig 57–1). Because of diffuse inhomogeneity seen on the CT scan, a liver-spleen scan was obtained on the same day (Fig 57–2); findings on this scan were considered normal. However, because the right upper quadrant pain persisted, ultrasonography (US) of the gallbladder also was performed that day (Fig 57–3), and showed two hypoechoic areas anterior to the portal vein within the liver parenchyma. What do these hypoechoic areas represent? Why did the CT scan fail to detect these lesions?

DISCUSSION

The CT examination demonstrates diffuse inhomogeneity in the liver parenchyma. Although no focal mass was identified, the diffuse "mottled" appearance with areas of lower density than surrounding areas suggests fatty infiltration of the liver; the subsequent liver-spleen scan shows no evidence of a photon-deficient area. The two studies were considered compatible with fatty infiltration of the liver.

Detection of focal abnormalities within the liver depends on contrast or density difference between the surrounding normal liver and the area of abnormality. A limitation of liver CT scans is encountered when the background liver is of lower than normal density. Such a finding is the result of either diffuse or focal fatty infiltration of the liver.

If the degree of fatty infiltration is severe, with a liver parenchymal CT number approximately that of water, structures of similar density within the liver parenchyma may be undetectable (Fig 57–4). Because bile has a CT number approximately that of water, dilated intrahepatic bile ducts may be overlooked in patients with severe fatty liver. Figure 57–5 demonstrates a dilated bile duct anterior to the portal vein on US. The CT scan shows severe fatty infiltration of the liver but no dilated intrahepatic bile ducts. Figure 57–4 shows an oval structure in the right upper quadrant; although the structure is isodense with the liver, it represents the dilated gallbladder. On more inferior sections (Fig 57–6) the pancreatic head mass producing the obstruction can be identified.

Quint and Glazer[1] reported 47 patients with

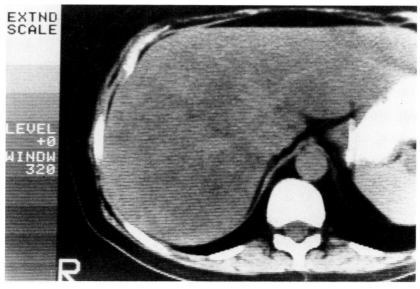

FIG 57–1.
Computed tomographic scan of the liver demonstrates diffuse "mottled" appearance with areas of slightly decreased density intermingled with normal appearing liver. No focal mass is identified. (From Halvorsen RA Jr, Foster WL Jr, Wilkinson RH Jr, et al: *Gastrointest Radiol* 1988; 13:135–141. Used by permission.)

fatty infiltration of the liver. In seven of these patients attenuation of the liver and bile differed by less than 10 Hounsfield units (HU). In two patients dilated intrahepatic bile ducts were invisible on CT scans because the bile was isodense with the fatty liver parenchyma. These authors suggested that for maximal accuracy scans should be obtained both before and after administration of intravenous contrast material in patients with severe fatty liver.

The detection of masses within the liver also may be difficult in patients with fatty infiltration. Metastatic lesions in the liver usually appear as areas of low density with an attenuation value 10 to 20 HU less than the surrounding normal liver paren-

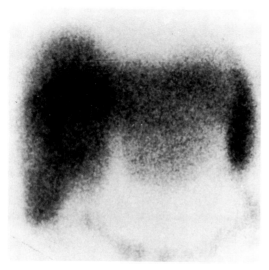

FIG 57–2.
Radionuclide liver-spleen scan, anterior view, is normal, with no evidence of photon-deficient area. (From Halvorsen RA Jr, Foster WL Jr, Wilkinson RH Jr, et al: *Gastrointest Radiol* 1988; 13:135–141. Used by permission.)

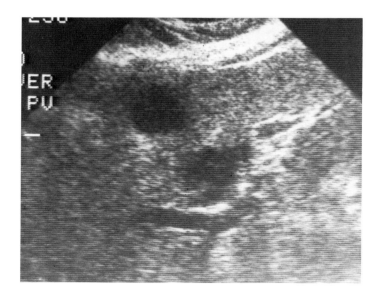

FIG 57–3.
Right upper quadrant ultrasonogram obtained the same day as the computed tomographic scan (Fig 57–1) and the liver-spleen scan (Fig 57–2) shows two hypoechoic areas anterior to the portal vein.

(From Halvorsen RA Jr, Foster WL Jr, Wilkinson RH Jr, et al: *Gastrointest Radiol* 1988; 13:135–141. Used by permission.)

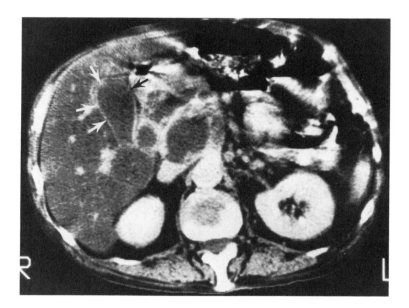

FIG 57–4.
Contrast-enhanced computed tomographic scan of the upper abdomen shows diffuse low density in the liver, with no evidence of dilated interhepatic bile ducts. Oval structure on the medial aspect of the liver represents dilated gallbladder *(arrows).*

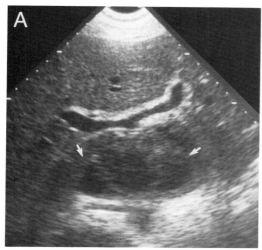

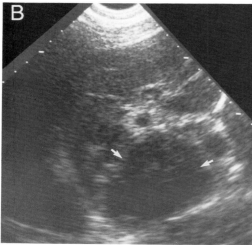

FIG 58–3.
Hepatic abscess. Transverse **(A)** and longitudinal **(B)** ultrasound studies show a mostly fluid-filled mass *(arrows)* in the caudate lobe, with thick irregular walls.

(e.g., echogenicity and relative attenuation values). In a series of 29 small (<5 cm) HCCs in 18 patients, sensitivity for radionuclide imaging was 39%, for ultrasonography 50%, for CT 56%, and for infusion hepatic arteriography 94%. Lesions larger than 3 cm could be detected by all studies; lesions between 2 and 3 cm usually were shown by ultrasound and CT but not nuclear medicine studies; and for those smaller than 2 cm infusion hepatic arteriography was necessary.[7]

Hemangioma, the most common benign hepatic tumor, occurs in all age groups, has a female predominance, and is found in 4% of autopsies. Be-

cause hepatic hemangiomas are benign and usually require no therapy, they must be distinguished from malignant tumors.[8] On ultrasonography most hemangiomas appear as well-defined hyperechoic lesions with posterior acoustical enhancement; less frequently they are hypoechoic or of mixed echogenicity, and may have a geographic appearance. The lesions in Figure 58–1 are typical of hemangioma. If suspicion of malignancy is low in a patient with such lesions (incidental detection, normal liver function test results, no known tumor), either no additional tests or a follow-up ultrasonogram is performed in a few months. When the clinical suspicion of malignancy is higher or when a definitive diagnosis is needed, additional imaging studies are indicated.

For many years arteriography was the "gold standard" for diagnosing hepatic hemangiomas. The arteriographic findings of hemangioma usually are characteristic (Fig 58–5) and include a normal sized feeding hepatic artery and early capillary staining in a ring or C-shaped configuration. The stain persists well into the venous phase, but arteriovenous shunting or prominent draining veins usually are absent.

The typical CT appearance of hepatic hemangioma is of a low-attenuation mass on noncontrast scans, peripheral contrast enhancement during the bolus phase, and isodensity in comparison with the normal surrounding hepatic parenchyma on delayed scans (Fig 58–6,A and B). However, in a series of 58 hemangiomas this "typical" appearance was seen in only 32 (55%).[9] Although some investigators believe that these criteria are too rigid, we have found that the false positive rate increases if less rigid criteria are used.

Hepatic scintigraphy with single photon emission CT (SPECT) imaging and ^{99m}Tc-labeled red blood cells is a highly sensitive and specific study for diagnosing 1 to 2 cm hepatic hemangiomas.[10–12] The lesion typically appears normal on initial scans but shows increased activity (becoming a "hot" lesion) compared with normal surrounding hepatic parenchyma on delayed scans (30 minutes to 24 hours after injection; Figs 58–7 and 58–8). Although HCC also may show increased activity on delayed scans, increased activity occurs on the initial or flow-phase study scans as well, but is not seen in hemangioma. Metastatic tumors show no increased activity on either initial or delayed scans. Using these criteria we have correctly diagnosed hepatic hemangioma in 85% to 90% of cases. Therefore this technique is now the procedure of choice at our institution when a suspected hemangioma is

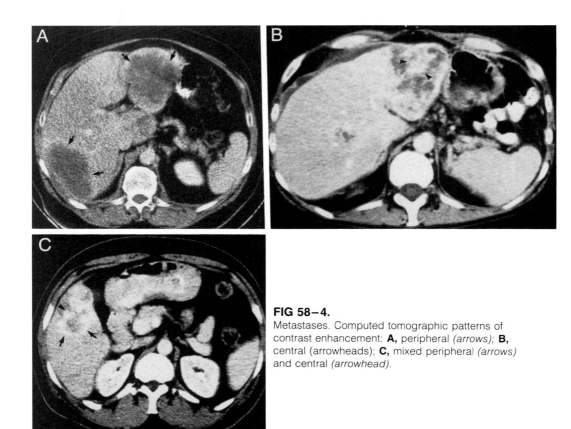

FIG 58–4.
Metastases. Computed tomographic patterns of
contrast enhancement: **A,** peripheral *(arrows);* **B,**
central (arrowheads); **C,** mixed peripheral *(arrows)*
and central *(arrowhead).*

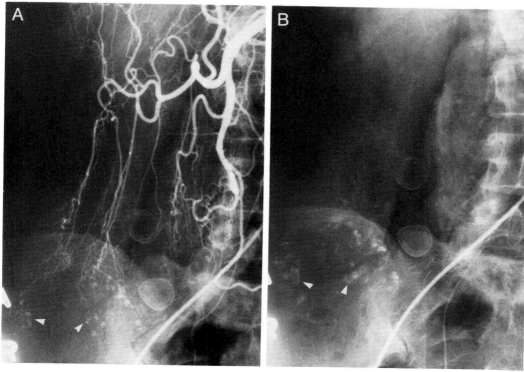

FIG 58–5.
Hemangioma. Typical arteriogram of hepatic hemangioma. **A,** normal sized feeding arteries, early capillary staining *(arrowheads).* **B,** persistent venous staining *(arrowheads).*

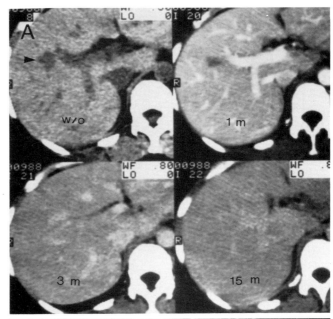

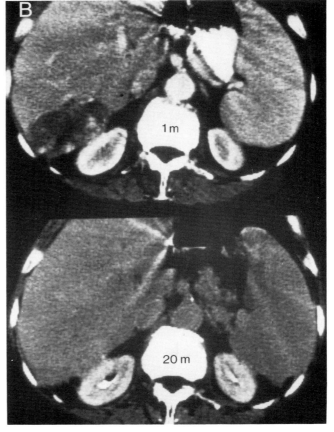

FIG 58–6.
Computed tomographic appearance of
hemangioma. **A,** small hemangioma
(arrowhead) has low attenuation on
scan without contrast; peripheral and
then central enhancement on bolus (1
minute) and 3-minute scans,
respectively; and isodense appearance
on delayed (15 minute) image. **B,**
larger hemangioma demonstrates more
focal intense peripheral enhancement
initially (1 minute) and isodense
appearance on delayed (20 minute)
scan.

of 30 HU led to sensitivity of 79% and specificity of 94%.

Focal fatty liver should be suspected when a low-density lesion is seen on a CT scan and if specific findings are present. In our study of 16 patients with focal fatty liver we noted four distinctive features[4] (Fig 59–2): (1) Focal fatty liver was never spherical. (2) No evidence of mass effect was present. On a CT scan mass effect appears as a bulge in the liver contour if the process is subcapsular, and displacement of normal vessels if it is within the liver parenchyma. (3) Distribution

of the focal fatty liver was predominately subsegmental (89%), and lobar in the remaining patients. (4) A poorly defined or indistinct margin of the areas of focal fatty liver was seen in 79% of the patients, and a well-defined margin was identified in 21%.

In all of our patients the regions of focal fatty liver were recognized because their attenuation value (density) was visibly lower than that of the surrounding "normal" liver and splenic tissue. In 10 of 11 patients who were examined without intravenous contrast medium the mean density of the focal

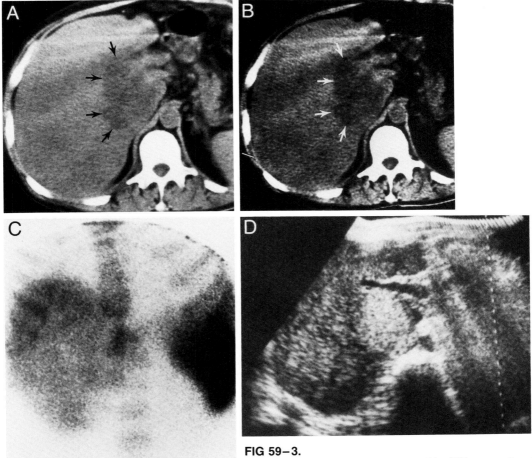

FIG 59–3.
A, unenhanced computed tomographic (CT) scan. Focal area of decreased attenuation in caudate lobe of the liver *(arrows).* **B,** CT scan. Narrow window setting of **A** better demonstrates lesion *(arrows).* **C,** radionuclide liver-spleen scan, anterior view. Decreased uptake in liver with shift to bone marrow and spleen but no focal photon-deficient area. **D,** sonogram of the liver. Hyperechoic area corresponds to area of fatty liver on CT scan.

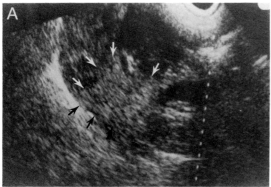

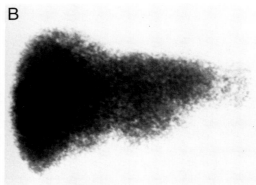

FIG 59–4.
A, sonogram. Oblique view of the right upper quadrant demonstrates hyperechoic area *(arrows)* in the liver, corresponding to areas of low density on computed tomographic scan. **B,** radionuclide liver-spleen scan, normal anterior view. (From Halvorsen RA, Korobkin M, Ram PC, et al: CT appearance of focal fatty infiltration of the liver. *AJR* 1982; 139:277–281. Used by permission.)

fatty liver tissue was at least 0 HU; in only one of the 11 patients did the attenuation value itself suggest that fatty tissue was present.

The degree of fatty infiltration correlates with the density on CT images. In general, because of the partial volume averaging of the fatty hepatocytes and other components of the liver, such as vessels and Kupffer cells, the CT number of the area involved will be above zero, even with severe fatty infiltration. Bydder et al.[12] compared liver biopsy findings, with quantitative measurement of fat content, with CT numbers and showed a strong inverse correlation between liver CT number and fatty change as observed histologically. Alpern et al.[11] also found that 0 HU measurements were uncommon in fatty infiltration, occurring on unenhanced studies in only three of their 23 patients. However, Bashist et al.[13] reported one case in which severe fatty infiltration initially presented with a CT number of −16 HU; the number increased during resolution of the fatty liver. Another study reported CT numbers below 0 HU in six patients with focal fatty liver.[14] The criterion for inclusion in that study was an area of the liver with a CT number less than zero. The areas of focal fatty liver had a mean value of −18 ± 15 HU. The authors stated that lack of vascular displacement (no mass effect) aids in the correct diagnosis of fatty liver but that homogeneity of the lesion is also a helpful differential point. Whereas metastatic lesions often demonstrate heterogeneous density, each small area of fatty infiltration tends to be homogeneous, even if the overall appearance of the liver is heterogeneous.[14]

The CT appearance of focal fatty liver can suggest the diagnosis, especially when a vessel extends across the area of low density with no evidence of mass effect; however, another study occasionally is required for confirmation (see Fig 59–2). Because fatty infiltration occurs within hepatocytes, often the reticuloendothelial system of the liver is normal. Therefore the Kupffer cells, which are studied with technetium 99m–sulfur colloid, should be undisturbed in the uncomplicated case of fatty liver.[4, 15] The liver-spleen scan should be normal, with no evidence of a photon-deficient area to correspond with the area of abnormality seen on the CT scan. In general a radionuclide liver scan usually resolves any confusion about the differential diagnosis of focal fatty infiltration: a well-defined focus of photon deficiency is due to neoplasm rather than to focal fatty liver.

Occasionally the appearance of focal fatty liver is atypical, with small rounded areas of low attenuation scattered throughout the liver and mimicking metastases. Three cases have been reported with this nodular appearance, and in all three patients results of the radionuclide liver-spleen scan were normal.[16, 17]

A normal liver-spleen scan, however, is not always seen in patients with fatty liver. Alcoholic cirrhosis may present as a diffuse abnormality within the liver parenchyma, suggesting hepatocellular disease (Fig 59–3). In such case the liver-spleen scan may be helpful, because there is no photon-deficient area to correspond with the abnormality on the CT scan. However, if liver uptake is so poor that the

TABLE 60–1.

Porta Hepatis/Hepatoduodenal Ligament Masses/Processes

Intrahepatic Benign	Intrahepatic Malignant
Hepatic cyst	Hepatocellular carcinoma
Cystadenoma	Cystadenocarcinoma
	Cholangiocarcinoma
	Hepatic metastases
Extrahepatic Benign	Extrahepatic Malignant
	Cholangiocarcinoma
Choledochal cyst	Metastatic disease (lymph nodes)
	Regional tumors (hepatic, biliary, gallbladder, pancreas, gastric, esophageal)
	Distant tumors (colon, breast, lung, melanoma)
	Lymphoma
Intramural/Mural	
Cholangitis	
Cholangiocarcinoma	
Metastatic disease	

Rarely metastatic disease can present as an intraluminal filling defect.[2]

Our patient's follow-up visit was to an oncologist. Six months earlier small cell carcinoma of the lung had been treated with radiation and chemotherapy. Therefore the findings represent metastases to the porta hepatis and pancreaticoduodenal lymph nodes.

The diagnosis was confirmed and treatment initiated. Had the patient had recognizable jaundice, the workup may have been different. A full discussion of the workup of jaundice is beyond the scope of this chapter, but some mention should be made

concerning the relative roles of US, CT, endoscopic retrograde cholangiopancreatography (ERCP), and percutaneous transhepatic cholangiography (PTC) in a patient with a suspected obstructing porta hepatis mass.[2, 3, 5–8]

For many, US is the initial screening examination in the evaluation of jaundice.[6–11] The normal structures of the hepatoduodenal ligament, the presence of intrahepatic biliary ductal dilation, and the caliber of the common bile duct can be demonstrated reliably with US. Furthermore, US is less expensive and does not require administration of intravenous contrast material or ionizing radiation.

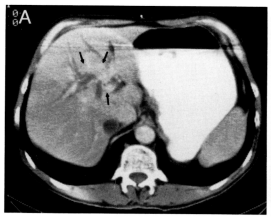
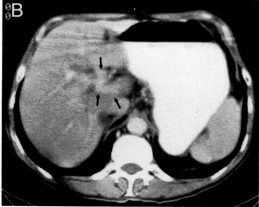

FIG 60–4.
A and **B,** enhancing infiltrative process due to cholangiocarcinoma. The bile ducts are dilated and the portal vein margin is obscured by the enhancing tumor *(arrows)* in the porta hepatis.

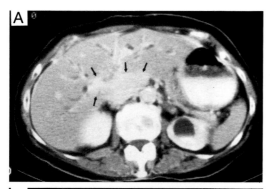

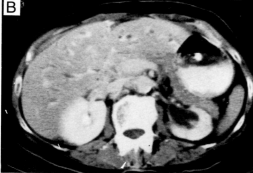

FIG 60–5.
A and **B,** enhancing infiltrative process due to metastatic disease of unknown origin. The bile ducts are dilated and the margin of the vein obscured by the enhancing tumor *(arrows).*

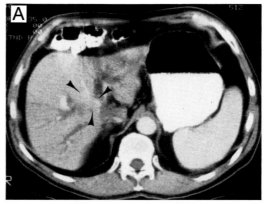

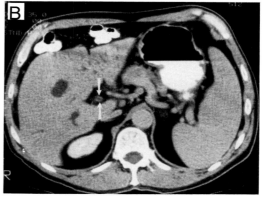

FIG 60–6.
Thickened common bile duct wall due to cholangiocarcinoma. **A,** enhancing infiltrative process *(arrowheads)* from cholangiocarcinoma obstructs the ducts at the level of the porta hepatis. **B,** common bile duct wall *(arrows)* is thickened.

When biliary ductal dilation is detected, US can provide helpful information as to the level and cause of obstruction.[6, 9, 10] The value of this technique is limited in large patients and in the presence of bowel gas. Furthermore, US may not detect early biliary obstruction.[11]

State-of-the-art US requires a meticulous scanning technique. We believe that the technique reported by Laing et al.[10] yields the most accurate information with the least number of inadequate studies. Their technique starts with examination of the distal common bile duct in the transverse plane through the head and uncinate process of the pancreas while the patient is semierect (60 degrees to vertical) and in the right posterior oblique position (45 degrees to vertical). If overlying gas limits evaluation, water is given to the patient, the patient is positioned to be semierect, and another scan is done. Transverse and longitudinal scans of the head and body of the pancreas are obtained with the pa-

tient remaining semierect. The proximal common bile duct and intrahepatic bile ducts are subsequently evaluated with the patient in the supine left posterior oblique position.

Preselection of patients prior to US examination is important. Patients most suitable for US are thin and young and have little subcutaneous and retroperitoneal fat. Patients who are large or who have an ileus probably should be initially evaluated with CT.

CT often is performed after the diagnosis of dilated ducts has been made with US.[6, 7, 12] In a patient with known or suspected malignant disease CT may be used as the first imaging study. As with US, meticulous technique is vital to ensure a high diagnostic yield. We routinely scan the liver and pancreas with an incremental dynamic technique.[13] We use an automated injector to give a bolus of 50 ml intravenous contrast material over 20 seconds (2.5 ml/sec), at which time scanning starts. The injection rate is then decreased to 1.2 ml/sec until the entire 200 ml is given. The liver and pancreas can be evaluated over 2 minutes with a GE model 9800 CT scanner (General Electric Medical Systems Division, Milwaukee) at 120 kVp and 170 Ma, with 2-second scans and a 7-second interscan delay. This technique yields the best lesion-liver-pancreas contrast. If primary pancreatic or biliary disease is suspected, contiguous 5 mm slices are obtained, proceeding from the level of the third portion of the duodenum cephalad toward the porta. Before dynamic scanning with intravenous contrast medium, we obtain test cuts through the second portion of the duodenum to ensure opacification of the sweep with either air or positive contrast.

In most cases, when US and CT findings are compared biliary obstruction is diagnosed and the cause and level are identified. With meticulous technique, modern rapid CT scanners, and phase focus US units are equivalent in their ability to diagnose obstruction and its level.[5-8] In our retrospective study of porta hepatis masses, CT appeared to detect the infiltrative soft tissue process more easily, whereas US more readily diagnosed small periportal and hepatoduodenal ligament lymph nodes.[2] In patients with a known primary malignant lesion CT has the advantage of surveying the entire abdomen.

ERCP and PTC generally are reserved for cases in which US and CT fail to detect the level and cause of obstruction, when internal or external drainage may be necessary or desirable, and when intrabiliary brushings or biopsy specimens are necessary for cytologic diagnosis.[6] The choice of ERCP or PTC depends on the institution. The success of ERCP depends on the skill and aggressiveness of the endoscopist and probably requires a greater expenditure of time and money per procedure. ERCP does have an advantage in that if the endoscopist is skillful an internal stent may be placed after sphincterotomy.[14]

In our patient ERCP was performed in the hope of placing such a stent. With radiation therapy there was concern that radiation-induced edema might obliterate the duct. The obstruction bridged the ductal confluence, and a stent could not be placed in one system without obstructing the other.

This case demonstrates the most common cause of obstruction in or around the porta hepatis—hepatoduodenal ligament: metastatic disease. In the unknown patient the described differential diagnosis and pattern recognition should be used to identify such a mass. Current noninvasive and invasive imaging techniques play a role in the diagnosis and treatment of this mass.

REFERENCES

1. Weinstein JB, Heiken JP, Lee JKT, et al: High resolution CT of the porta hepatis and hepatoduodenal ligament. *Radiographics* 1986; 6:55–74.
2. Baker ME, Silverman PM, Halvorsen RA, et al: Computed tomography of masses in periportal/hepatoduodenal ligament. *J Comput Assist Tomogr* 1987; 11:258–263.
3. Reiman TH, Balfe DM, Weyman PJ: Suprapancreatic biliary obstruction: CT evaluation. *Radiology* 1987; 163:49–56.
4. Zeman RK, Schiebler M, Clark LR, et al: The clinical and imaging spectrum of pancreaticoduodenal lymph node enlargement. *AJR* 1985; 144:1223–1227.
5. O'Connor KW, Snodgrass PJ, Swonder JE, et al: A blinded prospective study comparing four current noninvasive approaches in the differential diagnosis of medical versus surgical jaundice. *Gastroenterology* 1983; 84:1498–1504.
6. Zeman RK, Burrell MI, Gold JA, et al: The intrahepatic and extrahepatic bile ducts in surgical jaundice: Radiological evaluation and therapeutic implications. *CRC Crit Rev Diagn Imaging* 1984; 21:1–36.
7. Baron RL, Stanley RJ, Lee JKT, et al: A prospective comparison of the evaluation of biliary obstruction using computed tomography and ultrasonography. *Radiology* 1982; 145:91–98.
8. Gibson RN, Yeung E, Thompson JN, et al: Bile duct obstruction: Radiologic evaluation of level, cause, and tumor resectability. *Radiology* 1986; 160:43–47.
9. Honickman SP, Mueller PR, Wittenberg J, et al: Ultrasound in obstructive jaundice: Prospective evaluation of site and cause. *Radiology* 1983; 147:511–515.
10. Laing FC, Jeffrey RB, Wing VW, et al: Biliary dilatation: Defining the level and cause by real-time US. *Radiology* 1986; 160:39–42.
11. Zeman RK, Lee C, Jaffee MH, et al: Hepatobiliary scintigraphy and sonography in early biliary obstruction. *Radiology* 1984; 153:793–798.
12. Pedrosa CS, Casanova R, Rodriguez R: Com-

puted tomography in obstructive jaundice: The level of obstruction. *Radiology* 1981; 139:627–634.

13. Alpern MB, Lawson TL, Foley WD, et al: Focal hepatic masses and fatty infiltration de-

tected by enhanced dynamic CT. *Radiology* 1986; 158:45–49.

14. Cotton PB: Duodenoscopic placement of biliary prostheses to relieve malignant obstructive jaundice. *Br J Surg* 1982; 69:501–503.

PART VII

Pancreas

CHAPTER 61

Worsening Acute Pancreatitis: Rule Out Pseudocyst or Abscess

Michael P. Federle, M.D.

Case Presentation

A 24-year-old alcoholic woman was admitted to the hospital with a complaint of severe epigastric pain radiating to her back. She had a history of several similar but milder attacks. During the physical examination she was writhing in pain and had a tender, guarded abdomen with palpable "fullness" or mass in the epigastrium. Her pulse was 100 beats per minute and temperature 39° C. Laboratory findings included leukocytosis (29,000 cells/mm^3) and hyperamylasemia (500 Somogyi units). Bed rest, nasogastric suction, and large volumes of intravenous fluids failed to produce clinical improvement within 36 hours of admission. Abdominal computed tomography (CT) was performed (Fig 61–1). What are the diagnostic considerations? What should be done to confirm the diagnosis?

DISCUSSION

Acute pancreatitis is common in the United States and is associated with considerable morbidity and mortality. The disease may occur as a single attack or as repeated and progressive episodes (acute relapsing or recurrent pancreatitis), but the pancreas usually resumes its normal morphologic and functional integrity after resolution of the acute inflammatory process. Chronic pancreatitis is not clearly the end product of repeated episodes of acute pancreatitis but is defined as irreversible inflammatory disease of the pancreas.

Acute pancreatitis may result from numerous causes, but alcohol abuse and cholelithiasis account for more than 90% of cases. Regardless of the cause, the pathologic and radiographic findings are similar and represent a spectrum of changes.[1]

INDICATIONS FOR IMAGING PROCEDURES

In many cases of pancreatitis the diagnosis and management of the disease are straightforward. If a patient with a recent history of heavy alcohol intake has stabbing upper abdominal pain radiating to the back and hyperamylasemia, acute pancreatitis is the probable diagnosis and no immediate imaging evaluation beyond plain radiography is necessary. Horizontal beam films (upright or decubitus) should be obtained to rule out free air; pancreatic and biliary calculi also may be identified. During a patient's first hospitalization with pancreatitis, sonography and an upper gastrointestinal series are also obtained during the convalescent period to rule out biliary calculi and peptic ulcer disease, respectively. We are reluctant to perform an upper gastrointestinal examination in an acutely ill and unstable patient with presumed pancreatitis. The result is likely to be a suboptimal study of the stomach and duodenum and exacerbation of nausea and vomiting. In addition, the retained barium or iodinated contrast medium may adversely affect a subsequent CT scan, angiogram, or sonogram that may be required to evaluate possible complications of pancreatitis.

Acute pancreatitis generally is a clinical diagnosis, but manifestations vary widely and the correct diagnosis may not be considered. Peterson and Brooks[2] reported that a premortem diagnosis was not made in 43% of 40 patients who died of severe pancreatitis. Other diseases may simulate the clinical, laboratory, and radiographic manifestations of acute pancreatitis; these include acute cholecystitis, peptic ulcer disease, and bowel infarction. Patients may be subjected to nontherapeutic laparotomy, considered contraindicated in most cases of acute pancreatitis. Even more serious is a delay in surgical intervention in cases of bowel infarction misdiagnosed as acute pancreatitis.

Thus the role of sonography and CT is to help substantiate the clinical diagnosis and to identify surgically correctable abnormalities that may be responsible for the disease (e.g., gallstones) or that may have resulted from the disease (e.g., pseudocyst or abscess).

Sonography is unsurpassed in screening for biliary disease. In patients with pancreatitis who are not alcohol abusers, sonography commonly shows gallbladder and common duct stones as the likely cause of the acute pancreatitis. Criteria such as altered pancreatic size and echogenicity along with peripancreatic fluid or mass effects have been proposed for the sonographic diagnosis of pancreatitis. In addition to the diagnostic uncertainty caused by normal variability in size and texture, technical factors such as ileus and abdominal tenderness limit sonographic access to the pancreas and limit the value of sonography in acutely ill patients. Sonography reveals most pseudocysts but is much more limited in evaluation of extensive fluid collections or abscesses.[3, 4]

When patients fail to respond to conservative management or deteriorate clinically despite therapy, CT usually demonstrates the pathologic process. Although unexpected processes, such as perforated ulcers or infarcted bowel, may be diagnosed, CT usually confirms the clinical diagnosis of pancreatitis and answers the important question of whether an abscess, fluid collection, or other complication is present. CT signs of pancreatitis include pancreatic swelling, peripancreatic edema and infiltration of fat, thickened fascial planes, and peripancreatic fluid collections.[5–7]

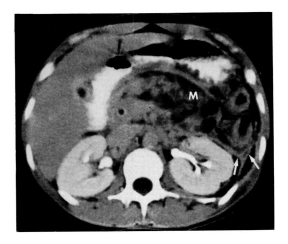

FIG 61–1.
Computed tomographic (CT) study in a 24-year-old woman with abdominal pain, fever, high white blood cell count, and a palpable mass. Heterogeneous mass *(M)* in the pancreatic bed displaces the stomach and duodenum. Note thickened renal and lateroconal fascia *(arrows)*. CT findings are consistent with phlegmon, early pseudocyst, or abscess.

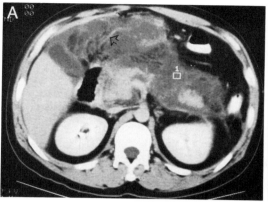
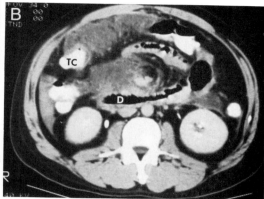

FIG 61–2.

Extensive pancreatitis, phlegmon. **A,** *cursor* marks part of a heterogeneous peripancreatic inflammatory process that fills the pancreatic bed, the left anterior pararenal space and the mesentery. Note the mesenteric vessel *(arrow).* **B,** inflammation envelops the duodenum *(D)* and the transverse colon *(TC)* by spreading along the transverse mesocolon. Phlegmonous masses such as this may resolve completely, evolve into pseudocysts, or become infected.

Semantic disputes have clouded our understanding of the natural history and significance of various complications of pancreatitis. Some authors describe most manifestations of extrapancreatic spread of inflammation as "fluid collections."[8] However, the majority of investigators prefer the term "phlegmon" to indicate an inflammatory mass arising from the pancreas that may go on to suppurate, liquefy, or resolve spontaneously. These are not fluid collections, as can be demonstrated by sonography or attempted needle aspiration, but represent boggy edematous mixtures of inflammation, exudate, and retroperitoneal fat. Phlegmonous extension is demonstrable by CT in 18% of unselected patients with pancreatitis[3] and in more than 50% of patients with more severe disease[4, 8] (Fig 61–2). Poorly encapsulated fluid accumulations do occur in pancreatitis, usually recognized as homogeneous, low-density, nonenhancing collections in the lesser sac or peritoneal cavity (Fig 61–3).

Pseudocysts are localized collections of necrotic tissue, old blood, and secretions that have es-

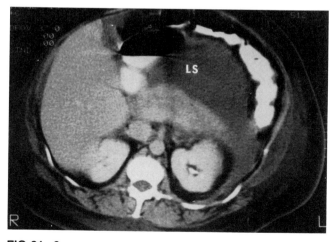

FIG 61–3.

Poorly encapsulated fluid collection distends the lesser sac *(LS).* Note extension of fluid or inflammation in the anterior pararenal space.

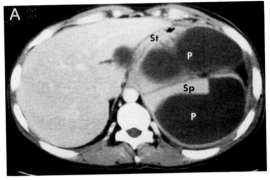

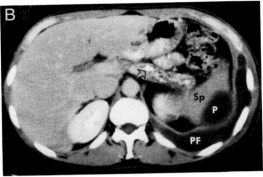

FIG 61-4.

Multiple extrapancreatic pseudocysts. **A,** complex pseudocysts *(P)* in the lesser sac displace the stomach *(St)* and the spleen *(Sp),* the latter due to subcapsular extension. **B,** subcapsular splenic pseudocyst *(P)* is again evident, along with pleural fluid *(PF)* and pancreatic calculi *(arrow).* Surgical drainage of the pseudocysts was unsuccessful. Percutaneous catheter drainage for 3 weeks resulted in complete resolution. *SP* = spleen.

caped from the pancreas damaged by acute inflammation.[9] These secretions, rich in proteolytic enzymes, may become loculated in the lesser sac or may extend along retroperitoneal tissue in any direction. Most pseudocysts are extrapancreatic and may dissect up into the mediastinum, liver, or spleen (Fig 61–4) or down as far as the groin. CT is the most accurate and useful means of showing the extent and number of pseudocysts as well as possible complications such as hemorrhage or obstruction of vessels or bile ducts (Fig 61–5). Pseudocysts are detected in about 10% of patients with acute pancreatitis.[5] CT and sonography may demonstrate evolution of a phlegmon into a pseudocyst by showing progressive liquefaction of the contents and development of a well-defined fibrous capsule. A pseudocyst may simulate a solid mass early in its formation, as blood and proteinaceous necrotic debris elevate the attenuation value. Sonography is useful in confirming the fluid nature of the contents of the developing cyst.

CT and sonography also are useful in following the course of phlegmons and pseudocysts. Within 6 weeks 20% to 44% of pseudocysts resolve sponta-

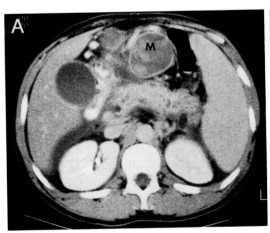
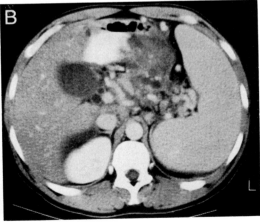

FIG 61-5.

Complications of pancreatitis. **A,** peripancreatic mass *(M)* is well encapsulated but contains heterogeneous high-density fluid characteristic of hemorrhage within a pseudocyst. Also note ascites and slight dilation of the pancreatic and common bile ducts. **B,** splenomegaly and numerous tortuous varices are caused by occlusion of the splenic vein by pancreatitis.

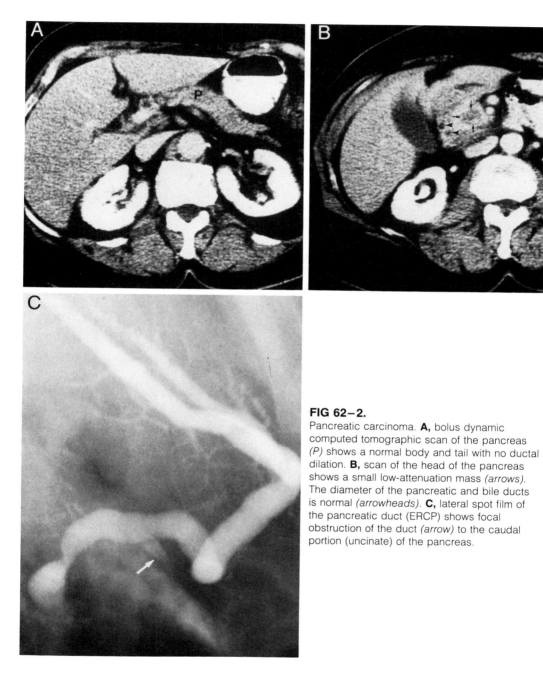

FIG 62–2.
Pancreatic carcinoma. **A,** bolus dynamic computed tomographic scan of the pancreas (P) shows a normal body and tail with no ductal dilation. **B,** scan of the head of the pancreas shows a small low-attenuation mass *(arrows)*. The diameter of the pancreatic and bile ducts is normal *(arrowheads)*. **C,** lateral spot film of the pancreatic duct (ERCP) shows focal obstruction of the duct *(arrow)* to the caudal portion (uncinate) of the pancreas.

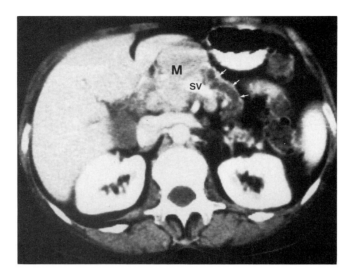

FIG 62–3.
Islet cell carcinoma. Bolus dynamic computed tomographic scan of the pancreas shows a large mass *(M)* in the mid-body. The mass is virtually isointense with the liver, suggesting a diagnosis of islet cell tumor rather than ductal carcinoma. The upstream pancreatic duct *(arrows)* is dilated and the surrounding parenchyma is atrophic. *SV* = splenic vein.

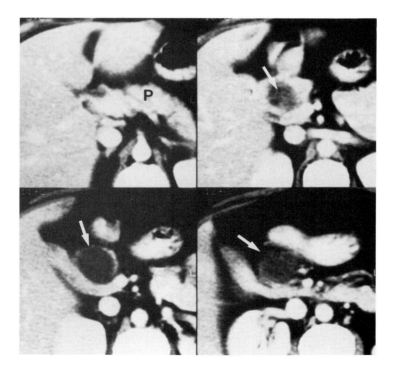

FIG 62–4.
Microcystic adenoma. Sequential bolus dynamic computed tomographic scans of the pancreas show a unilocular cystic mass *(arrows)* in the head of the pancreas. The body and tail of the pancreas *(P)* are normal. Surgical resection showed a benign, unilocular cystadenoma.

Inflammatory pancreatic masses. Problems in differentiating focal pancreatitis from carcinoma. *Radiology* 1984; 150:35–38.

14. Itai Y, Moss AA, Goldberg HI: Pancreatic cysts caused by carcinoma of the pancreas: A pitfall in the diagnosis of pancreatic carcinoma. *J Comput Assist Tomogr* 1982; 6:772–776.

15. Siegelman SS, Copeland BE, Saba GP, et al: CT of fluid collections associated with pancreatitis. *AJR* 1980; 134:1121–1132.

16. Torres WE, Evert MB, Baumgartner BR, et al: Percutaneous aspiration and drainage of pancreatic pseudocysts. *AJR* 1986; 147:1007–1009.

CHAPTER 63

Cystic Pancreatic Masses

Alec J. Megibow, M.D.

Case Presentation

A 60-year-old previously healthy woman had a 1-month history of epigastric fullness and the suggestion of a palpable mass in the left upper quadrant. A computed tomographic (CT) scan was ordered (Fig 63–1). What are the findings? Is this a benign or malignant lesion? What is the differential diagnosis? How should this lesion be managed?

DISCUSSION

The CT scan in Figure 63–1 reveals a well-marginated mass arising from the tail of the pancreas. There is minimal enhancement of the wall and dense central calcification. A radiating pattern due to the multiple fibrous septation within the mass is also present. Portions of the mass appear cystic; other areas are of higher density. The CT appearance is most consistent with a microcystic serous cystadenoma. However, a number of other lesions should be considered as well.

A wide variety of cystic masses can occur in the pancreas. In a group of 205 patients (mostly adults) who underwent surgery because of pancreatic cysts the most common types of cysts found were pseudocyst (168), neoplastic (21), retention (13), and congenital (3) cysts.[1] Pancreatic cystic masses can be classified into five broad categories: congenital, retention, pseudocyst, cystic neoplasm, and miscellaneous. Major pathologic entities within each of these categories are listed in Table 63–1.

This chapter reviews the characteristics of the clinically important pathologic and radiologic features of cystic pancreatic lesions and provides a differential diagnosis of other cystic masses that can arise around the pancreas. A radiologic approach to the characterization of these lesions is presented as well.

BENIGN CYSTIC PANCREATIC NEOPLASMS (FIGS 63–1, 63–2, 63–3)

Benign cystic tumors of the pancreas include the serous and mucinous cystadenomas and mucinous ductectatic cystadenoma as well as solid and cystic (papillary cystic) tumors.

Serous Cystadenomas

The serous cystadenoma (microcystic adenoma, microcystic tumor) is a multiloculated lesion that occurs more commonly in the pancreatic body and tail. Some series report slight female predominance, although other series find no sex predilection. These tumors tend to occur in the elderly. Serous cystadenomas account for 4% to 10% of all pancreatic cystic lesions. Gross examination of the cut surface reveals a multiloculated tumor with a characteristic central fibrous, occasionally calcified, stellate scar. Radiating bands of fibrous stroma di-

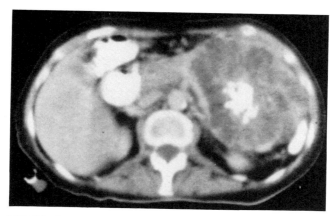

FIG 63–1.
Computed tomographic scan through the level of the pancreas.
What are the findings?

vide the lesion into innumerable microcysts, giving it a characteristic honeycomb appearance (see Figs 63–2 and 63–3). Histologic analysis shows the cysts to be lined with a flattened to cuboid epithelium. A clear, glycogen-rich cytoplasm that stains positive with periodic acid–Schiff stain is characteristic. Malignant transformation does not appear to occur in these tumors.[2–4]

Preoperative recognition of these tumors is important. In Compagno and Oertel's[2] series 21 of 34

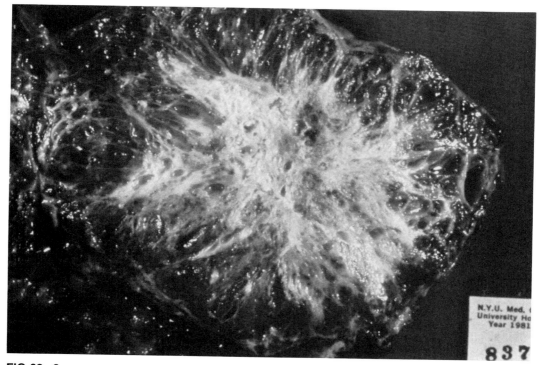

FIG 63–2.
Microcystic serous cystadenoma. Pathologic specimen from patient in Figure 63–1. Notice the innumerable tiny cysts but the predominance of fibrous tissue, which makes it impossible to register a water density reading on computed tomography.

TABLE 63–1.

Classification of Cystic Masses Within and Adjacent to the Pancreas*

Congenital
    Simple
    Polycystic diseases
    Cystic fibrosis
    Duodenal enteric (duplicative)
    Intrapancreatic choledochal cyst
    Cystic biliary and pancreatic duct
    Anomalies
    Miscellaneous
Retention
    Pancreatic cancer
    Pancreatic lithiasis
    Pancreatitis: acute and chronic
    Cholelithiasis and cholecystitis
    Parasitic
    Echinococcus
    Amoeba
    Ascaris
    Clonorchis sinensis
    Miscellaneous
Pseudocyst
    Postinflammatory
    Posttraumatic
    Postsurgical
    Unknown cause
Cystic neoplasms
    Duct cancer
    Cystadenoma and cystadenocarcinoma
    Leiomyosarcoma
    Dermoid
    Vascular
    Lymphangioma
    Hemangioma
    Other
Miscellaneous
    Nutritional fibrocalcific pancreatitis
    Solitary

*Data from Cubilla AL, Fitzgerald PJ: Surgical pathology of tumors of the exocrine pancreas, in Moosa AR (ed): *Tumors of the Pancreas.* Baltimore, Williams & Wilkins Co, 1980, pp 159–218.

elderly patients died of causes other than metastatic disease or local invasion; in the remaining 13 patients, median disease-free survival was more than 4 years. Therefore surgical benefit afforded by resection is unclear in the elderly.

Mucinous Cystadenomas (Fig 63–4)

Compared with serous lesions, mucinous cystadenomas are unilocular or macrocystic. Although they may be lined with a simple cuboid columnar epithelium without overt features of malignancy, these mucinous tumors have a high potential for malignancy and should be considered carcinomatous.

Recently a form of apparently benign mucinous cystic pancreatic neoplasm was described in Japan. This so-called ductectatic neoplasm communicates with the secondary pancreatic duct and usually is found in the region of the uncinate process. Pathologic appearance in four of five patients was characterized by dilated pancreatic ducts lined with atypical epithelium. In one patient overt cancer cells were detected.[5]

Solid and Papillary Epithelial Neoplasms (Fig 63–5)

The solid and papillary neoplasm has a striking female predominance.[6] This lesion characteristically occurs in adolescents, and only a few cases occur in women older than 35 years.[3] A recent report of six patients (five women, one man) documented one case of metastatic deposits in liver and lymph nodes.[7] In another series three recurrences were described in 74 collected lesions.[8] These large round masses (average diameter 8 cm) are well demarcated from the remaining pancreas. The cut surface of the tumor reveals lobulated light brown cystic zones of hemorrhage and tissue necrosis. Histologic analysis of preserved tissue exhibits variable sclerosis; the epithelial tissue shows pseudopapillary and microcystic changes. These cells are arranged in a perithelial pattern around hyalinized fibrovascular stalks or papillary projections and characteristically stain immunocytochemically with antitrypsin.[9]

MALIGNANT CYSTIC NEOPLASMS

Mucinous Cystadenocarcinomas (Figs 63–6, 63–7)

The most common cystic malignant tumors are mucinous cystadenocarcinomas. Mucinous cystic neoplasms account for about 1% or 2% of pancreatic exocrine tumors, with a female-to-male ratio of 6 : 1. In most cases the tumors are large, bulky, and arise in the tail of the pancreas. The cut surface reveals a unilocular or multilocular cystic lesion filled with sticky mucin (see Fig 63–6,B). The cysts are lined with mucinous columnar epithelium, which may form intracystic papillary projections. Compagno and Oertel[10] found that of their 75 cases of cystadenoma and cystadenocarcinoma 55% were of the mucinous cystic variety. In only 5% of these

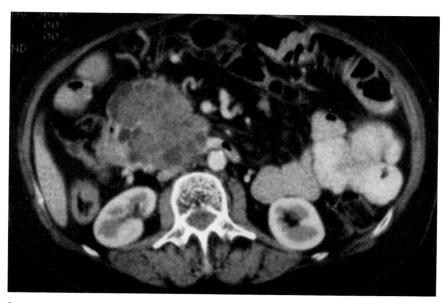

FIG 63–3.

Mixed appearance benign cystadenoma. A well-defined mass arises in the head of the pancreas. Centrally a radiating pattern of dense fibrous stroma is seen; peripherally large macrocysts are present. This lesion has obstructed the superior mesenteric vein, and multiple collateral vessels are present in the transverse mesocolon. This lesion has remained stable over 4 years of observation.

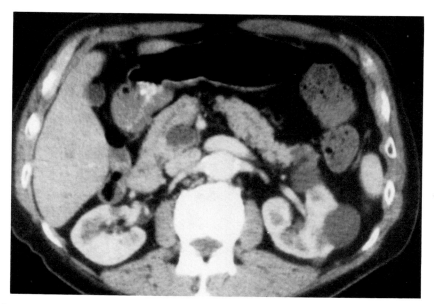

FIG 63–4.

Ductectatic mucinous cystadenoma. A well-defined water density unilocular mass is identified in the uncinate process of the pancreas. There is no evidence of chronic pancreatitis. On endoscopic retrograde cholangiopancreatography this lesion was seen to communicate with a side branch of the pancreatic duct. Although not proved, this lesion remains unchanged over 3 years of observation.

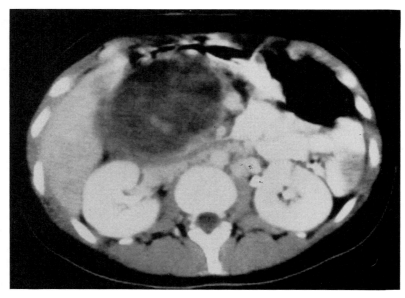

FIG 63–5.
Solid and papillary epithelial pancreatic neoplasm in an 18-year-old female patient. A large low-density mass is seen in the head of the pancreas. Poorly de- fined internal areas of increased density represent hemorrhage, tissue necrosis, and remnants of papil- lary projections.

was the head of the pancreas involved. The epithe- lium varied from cyst to cyst and even within the same section. In 81% of cases tissue atypical of car- cinomatous epithelium was demonstrated only after many blocks of tissue were examined. Treatment is by surgical excision. If the entire tumor is resected, survival rate is excellent, averaging 6.7 years.

Occasionally adenocarcinoma presents as a cystic mass. These mucinous adenocarcinomas are rare. Cystic spaces filled with mucin surrounded by collagenous septae are present. No cells line the wall, but signet ring cells are seen floating within the mucin (Fig 63–8).

Recently the mucinous hypersecreting carci- noma was described.[12] In these lesions the pancre- atic duct becomes engorged by thick mucin secreted by the neoplasm, which arises along the surface of the pancreatic duct. These tumors rarely metastasize but are considered malignant.

RADIOLOGIC FEATURES OF PANCREATIC NEOPLASMS

The radiologic findings in cystic pancreatic neoplasms are reported extensively in the literature. The major reason for the continuing interest in this group of lesions is that as experience in cross-sec- tional imaging (particularly CT) increases, certain morphologic patterns are being recognized with in- creasing frequency, allowing a more confident diag- nosis of benign versus malignant lesion. The radio- logic features of these neoplasms as a group, are re- viewed, as seen on indirect radiologic imaging tech- niques including upper gastrointestinal series, an- giography, and endoscopic retrograde cholangiopan- creatography (ERCP); and ultrasonography and CT.

Indirect Imaging Techniques

Indirect imaging techniques have taken a sec- ondary role to direct cross-sectional imaging meth- ods in the evaluation of pancreatic lesions. The most frequent clinical finding in these patients is a palpable abdominal mass. Virtually all palpable ab- dominal masses initially are studied with either ul- trasonography (US) or CT, bypassing the upper gas- trointestinal series. Barium studies show only ex- trinsic displacement of the stomach or duodenum. Unless calcifications in a microcystic tumor are present on the plain film, these studies seldom add new information.

Only a few cases have been studied by ERCP and reported in the literature. In microcystic neo-

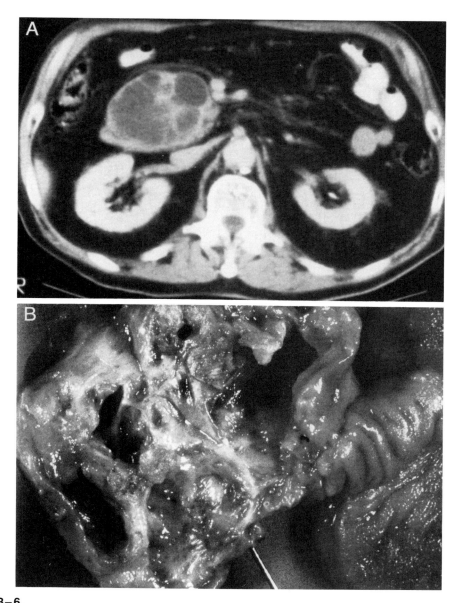

FIG 63–6.

Macrocystic mucinous cystadenocarcinoma. **A,** computed tomographic scan reveals well-demarcated mass arising in the head of the pancreas. Note the well-defined fluid density spaces separated by variably thickened curvilinear septae. No radiating pattern is identifiable. **B,** pathologic specimen from patient in **A.** Note the thickened septae, large spaces, and glistening appearance due to the presence of mucin.

plasms, only duct displacement has been reported, with no other abnormalities seen. Microcystic tumors rarely communicate with the pancreatic duct[13]; this is to be expected, because pathologic examination does not reveal that cystic neoplasms display true ductal continuity. Ductal obstruction as seen in adenocarcinoma is not found in these cases. If duct obstruction is noted the possibility of retention cyst associated with a pancreatic neoplasm should be considered.

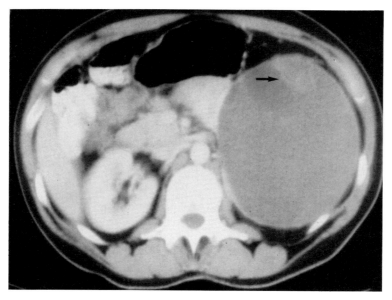

FIG 63–7.
Mucinous cystadenocarcinoma. A large unilocular mass arises from the tail of the pancreas. A papillary excrescence along the ventral margin *(arrow)* differentiated this lesion from a simple cyst.

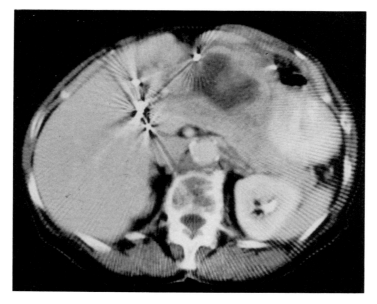

FIG 63–8.
Mucoid adenocarcinoma of the pancreas. There is a moderately well-defined mass in the body of the pancreas. A macrocystic cystadenocarcinoma could have a similar appearance. The wall of this lesion is lined with fibrous tissue, with signet ring cells floating in the central mucoid matrix.

Conversely, ductectatic cystic neoplasm of the pancreas characteristically communicates with a side branch of the main pancreatic duct. ERCP demonstrates filling of multiple loculated spaces within the neoplasm. Filling defects due to inspissated mucoid material may be seen. A morphologically normal main pancreatic duct rules out chronic pancreatitis and is diagnostic of this neoplasm.[5]

Angiography

Freeny et al.[14] compiled data on the important angiographic findings in both cystadenoma and cystadenocarcinoma. The primary angiographic manifestations of the microcystic adenomas include arterial displacement, dilation, and neovascularity. Arterial encasement is rarely seen. Obstruction or compression of the splenic or superior mesenteric veins is seen in approximately 50% of patients. The tumors usually are hypervascular or moderately vascular; conversely, mucinous cystadenocarcinomas usually are hypovascular. Arterial dilation and neovascularity are less frequently seen than with the microcystic variety; however, angiographic findings of malignancy (either arterial encasement or obstruction) are seen in all cases. When these findings are associated with metastases or organ invasion they are helpful in differentiating malignant from benign lesion.[15]

Cross-sectional Imaging Techniques

Ultrasonography

The US findings in mucinous and microcystic tumors have been reported.[16–18] The mucinous tumors are multilocular with fixed septations and nodular tumor papillary excrescences. At high gain settings complex echo patterns are seen. The microcystic adenoma is a more complex mass, with numerous internal echoes resembling a solid lesion. This is attributable to the tiny cysts and dense radiating septae, which result in numerous acoustic interfaces.

Computed Tomography

Multiple reports in the literature describe the CT findings in cystic pancreatic neoplasms. This method has become increasingly important in the evaluation of pancreatic lesions, because many features on CT can predict the gross and histologic appearance of resected tumors. Itai et al.[19] evaluated the role of CT in distinguishing benign cystadenoma from cystadenocarcinoma. They retrospectively reviewed and evaluated 10 lesions (three serous cyst-

adenomas, seven mucinous tumors). All of the cystadenomas had stellate septae, contrast enhancement in the septal and cyst wall, and a honeycomb appearance. Cysts had variable density within the same tumor. Two of the three lesions had central calcifications (see Fig 63–1). None of the mucinous lesions had central stellate septae, but three had curvilinear septae. Mural projections and localized thickening of cyst walls were seen in three of the lesions. None had a honeycomb appearance (see Figs 63–6 and 63–7). Friedman et al.[20] evaluated 35 primary cystic pancreatic neoplasms (15 microcystic adenomas, 20 mucinous cystic neoplasms). Their findings concurred with those of Compagno and Oertel[10] and classified all mucinous lesions as either frankly or potentially malignant. Four patients with microcystic adenomas underwent CT; two of these had central calcification. Peripheral enhancement of the cyst wall was present in one patient examined with dynamic enhancement. CT scans of four mucinous tumors were available and showed larger areas of low density. CT scans of three of seven multilocular neoplasms were available; septae were seen in two and missed in one. However, these cases were not uniformly studied with thin-section CT or with present-day state-of-the-art equipment.[20] Both groups believe that correct preoperative radiologic diagnosis should be possible in most cases of cystic pancreatic neoplasms.

In our experience, volume averaging precludes accurate water density readings in microcystic cystadenomas, because of the preponderance of fibrous stroma and the smallness of the cysts. Furthermore, many lesions we see actually have a mixed morphologic pattern on CT. Both microcystic portions intermingle with relatively large (macrocystic) septated areas. Of three lesions seen at our institution, two were resected. These were glycogen-rich serous cystadenomas despite the presence of scattered macrocyst. Surgical resection of the third lesion was impossible because of encasement of the superior mesenteric vein. This lesion has not changed in size or character over 4 years of follow-up and is presumed to be benign.

Ductectatic mucinous cystadenoma and cystadenocarcinoma appear as a unilocular mass on CT and on US. Septae are not recognized within the mass. The size of the pancreatic duct appears normal (see Fig 63–4).

Solid and papillary epithelial pancreatic neoplasms of the pancreas appear on CT as well-defined round lobular masses containing both cystic and solid portions, with variable ratios of cystic to solid material. After intravenous contrast administration there is little enhancement either in the central portion of the cyst or in the periphery of the lesion. As experience with this lesion accumulates there are more reports of calcifications within the actual central portion of the lesion, a finding previously believed to be rare[7, 8] (Fig 63–5).

OTHER CYSTIC PANCREATIC LESIONS

Other entities can produce cysts in the pancreas but generally cause no problem in the differential

diagnosis. Simple cysts, multiple cysts in polycystic disease,[21] von Hippel-Lindau disease,[22] and cystic fibrosis may be seen. Rare forms of cysts such as those due to *Echinococcus, Amoeba,* and *Ascaris* are unusual in the western hemisphere. Other neoplasms of the pancreas, such as leiomyosarcoma, dermoid tumors, lymphangiomas, the rare mucoid adenocarcinoma (see Fig 63–8), and hemangiomas, may present as cystic neoplasms (see Table 63–1).

An important cystic lesion is the retention cyst, which can occur secondary to the obstruction of the pancreatic duct system, usually from carcinoma of the pancreas. In one autopsy series these cysts were found in 15 of 100 patients and were of appreciable

FIG 63–9.
Retention cyst. **A,** unilocular smooth-walled cystic mass arises from the body of the pancreas. Note the atrophic distal pancreas with evidence of dilated main pancreatic duct *(arrow).* **B,** scan 1 cm lower. A mass *(arrow)* is seen in the body of the pancreas. There is evidence of retropancreatic extension. **C,** Endoscopic retrograde cholangiopancreatography reveals complete obstruction of the main pancreatic duct, compatible with adenocarcinoma. The common bile duct is dilated as well.

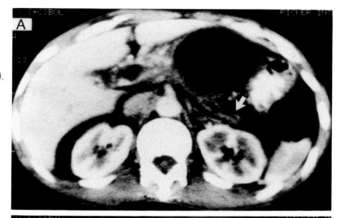
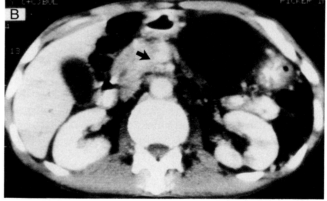
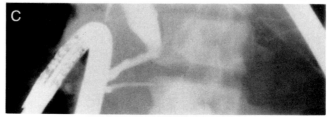

CHAPTER 64

Abnormal Pancreatogram

Howard J. Ansel, M.D.
Charles A. Rohrmann, Jr., M.D.

Case Presentation

A 65-year-old man had a 6-month history of boring abdominal pain radiating to the back, weight loss, and onset of jaundice. In the course of examination endoscopic retrograde cholangiopancreatography (ERCP) was performed (Fig 64–1). What is the finding? What is the differential diagnosis?

DISCUSSION

The pancreas is embryologically formed from dorsal and ventral buds that protrude from the gut at the level of the duodenum. The ventral bud, with the associated bile duct, swings behind the duodenum to fuse with the dorsal bud to form the mature pancreas. The ventral duct and the common bile duct enter the duodenum at the major papilla. The dorsal duct drains through the minor papilla. When fused the ventral duct forms the duct of Wirsung in the head of the pancreas; the dorsal duct forms the duct of Santorini (from the minor papilla to the main pancreatic duct) and the portion of the main pancreatic duct in the body and tail[1, 2] (Fig 64–2).

The normal pancreatic duct tapers from its largest diameter in the head to a progressively smaller diameter in the tail. Several major branches or numerous small side branches may project off the main pancreatic duct (Fig 64–3). The side branches also taper smoothly from the main duct peripherally. If the pancreatic duct is overfilled with contrast material a parenchymal blush (acinarization) may result.[3–7]

ERCP is indicated to evaluate complications of pancreatitis such as pseudocysts, ascites, and pancreatic abscess, to define the ductal abnormalities of

neoplasm, and to evaluate duct disruption from trauma.

A 1963 symposium on pancreatitis at Marseille classified pancreatitis into four categories: acute, relapsing acute, chronic relapsing, and chronic pancreatitis.[8] During an international workshop at Kings College, Cambridge, England, in 1983 the classification was modified to recognize two types of pancreatitis: acute pancreatitis and chronic pancreatitis with residual damage.[9]

The pancreatographic findings of chronic pancreatitis were defined and classified at the Kings College workshop. Mild changes of chronic pancreatitis include loss of tapering, clubbing, and ectasia of at least three side branches of the main pancreatic duct; the main pancreatic duct remains normal. If fewer than three side branches are involved the duct is classified as equivocal or normal. As the disease progresses the main pancreatic duct becomes involved. The duct loses smooth tapering and develops areas of stenosis and proximal dilation (Fig 64–4). The disease may be localized to a single portion of the gland, such as the tail, or may involve the entire pancreas. The combination of side branch abnormalities and an abnormal main pancreatic duct is classified as moderate change. In later stages of the disease inflammatory response leads to

545

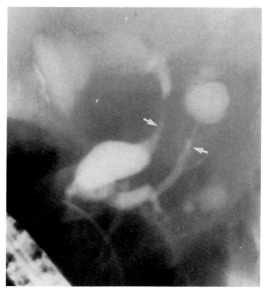

FIG 64–1.
Injection of contrast material through the major papilla fills both a portion of the common bile duct and the main pancreatic duct. A short distance from the papilla narrowing of both ducts is observed *(arrows)*. Proximal to these areas of narrowing a small amount of contrast partially outlines the dilated pancreatic and biliary ducts.

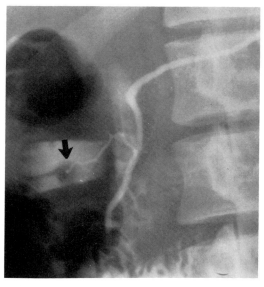

FIG 64–2.
On this normal pancreatogram a small duct of Santorini is seen connecting the main pancreatic duct with the minor papilla *(arrow)*, outlined by contrast in the duodenum. The main duct gradually tapers from the major papilla as it progresses toward the tail.

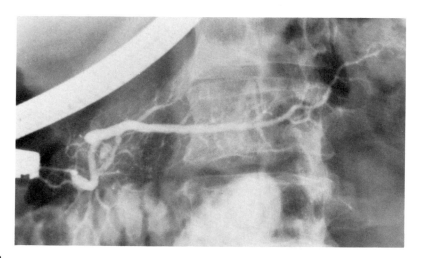

FIG 64–3.
Injection of contrast material in this normal pancreas demonstrates a main pancreatic duct that gradually tapers from papilla to tail. In addition, multiple side branches of various sizes taper gradually to form a delicate branching pattern.

CHAPTER 65

Rule Out Functioning Pancreatic Tumor

Steven M. Genkins, M.D.
N. Reed Dunnick, M.D.

Case Presentation

A 30-year-old woman had a 2-month history of late morning drowsiness relieved by food. If she missed lunch she noted blurred vision in the afternoon. The fasting serum glucose level was 34 mg/dl, and the serum insulin level inappropriately elevated at 8 μU/ml. What are the possible diagnoses and what imaging studies would you recommend?

DISCUSSION

Insulinoma

The many possible causes of fasting hypoglycemia include factitious injection of insulin, alcoholism, diffuse liver disease, malnourishment, severe congestive heart failure, and decreased circulating levels of cortisol or glucagon.[1] However, insulinoma, a tumor of pancreatic islet beta cells, is the most common cause of fasting hypoglycemia in adults.[2] Many other nonpancreatic tumors occasionally cause hypoglycemia by secreting insulinlike substances; these include retroperitoneal fibrosarcoma, pleural mesothelioma, hepatoma, gastrointestinal carcinoma, adrenal cortical carcinoma, lymphoma, bronchogenic carcinoma, ovarian neoplasm, neuroblastoma, Wilms' tumor, and hemangiopericytoma.[1,2] Hypoglycemic symptoms, which may be accentuated by fasting or exercise, include disturbances of consciousness, seizures, blurred vision, paresthesias, diaphoresis, tremulousness, anxiety, and palpitations.[1,2]

Most nonneoplastic causes of fasting hypoglycemia may be ruled out by the medical history, physical examination, and measurement of serum levels of such hormones as cortisol and glucagon. Subsequently, possible neoplastic causes may be pursued, the most important of which is insulinoma.

In 1927 Wilder et al.[3] first described severe hypoglycemia in association with a metastatic islet cell tumor. Eleven years later, in association with an insulinoma, Whipple described the classic triad of spontaneous hypoglycemia, associated central nervous system and vasomotor symptoms, and resolution of symptoms on oral or intravenous administration of glucose.[4] Such findings, as manifested in our patient, associated with an inappropriately or absolutely elevated serum insulin level, mandate the search for an underlying insulinoma.

Insulinomas are slightly more common in women than in men, with an average age of presentation in the fifth decade, although they have been reported in all age groups. Coming to clinical attention early because of the insulin they secrete, these tumors are typically quite small at the time of diagnosis, averaging 0.5 to 4 cm in diameter.[2, 5-12]

As a consequence they are difficult to image.

Ninety percent of insulinomas are solitary, 5% to 8% of the time they are multiple, and in 2% to 5% of cases hyperinsulinism is due to focal or diffuse islet cell hyperplasia or microadenomatosis. Multiple tumors or diffuse hyperplasia often occurs in association with pituitary and parathyroid adenomas or hyperplasia in the dominantly inherited familial multiple endocrine neoplasia type I (MEN I; Wermer's syndrome).

Ninety-nine percent of insulinomas are intrapancreatic, occurring with equal frequency in the pancreatic head, body, and tail. Metastases to peripancreatic lymph nodes or the liver are present at diagnosis in only 10% of patients. Thus if diagnostic imaging can localize the tumor, surgery is likely to result in cure.[1, 2, 5, 8, 9, 13]

The imaging workup of a possible insulinoma should begin with an abdominal computed tomographic (CT) examination (Fig 65–1). Scanning technique must be meticulous if small tumors are to be detected. At least 1,000 ml of oral contrast is administered, with the last 400 ml given just before scanning to ensure gastric and duodenal distention. Scans are obtained incrementally during intravenous contrast infusion. In our protocol, 20 seconds after the mechanical injection of 60% water-soluble contrast material at a rate of 2.5 ml/sec is begun, scanning is initiated just caudal to the uncinate process of the pancreas. The remainder of the 200 ml contrast infusion is delivered at a rate of 1.2 ml/sec. Contiguous 5 mm sections are obtained through the pancreas, followed by 1 cm slices through more cephalad portions of the liver.

Because of their small size, only 40% to 60% of insulinomas are detected by CT. Diagnosis of this and other types of islet cell tumors is based on a focal contour bulge of the pancreas or the presence of a soft tissue mass that enhances to a greater extent (10 to 50 Hounsfield Units, HU) than the remainder of the gland[2, 6, 8, 13–17] (Fig 65–2). CT is also useful for identifying metastatic disease and for preoperative staging. Enlarged peripancreatic lymph nodes, invasion of adjacent retroperitoneal structures, and hepatic metastases are all well delineated. Large tumor size and tumor necrosis or calcification correlate with a greater frequency of malignancy in this and other types of islet cell tumors.[2, 8, 18]

The small size of insulinomas coupled with the frequent obesity of these patients due to constant eating to avoid hypoglycemic symptoms make transabdominal ultrasonographic (US) localization of these tumors difficult. However, 30% to 60% of insulinomas may be imaged with this technique, and lesions as small as 7 mm have been reported.[2, 9, 11–16] We use 3 or 5 MHz transducers for transabdominal studies. Patients fast overnight to decrease the amount of epigastric gas that might ob-

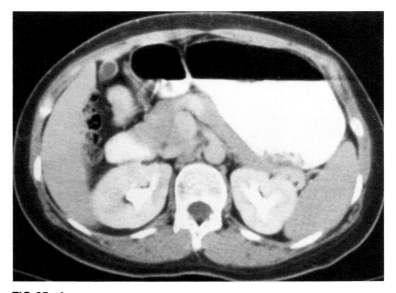

FIG 65–1.
Computed tomographic scan through the pancreas fails to reveal an insulinoma.

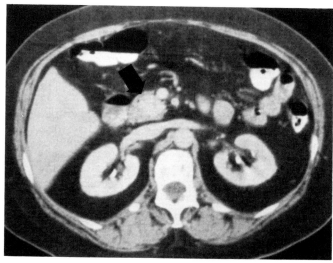

FIG 65–2.
Computed tomographic scan at the level of the pancreatic head and uncinate process reveals a subtle 2 cm insulinoma *(arrow).*

scure the pancreas. Supine and upright positions are the most useful for imaging. Examination is aided by the administration of a fatty meal and water, which provides a fluid-filled stomach as a sonic window to the pancreas, allowing improved visualization, particularly of the pancreatic tail.

Insulinomas and other types of islet cell tumors typically are well demarcated, homogeneously hypoechoic, round or oval masses. Occasionally a thin hyperechoic capsule is noted. Rarely insulinomas are cystic.[12]

US is useful in staging insulinomas. Hepatic metastases are typically echogenic, or may be "target lesions" with an echogenic center and a hypoechoic rim. Peripancreatic lymph node enlargement and invasion of retroperitoneal structures by tumor, as well as tumor necrosis or calcification, also may be detected.

Regardless of the results of CT and US examinations, arteriography should be performed in all patients with suspected insulinoma. Knowledge of vascular anatomy aids preoperative planning. In addition, multiple primary tumors, hepatic metastases, and invasion of adjacent structures may be demonstrated.

Conventional arteriography is preferred, although both intravenous and intra-arterial digital subtraction angiography have been used to detect insulinomas[14, 19] (Fig 65–3). Celiac, splenic, proper hepatic, gastroduodenal, and superior mesenteric ar-

tery injections may be required. In addition, superselective injections of the superior and inferior pancreaticoduodenal arcades and dorsal pancreatic and pancreatica magna arteries may increase diagnostic yields. Subtraction, magnification, and oblique views also may improve tumor localization.[1, 7, 13]

Arteriography localizes 70% to 90% of insulinomas, although detection rates as low as 18% are reported.[1, 6–8, 11, 13, 20] Tumors as small as 5 mm

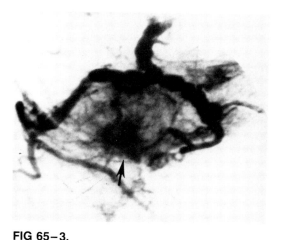

FIG 65–3.
Intra-arterial digital subtraction angiogram (same patient as in Fig 65–1) demonstrates a homogeneous vascular blush in the pancreatic head region compatible with an insulinoma *(arrow).*

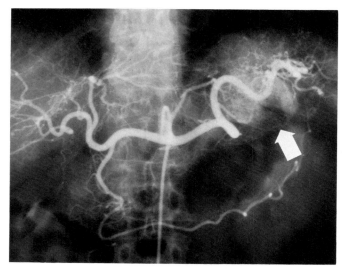

FIG 65–4.
Celiac injection from a conventional arteriogram reveals a hypervascular insulinoma of the pancreatic tail *(arrow).*

may be imaged. Typically insulinomas and other islet cell tumors are hypervascular, with a well-circumscribed homogeneous capillary blush slightly denser than the surrounding pancreatic parenchyma, which may persist well into the venous phase (Fig 65–4). Rarely insulinomas are hypovascular.[21] Larger tumors may demonstrate enlarged feeding vessels and tumor neovascularity. Adjacent vessels may be displaced or encased, and venous occlusion and shunting may occur.[2, 13, 20] Hepatic metastases are usually hypervascular and may be demonstrated up to 100% of the time with angiography.

Despite its central role in tumor localization and staging, there are many problems with arteriographic localization of insulinomas.[2, 7, 13, 14, 21, 22] Small tumors, those in ectopic locations or overlying the spine, and focal or diffuse islet cell hyperplasia or microadenomatosis may remain undetected by this technique. Peripancreatic lymph nodes, accessory spleens, normal lobulations in pancreatic contour, and the pancreatic tail seen on end all can be mistaken for tumor. Even when an insulinoma is angiographically localized, its precise relationship to adjacent structures, such as the pancreatic or common bile ducts, is not established. CT and US are complementary studies used to clarify such relationships.[16]

When CT, US, and arteriography fail to localize a suspected insulinoma, the more invasive and time-consuming technique of transhepatic pancreatic venous sampling developed by Ingemansson and Lunderquist in Sweden in the mid-1970s may be utilized. This procedure involves obtaining venous blood samples at 1 to 2 cm intervals along the splenic, superior, and inferior mesenteric veins. Subselective sampling from as many small veins draining the pancreatic bed as is technically possible is recommended. Insulin gradients between samples localize tumors[6, 14, 23] (Fig 65–5).

When properly performed, pancreatic venous sampling is safe and localizes insulinomas in 95% to 100% of cases.[2, 6, 17, 22, 23] In addition, multiple tumors and focal hyperplasia or microadenomatosis may be detected.[14, 23] In two reported series totaling 80 patients only one serious complication occurred; accidental gallbladder perforation requiring cholecystectomy.[6, 23] Other possible complications of this procedure include intrahepatic or intraperitoneal bleeding, creation of portosystemic fistulas, venous thrombosis, and bile peritonitis.[14]

As with arteriography, even when a tumor is localized with pancreatic venous sampling, it is not exactly defined in relationship to adjacent structures.[14] In addition, successfully localized tumors, particularly those within the pancreatic head, may not be palpable at surgery. However, at least a directed partial pancreatectomy may be performed on the basis of findings obtained at pancreatic venous sampling.[20]

Venous sampling may fail to resolve two

solitary and larger than 3 cm, occurring with greatest frequency in the pancreatic body and tail. Five percent of vipomas are ectopic. Fifty percent to 60% are malignant, 30% are benign adenomas, and 15% are due to islet cell hyperplasia.[2, 8]

Upper gastrointestinal tract examination may demonstrate dilated small bowel loops with increased intraluminal fluid and increased transit time.[2] Primary tumors and metastases typically are hypervascular at angiography. Microaneurysms have been noted in some cases.[2, 29] Although there are insufficient reports to determine the utility of specific imaging methods in localizing vipomas, their relatively large size and low incidence of ectopic location imply that they should be easy to detect. Scattered case reports confirm this suspicion.[2, 8, 11, 29]

Somatostatinoma

The rarest of the functioning islet cell tumors is the somatostatinoma, with nine cases reported in the literature. Signs and symptoms include mild diabe-

tes, steatorrhea, diarrhea, weight loss, hypochlorhydria or achlorhydria, and gallstones. Increased somatostatinlike immunoreactivity may be detected in the serum, especially after tolbutamide administration.[2, 8, 29–31]

Somatostatinomas arise from pancreatic islet delta cells. They occur most frequently in the pancreatic body and tail, and range in size from 3 to 10 cm (Fig 65–8). Two thirds are metastatic to the liver at the time of diagnosis. Because of the rarity of these tumors, meaningful statements cannot be made about the relative abilities of specific imaging methods to localize them.[2, 11, 22, 30] Because most somatostatinomas are metastatic at the time of diagnosis, curative surgery seldom is possible.

TREATMENT OF ISLET CELL TUMORS

The mainstay of treatment for functioning islet cell tumors is surgery. Cure can be effected by low

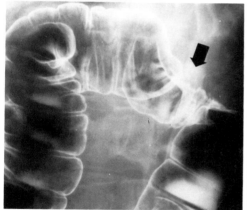

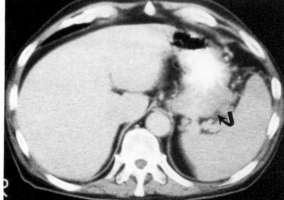

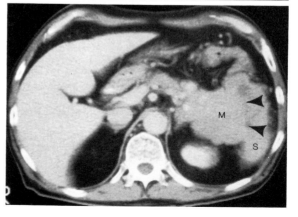

FIG 65–8.
A, steep right posterior oblique view from an air contrast barium enema study reveals extrinsic compression on the splenic flexure of the colon by a somatostatinoma of the pancreatic tail *(arrow).* **B,** computed tomographic (CT) scan demonstrates the superior extension of the tumor *(curved arrow)* to be inseparable from the gastric fundus. **C,** CT scan shows the main tumor mass *(M)* abutting the spleen *(S)* and the splenic flexure of the colon *(arrowheads).* (From Roberts L Jr, Dunnick NR, Foster WL Jr, et al: *J Comput Assist Tomogr* 1984; 8:1015–1018. Used by permission.)

morbidity enucleation of localized solitary tumors. Subtotal distal pancreatectomy is performed when a tumor is not localized either preoperatively or at exploratory laparotomy. The twofold rationale for this procedure is that most islet cell tumors are located in the pancreatic body and tail, and these portions of the gland are most easily resected.

Because the majority of nonbeta islet cell tumors are metastatic or locally invasive at the time of diagnosis, surgery often is limited to a debulking procedure. Long-term survival is not precluded in such cases, however, because of the slow growth typical of islet cell tumors and because residual tumor often responds to systemic or intra-arterial chemotherapy with such agents as streptozotocin or 5-fluorouracil.[2, 8, 13, 23]

Total gastrectomy is a surgical option in Zollinger-Ellison syndrome when curative tumor resection is not possible. This removes the target organ of the gastrin secreted and cures the debilitating gastrointestinal symptoms. Medical therapy with gastric histamine receptor blockers such as cimetidine or ranitidine is an alternative to gastrectomy. Medical therapy also can sustain patients with islet cell tumors who are awaiting surgery. Examples include glucose administration to patients with insulinoma and electrolyte replacement in patients with WDHA syndrome.

REFERENCES

1. Clinical Conferences at the Johns Hopkins Hospital. *Johns Hopkins Med J* 1980; 146:118–123.
2. Dodds WJ, Wilson SD, Thorsen MK, et al: MEN I syndrome and islet cell lesions of the pancreas. *Semin Roentgenol* 1985; 20:17–63.
3. Wilder RM, Allan FN, Power MH, et al: Carcinoma of the islands of the pancreas. *JAMA* 1927; 89:348–355.
4. Whipple AO: The surgical therapy of hyperinsulinism. *J Int Chir* 1938; 3:237–240.
5. Charboneau JW, James EM, Van Heerden JA, et al: Intraoperative real-time ultrasonographic localization of pancreatic insulinoma: Initial experience. *J Ultrasound Med* 1983; 2:251–254.
6. Cho KJ, Vinik AI, Thompson NW, et al: Localization of the source of hyperinsulinism: Percutaneous transhepatic portal and pancreatic vein catheterization with hormone assay. *AJR* 1982; 139:237–245.
7. Clouse ME, Costello P, Legg MA, et al: Subselective angiography in localizing insulinomas of the pancreas. *AJR* 1977; 128:741–746.
8. Dunnick NR, Doppman JL: Computed tomography of islet cell tumors. *Clin Comput Tomogr* 1983; 1:179–198.
9. Kuhn F-P, Gunther R, Ruckert K, et al: Ultrasonic demonstration of small pancreatic islet cell tumors. *J Clin Ultrasound* 1982; 10:173–175.
10. Lane RJ, Coupland GAE: Operative ultrasonic features of insulinomas. *Am J Surg* 1982; 144:585–587.
11. Shawker TH, Doppman JL, Dunnick NR, et al: Ultrasonic investigation of pancreatic islet cell tumors. *J Ultrasound Med* 1982; 1:193–200.
12. Pogany AC, Kerlan RK Jr, Karam JH, et al: Cystic insulinoma. *AJR* 1984; 142:951–952.
13. Dunnick NR, Long JA Jr, Krudy A, et al: Localizing insulinomas with combined radiographic methods. *AJR* 1980; 135:747–752.
14. Gunther RW, Klose KJ, Ruckert K, et al: Localization of small islet-cell tumors: Preoperative and intraoperative ultrasound, computed tomography, arteriography, digital subtraction angiography, and pancreatic venous sampling. *Gastrointest Radiol* 1985; 10:145–152.
15. Gunther RW, Klose KJ, Ruckert K, et al: Islet-cell tumors: Detection of small lesions with computed tomography and ultrasound. *Radiology* 1983; 148:485–488.
16. Krudy AG, Doppman JL, Jenson RT, et al: Localization of islet cell tumors by dynamic CT: Comparison with plain CT, arteriography, sonography and venous sampling. *AJR* 1984; 143:585–589.
17. Stark DD, Moss AA, Goldberg HI, et al: CT of pancreatic islet cell tumors. *Radiology* 1984; 150:491–494.
18. Wolf EL, Sprayregen S, Frager D, et al: Calcification in an insulinoma of the pancreas. *Am J Gastroenterol* 1984; 79:559–561.
19. Baert AL, deSomer FM, Wilms GE: Value of intravenous digital subtraction angiography to demonstrate hypervascular endocrine tumors: Report of two cases. *Cardiovasc Intervent Radiol* 1984; 7:193–195.
20. Doppman JL, Brennan MF, Dunnick NR, et al: The role of pancreatic venous sampling in the localization of occult insulinomas. *Radiology* 1981; 138:557–562.
21. Fink IJ, Krudy AG, Shawker TH, et al: Demonstration of an angiographically hypovascular insulinoma with intraarterial dynamic CT. *AJR* 1985; 144:555–556.
22. Lunderquist A, Eriksson M, Ingemansson S, et al: Selective pancreatic vein catheterization for hormone assay in endocrine tumors of the pancreas. *Cardiovasc Radiol* 1978; 1:117–124.
23. Roche A, Raisonnier A, Gillon-Savouret M-C:

Pancreatic venous sampling and arteriography in localizing insulinomas and gastrinomas: Procedure and results in 55 cases. *Radiology* 1982; 145:621–627.

24. Mills SR, Doppman JL, Dunnick NR, et al: Evaluation of angiography in Zollinger-Ellison syndrome. *Radiology* 1979; 131:317–320.
25. Dunnick NR, Doppman JL, Mills SR, et al: Computed tomographic detection of nonbeta pancreatic islet cell tumors. *Radiology* 1980; 135:117–120.
26. Breatnach ES, Han SY, Rahatzad MT, et al: CT evaluation of glucagonomas. *J Comput Assist Tomogr* 1985; 1:25–29.
27. Wawrukiewicz AS, Rosch J, Keller FS, et al: Glucagonoma and its angiographic diagnosis. *Cardiovasc Intervent Radiol* 1982; 5:318–324.

28. Inamoto K, Yoshino F, Nakao N, et al: Angiographic diagnosis of a pancreatic islet tumor in a patient with the WDHA syndrome. *Gastrointest Radiol* 1980; 5:259–261.
29. Galmiche JP, Chayvialle JA, Dubois PM, et al: Calcitonin-producing pancreatic somatostatinoma. *Gastroenterology* 1980; 78:1577–1583.
30. Gerlock AJ Jr, Muhletaler CA, Halter S, et al: Pancreatic somatostatinoma: Histologic, clinical and angiographic features. *AJR* 1979; 133:939–943.
31. Roberts L Jr, Dunnick NR, Foster WL Jr, et al: Somatostatinoma of the endocrine pancreas: CT findings. *J Comput Assist Tomogr* 1984; 8:1015–1018.

when displacement is in an anteroposterior diameter, and the latter may be difficult to distinguish from normal bowel gas. Ultrasonography (US) is unreliable for abscess detection because it is highly operator dependent and is limited by bone and bowel gas.[11] The best method for abscess detection is the CT scan, which should yield an accuracy in excess of 95% overall[11, 12] and has a sensitivity of 97% in detection of liver abscesses.[6] Aside from its accuracy in abscess detection, CT is the best method for route planning because of the detail with which it shows all of the surrounding viscera.

DIFFERENTIAL DIAGNOSIS

There is no sign entirely specific for intra-abdominal abscesses, particularly in the postoperative abdomen, in which a wide variety of fluid collections may occur. The differential diagnosis must include simple cysts originating from any organ, pancreatic pseudocysts, localized ascites, and any fluid-filled loop of bowel that has not opacified with oral contrast material. In addition, the clinician must consider several specific postoperative fluid collections: biloma, lymphocele, urinoma, seroma, and hematoma (mnemonic: BLUSH).[13] Dilated fluid-filled loops of colon just proximal to a new colostomy as well as the Hartman rectal pouch may closely resemble an abscess (enhancing wall, fluid center, gas bubbles). To be certain that a catheter is not precipitously inserted into a sterile fluid collection or loop of bowel one must carefully correlate clinical history, physical examination, and CT scan prior to confirmation by needle aspiration.

PLANNING A PERCUTANEOUS DRAINAGE ROUTE

The best drainage route usually is the shortest, safest direct route from the skin. No attempt should be made to provide "dependent" drainage, because manual syringe decompression of an abscess and the effect of intra-abdominal pressure on any remaining fluid do not require this. When intervening vital structures are found, oblique or angled approaches in a variety of planes may be necessary.[14] This most commonly occurs in the subphrenic space, where angulation from below upward is necessary to avoid the costophrenic sulcus. Diagnostic aspiration of a sterile fluid collection or sterile pancreatitis across the colon may result in iatrogenic infection and

should be meticulously avoided.[15] After route planning, the patient may remain in the CT room or be transferred to an ultrasound or fluoroscopy room for the drainage procedure, depending on the exact anatomy, abscess location, and physician preference.

There are three aspects to the planned route: the entry site on the skin, the center of the abscess, and the angle of the line connecting these two points.[13] Once these are planned from the CT scan, they should be transposed to the patient as meticulously as possible. We place a small barium mark on the skin at the entry site and confirm this with a CT scan. From that point the angle of entry and the depth are measured. When angulation is required we use a goniometer with arms fixed at the appropriate angle to guide the aspiration needle.

NEEDLE ASPIRATION

We prefer a 20 cm 20-gauge Teflon sleeve needle for diagnostic aspiration. It is large enough to allow recovery of even thick purulent material but is somewhat flexible. When using an angled approach to the subphrenic space, we prefer an 18-gauge Teflon sleeve needle, which is stiff enough to resist bending when angling cephalad. Only if infection is confirmed by Gram stain is a drainage catheter inserted. Sterile fluid collections are evacuated entirely and the Teflon sleeve is removed. Samples of the aspirate are sent for anaerobic, aerobic, and fungal cultures whether or not the Gram stain shows infection.

CATHETER INSERTION

Several commercially available catheters can be used for abscess drainage. Most are used with either the Seldinger or modified trocar technique. The advantage of the Seldinger technique is that a catheter follows a preplaced guidewire. This is useful in small deep abscesses to avoid the dangers of multiple passes with a large trocar catheter. Modified trocar catheters are useful in larger superficial abscesses because of their ease of insertion and because they allow a larger bore catheter than does the Seldinger technique. Success and complication rates with both techniques are similar. The choice of technique should depend on the accessibility of the abscess and the danger of damage to surrounding

anto...

structures. All of the side holes of the drainage catheter should be positioned within the abscess cavity to avoid intraperitoneal leakage.

MANAGEMENT STRATEGY

The abscess should be completely evacuated by manual syringe suction. Most abscesses collapse immediately, with little significant residual fluid (Fig 66–4). When the abscess has been emptied the pus develops a bloody tinge due to syringe suction on the abscess wall.

Some clinicians lavage the abscess gently with sterile saline solution to remove any residual fluid or debris.[16] We prefer not to do so, because of the risk of increasing pressure within the abscess, extravasating fluid, and either disseminating sepsis locally or creating intravasation of infected fluid, with resulting septicemia.[17] Comparison of abscesses that have been lavaged with those that have not shows little difference in success or complication rate, although resolution may be slightly earlier with lavage.

Comparison of the volume of the aspirate with the volume estimated from the CT scan can assure that the entire abscess has been drained. Any discrepancy should prompt a repeat CT scan to exclude any undrained residuum that may require a second catheter. This may be critical, because an undrained

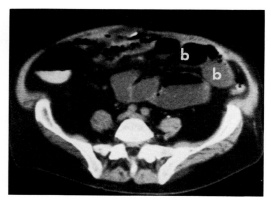

FIG 66–4.
Follow-up computed tomographic scan immediately after percutaneous drainage of 1,650 ml of pus. The abscess is completely decompressed and the loops of bowel *(b)* have returned to their normal location. If a catheter had not been inserted prior to decompression (at a lower level, not shown), this return of bowel loops to normal position would prevent further attempt at catheter insertion.

loculation leaves the patient at risk for continued septicemia.

The catheter should be sutured or taped carefully to the skin to prevent inadvertent removal. Removal may be serious, because after the abscess is decompressed there may no longer be a safe route for cutaneous entry and reinsertion of the catheter may not be possible until the fluid reaccumulates. Most patients require intravenous antibiotic therapy and hospitalization during the drainage period. However, selected patients may be discharged with catheters in place to reduce hospital stay and cost.[18]

CATHETER REMOVAL

The drainage catheter can be removed when the abscess has resolved. Resolution is judged by recording daily drainage volumes, temperatures, and white blood cell count. In most patients simple abscesses defervesce within 48 hours, but normalization of the white blood cell count generally requires 1 week. A repeat CT scan is not mandatory to confirm resolution; if the drainage has decreased to almost nil and there is no fever or leukocytosis, a significant septic focus is most unlikely. However, CT does provide clear confirmation of the effectiveness of percutaneous drainage.

Abscessograms or sinograms seldom are indicated unless the volume or character of persistent drainage suggests a communication with the bowel. These studies are best performed by a radiologist familiar with the initial drainage and only under close fluoroscopic control. Any increased pressure may cause rupture or intravascular dissemination of pus, with severe septicemia.[17] Communication with the gastrointestinal tract usually indicates the initial source of the abscess, although the possibility of iatrogenic catheter trauma to the bowel is sometimes raised. By that time the catheter has created a "controlled fistula," the vast majority of which will heal spontaneously. However, healing may take 2 to 4 weeks longer than the drainage time required for a simple abscess (usually 7 to 10 days).[19]

INDICATIONS FOR PERCUTANEOUS ABSCESS DRAINAGE

The initial criteria for percutaneous drainage included only well-defined unilocular abscesses, for which cure was achieved in about 90% of cases.[20]

These are now termed "simple" abscesses. Experience has expanded indications to include complex abscesses with enteric fistulas, diverticular and appendiceal abscesses, and septate abscesses. In these complex abscesses the cure rate decreases to about 45%.[21] However, because there are no absolute predictors of success, percutaneous drainage should be tried in all intra-abdominal abscesses.[22]

In the case presented (see Fig 66–1) the multiple liver abscesses were due to hematogenous spread via the portal veins from diverticulitis. Recently it was demonstrated that diverticular abscesses are amenable to percutaneous drainage.[23] Prior to the introduction of percutaneous drainage the usual operative treatment involved two or three stages: (1) abscess drainage and diverting proximal colostomy; (2) resection of the sigmoid colon with end-to-end anastomosis; (3) closure of the colostomy. This sequence requires about 6 months and includes three major operations, with compounded morbidity and mortality. Percutaneous drainage controls the initial diverticular abscess and can be followed within 10 days to 2 weeks by an operative resection and primary end-to-end anastomosis. In a series of 24 patients, 14 underwent a single-stage procedure within 10 days of percutaneous drainage.[23]

Similarly, in patients who have well-developed appendiceal abscesses percutaneous drainage has been curative.[24, 25] It now remains questionable whether interval appendectomy is needed. It should be emphasized that percutaneous drainage in both appendiceal and diverticular abscesses is restricted to patients who already have formed an abscess and is not indicated in those with spreading peritonitis.

CONTRAINDICATIONS TO PERCUTANEOUS DRAINAGE

Contraindications to percutaneous drainage must be considered relative to the risks and benefits. When the patient needs surgery to repair the underlying disease process but is a poor operative risk, percutaneous drainage can be used as a temporizing measure until the patient can better tolerate surgery.[20, 26] Currently our only contraindications are relative and include absence of a safe percutaneous route, coagulopathy, and the presence of a foreign body, such as a retained sponge. Even with a foreign body percutaneous drainage may provide a temporizing effect, and most coagulopathy can be corrected, at least for the duration of the procedure.

Ultimately the safety of percutaneous drainage must be viewed in light of alternative therapies. Given that the patient has an abscess and that surgery is the only other treatment, the radiologist can only improve the patient's condition. In the event of failure or complication, the abscess is treated surgically.

There are a number of documented comparisons between percutaneous and operative drainage. In two series the complication rate was lower for percutaneous drainage than for operative drainage (4% to 8% versus 16% to 21%), as was the morbidity rate (0% to 11% versus 12.5% to 21%); the postdrainage hospitalization stay was shorter (11 to 17 days versus 21.2 to 29 days).[27, 28] In addition, the nature of the complications was far less serious for percutaneous drainage than for operative drainage.[21, 22]

Percutaneous drainage is best utilized when radiologists, surgeons, and infectious disease specialists cooperate in management. In many complex cases the judicious application of percutaneous drainage combined with surgery offers the best chance for cure. Timing of an operation after percutaneous drainage has become a difficult decision, and relatively few guidelines are available.

REFERENCES

1. Case Records of the Massachusetts General Hospital. *N Engl J Med* 1977; 296:1051–1057.
2. Read DR, Hambrick E: Hepatic abscesses in diverticulitis. *South Med J* 1980; 73:881–883.
3. McKenzie CG: Pyogenic infection of liver secondary to infection of the portal drainage area. *Br Med J* 1964; 2:1558–1563.
4. Herbert DA, Rothman JR, Simmons F, et al: Pyogenic liver abscesses: Successful nonsurgical therapy. *Lancet* 1982; 1:134–136.
5. Gerzof SG, Robbins AH, Birkett DH: CT in the diagnosis and management of abdominal abscesses. *Gastrointest Radiol* 1978; 3:287–294.
6. Halvorsen EA, Korobkin M, Foster WL, et al: The variable CT appearance of hepatic abscesses. *AJR* 1984; 142:941–946.
7. Gerzof SG, Johnson WC, Robbins AH, et al: Intrahepatic pyogenic abscess: Treatment by percutaneous drainage. *Am J Surg* 1985; 149:482–494.
8. Bernardino ME, Berkman WA, Plemmons M, et al: Percutaneous drainage of multiseptated hepatic abscess. *J Comput Assist Tomogr* 1984; 8:38–41.

9. Percutaneous drainage of the abdominal abscess (editorial). *Lancet* 1982; 8277:889–890.

10. Johnson RD, Mueller PR, Ferrucci JT Jr, et al: Percutaneous drainage of pyogenic liver abscesses. *AJR* 1985; 144:463–467.

11. Mueller PR, Simeone JF: Intraabdominal abscess. Diagnosis by sonography and computed tomography. *Radiol Clin North Am* 1983; 21:425–554.

12. Gerzof SG, Oates ME: Imaging techniques for infections in the surgical patient. *Surg Clin North Am* 1988; 68:147–165.

13. Gerzof SG, Spira R, Robbins AH: Percutaneous abscess drainage. *Semin Roentgenol* 1981; 16:62–71.

14. Gerzof SG: Triangulation for indirect CT guidance. *AJR* 1981; 137:1080–1081.

15. Gerzof SG, Banks PA, Robbins AH, et al: Early diagnosis of pancreatic infection by CT guided aspiration. *Gastroenterology* 1987; 93:1315–1320.

16. vanSonnenberg E, Ferrucci JT, Mueller PR: Percutaneous drainage of abscesses and fluid collections: Technique, results and applications. *Radiology* 1982; 142:1–10.

17. Gerzof SG: Results and clinical correlations of percutaneous abscess drainage. *ARRS Categorial Course on Interventional Radiology.* Boston, April 21–25, 1985. American Roentgen Ray Society, 1985, pp 173–178.

18. Rifkin MD, Heffelfinger D, Kurtz AB, et al: Outpatient therapy of intraabdominal abscesses following early discharge from the hospital. *Radiology* 1984; 155:333–334.

19. Kerlan RK, Jeffrey RB, Pogany AC, et al: Abdominal abscess with low output fistula: Successful percutaneous drainage. *Radiology* 1985; 155:73–75.

20. Gerzof SG, Robbins AH, Birkett DH, et al: Percutaneous catheter drainage of abdominal abscesses guided by ultrasound and computed tomography. *AJR* 1979; 133:1–8.

21. Gerzof SG, Johnson WC, Robbins AH, et al: Expanded criteria for percutaneous abscess drainage. *Arch Surg* 1985; 120:227–232.

22. Jaques P, Mauro M, Safrit H, et al: CT features of intraabdominal abscesses: Prediction of successful percutaneous drainage. *AJR* 1986; 146:1041–1045.

23. Mueller PR, Saini S, Wittenberg J, et al: Sigmoid diverticular abscesses: Percutaneous drainage as an adjunct to surgical resection in 24 cases. *Radiology* 1987; 164:321–325.

24. Jeffrey RB Jr, Tolentino CS, Federle MP, et al: Percutaneous drainage of periappendiceal abscesses: Review of 20 patients. *AJR* 1987; 149:59–62.

25. vanSonnenberg E, Wittich GR, Casola G, et al: Periappendiceal abscesses: Percutaneous drainage. *Radiology* 1987; 163:23–26.

26. vanSonnenberg E, Wing VW, Casola G, et al: Temporizing effect of percutaneous drainage of complicated abscesses in critically ill patients. *AJR* 1984; 142:821–826.

27. Johnson WC, Gerzof SG, Robbins AH, et al: Treatment of abdominal abscesses— Comparative evaluation of operative drainage versus percutaneous catheter drainage guided by computed tomography or ultrasound. *Ann Surg* 1981; 194:510–520.

28. Brolin RE, Nosher JL, Leiman S, et al: Percutaneous catheter versus open surgical drainage in the treatment of abdominal abscesses. *Am Surg* 1983; 50:102–108.

CHAPTER 67

Percutaneous Abdominal Biopsy

Janis Gissel Letourneau, M.D.

Case Presentation

A 56-year-old man was seen in the oncology clinic for follow-up evaluation of known non-Hodgkin's lymphoma. He had completed chemotherapy within the past 12 months and was considered to be in complete remission. His current symptoms were mild and constitutional. A computed tomographic (CT) scan was obtained on the day of the clinic appointment (Fig 67–1). What diagnostic considerations must be made and how might they be approached?

DISCUSSION

CT sections through the upper abdomen in this patient reveal multiple small poorly marginated regions of low attenuation within the liver parenchyma. In the setting of non-Hodgkin's lymphoma primary diagnostic considerations include recurrent lymphoma, opportunistic infection, and metastatic foci from a second, undiagnosed malignancy. Histopathologic material is required for this determination and can be obtained by percutaneous needle biopsy of the liver.

Guided percutaneous needle biopsy of abdominal and pelvic masses has become a commonplace radiologic procedure.[1, 2] It can be performed in a variety of clinical situations, but is most commonly done when a malignant process is suspected. Biopsy can be used to establish the primary diagnosis, document the presence of metastases, and confirm the presence of recurrent neoplasm. Both cytologic and histologic specimens can be obtained with conventional techniques. Needle biopsy can also provide material for microbiologic analysis when infection is a diagnostic consideration.

Percutaneous needle biopsy was first routinely applied to pulmonary lesions and utilized fluoroscopic target localization. Fluoroscopy was subsequently used for target localization in biopsy of abdominal lesions, usually when coupled with some type of contrast administration. Fluoroscopy is still used for abdominal biopsy following intravenous or intra-arterial, biliary, gastrointestinal, or lymphangiographic opacification. The widespread availability of cross-sectional imaging techniques, such as sonography and CT, has, however, led to increased use of percutaneous needle biopsy of abdominal lesions. Regardless of the means of target localization, precise localization remains essential for successful percutaneous biopsy.

Different means of target localization present specific advantages and disadvantages. Although fluoroscopy cannot be used for biopsy of most small or deep abdominal lesions, it is inexpensive and usually readily available and permits continuous monitoring of needle position. Sonography allows biopsy to be performed without the use of ionizing radiation and, like fluoroscopy, permits continuous monitoring of needle position. Its use is especially

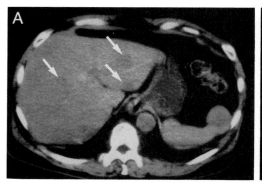
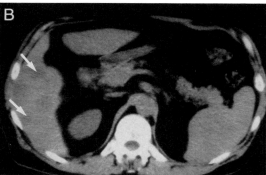

FIG 67–1.
A, multiple low dense foci *(arrows)* are seen within both lobes of the liver parenchyma on this enhanced computed tomographic scan. **B,** additional lesions *(arrows)* are seen in the inferior aspect of the right hepatic lobe.

valuable when a needle course angled from the sagittal or horizontal plane is desired. Some lesions, however, are not optimally visualized by sonography. CT is an excellent means of target localization, particularly for lesions that are small or deep to the skin surface (Fig 67–2). However, CT is an expensive means of biopsy guidance and does not allow continuous monitoring of needle position. Physical

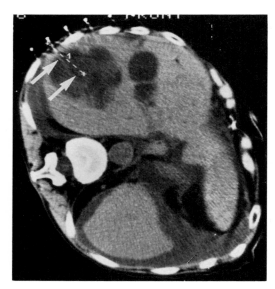

FIG 67–2.
The needle course can be easily planned with computed tomography localization using the computer software packages available. The angle that the needle should take in relation to the horizontal plane and the depth of the target from the skin surface are calculated by the scanner *(arrows).*

constraints of CT localization requiring the biopsy needle to stay within the horizontal plane can be partially obviated by triangulation methods or by gantry angulation.[3, 4]

Three basic types of biopsy needles are commercially available for percutaneous needle biopsy: simple aspiration, cutting, and screw-tip varieties. Cutting needles have a tip modification that permits cutting of a tissue core by rotation of the needle or by closure of a biopsy window. A screw-tip biopsy needle extracts the pathologic specimen by advancing the tip into the lesion and then sliding a cutting sheath over the tip. Biopsy needles are available either in fine bore (20, 21, and 22 gauge) or larger (14, 16, 18, and 19 gauge) sizes and also in a variety of lengths. Selection of a biopsy needle depends in part on the target location and proximity to vital organs, on its depth, and on its suspected character. For example, a large cutting needle would not be selected for biopsy of a large retrocolonic pancreatic mass that is inseparable on CT from the superior mesenteric artery and vein.

Just as there are several approaches to target localization, there are also a number of technical approaches to percutaneous needle biopsy. In the simplest form, multiple individual passes of the biopsy needle can be made. This is most valuable when it is considered safest to use a thin (21 or 22 gauge) needle for biopsy. A tandem biopsy approach permits fine-needle localization and parallel biopsy of the target lesion with a larger needle (Fig 67–3). Multiple passes of the biopsy needle can be made, keeping the fine localizing needle in place. A coaxial biopsy can be performed when little risk is anticipated for initial placement of a larger needle (18 or

biopsy procedures, and intracanalicular radiation therapy.

The traditional therapy for malignant biliary obstruction has been surgical creation of a biliary enteroanastomosis. This technique has a significant morbidity and carries an operative mortality as high as 50% to 60%, depending on the severity of the liver disease.[13–16] Knowledge of the anatomy of the biliary tree in patients with malignant obstruction helps to determine whether surgical decompression is advisable or whether percutaneous drainage is indicated instead. For example, high obstructions of the common hepatic duct should be managed by percutaneous techniques, because in such cases surgical decompression is extremely difficult if not impossible. For example, in this patient with a tumor involving the bifurcation of the common hepatic duct and the proximal segment of the right and left hepatic ducts, surgical decompression would have been difficult because of the high level of the obstruction. Using a dual approach, both lobes were drained (see Fig 68–1). In patients with terminal malignancy an endoprosthesis can be placed, either from a single or dual approach (Fig 68–2). In addition, patients with short life expectancy are probably also better served by the less invasive percutaneous techniques. In some cases percutaneous techniques can be used to stabilize a patient's clinical condition prior to a surgical procedure, as was the case in this patient with cholangitis secondary to obstruction by common bile duct stones (Fig 68–3). After stabilization the patient underwent a cholecystectomy and bile duct exploration.

Percutaneous biliary drainage procedures can be divided into two broad categories:

1. Internal drainage with internal-external drainage catheters, is commonly preferred in patients who have an expected survival of more than a year. This group includes patients with cholangiocarcinoma and ampullary carcinoma, with a survival rate of 33% at 5 years.[17, 18] This type of drainage is also used as a preliminary staging technique before placement of an endoprosthesis in patients with short life expectancy.

2. Endoprostheses, or internalized stents with no exteriorized catheter, are commonly used in patients with short life expectancy.

Internal-External Drainage

Internal-external drainage is most commonly used in patients with malignant obstructions because

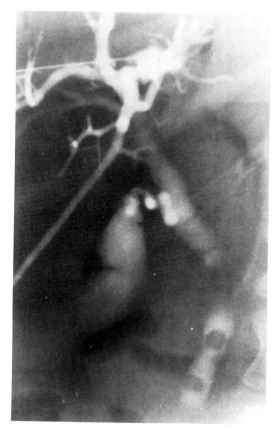

FIG 68–3.
Fine-needle cholangiogram shows two round filling defects within the distal common bile duct in a patient with cholangitis. An external drainage catheter was placed to stabilize the patient's clinical condition before surgical exploration.

it allows internal drainage of bile while preserving access to the biliary tree. It is preferably used in patients in whom longer life expectancy is expected, for example, those with ampullary carcinoma or cholangiocarcinoma,[17, 18] as in our patient (see Fig 68–1) with a tumor involving the bifurcation and the proximal segments of the right and left hepatic ducts. After dilation of the tract number 12 French internal-external stents were placed across the obstruction, with their tips in the distal common bile duct (see Fig 68–1). In addition, in patients with cholangiocarcinoma iridium seeds can be easily placed using the percutaneous tract (Figs 68–4 and 68–5), while at the same time externally draining the biliary tree.

Both free catheters and fixed catheters can be

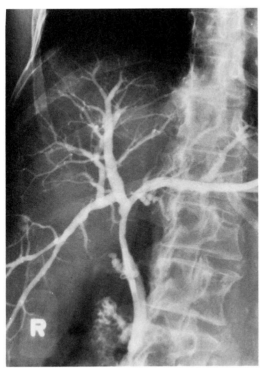

FIG 68–4.
Metastatic carcinoma at the level of the porta hepatis in a 72-year-old patient. A 12 French malecot internal-external stent was placed across the obstruction, with the distal tip in the distal common bile duct.

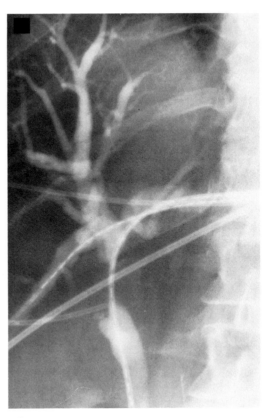

FIG 68–5.
After placement of a second catheter into the right biliary radicles, iridium seeds were placed across the drainage catheters for intracanalicular radiation therapy.

used for internal-external drainage. Free catheters have minimal self-retaining capabilities, and include pigtail, ring, and universal drainage catheters; fixed catheters include all those with a self-retaining mechanism, such as Cope, Hawkins, and Sachs catheters and any catheter with a retention balloon. Another important consideration in the selection of the internal-external drainage catheter is the material from which it is made. Materials used today include polyethylene, Teflon, polyurethane, C-flex, and Silastic.

The long-term patency of the drainage catheter is related to several factors, including internal lumen dimensions, distal tip opening diameter, material from which the catheter is made, and the site where the distal tip is placed. Catheters with larger interior lumens have a longer patency rate than do catheters with smaller internal diameters.[19] Percuflex material seems to provide the best internal dimensions of the available catheters. Silastic probably has the longest patency rate of the materials available[19, 20]; its major disadvantage is a high fric-

tion coefficient, which makes introduction difficult. Percuflex probably has the second highest patency rate of the materials available, followed closely by Teflon.[19] A large distal opening helps to improve the patency rate,[19] and in this respect Cragg's[20] warhead tip is particularly useful to provide a large diameter at the distal end of the catheter (Fig 68–6). Finally, better patency rates are obtained when the distal end of the catheter is maintained within the distal bile duct beyond the obstruction; placement of the tip within the duodenum leads to reflux of gastrointestinal contents, sepsis, and obstruction of the catheter.

Endoprostheses

Endoprostheses are commonly used in patients with malignant disease with short life expectancy,

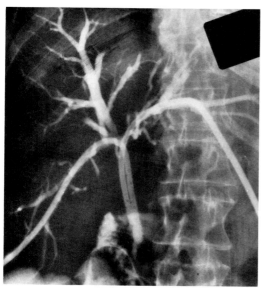

FIG 68–6.
Cragg's warhead catheters placed across a proximal obstruction of the common hepatic duct. Observe the blunt end and tip of the catheters are placed within this common bile duct.

because they tend to become obstructed at 3 to 6 months, depending on the internal lumen diameter and on the material they are made of.[1] Endoscopic management of biliary obstruction, as a general rule, calls for internal stents.

Internal stents of different designs have been described. The most commonly used currently include the Amplatz, the Carey-Coons, and Silastic malecot stents. The Carey-Coons stent is made of Percuflex (12 French), with a tapered tip and multiple side holes at the proximal and distal ends of the stent (Fig 68–7). The main advantage of this stent is the wide internal lumen of the tubing and the low friction coefficient of Percuflex. The main disadvantages are its tapered tip and length, which places the tip of the stent deep into the duodenum. This causes reflux of gastrointestinal contents, with premature closure of the stent[19] and a higher incidence of cholangitis.[19] The stent can be modified following the Cragg warhead technique[20] to improve its long-term patency rate, leaving the tip of the stent in the distal common bile duct.

The Amplatz stent is made of C-flex, with an introducing system that makes placement easier and more accurate. The S-curve in the stent helps to prevent migration (Fig 68–8). This catheter is available in 10 and 12 French sizes. Its main disadvan-

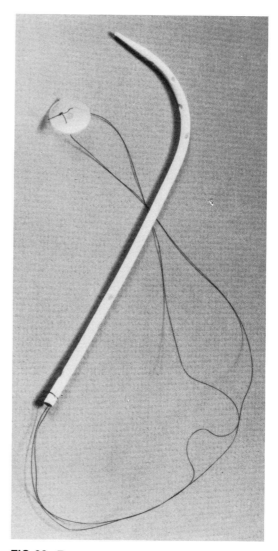

FIG 68–7.
Carey-Coons stent.

tages are the smaller internal diameter of C-flex and the tapered distal end, which causes early occlusion of the stent. The distal end of the stent can be modified using the warhead technique to improve patency rate by leaving the tip of the catheter in the common bile duct and having a wide open end. A 12 or 14 French Silastic stent (USCI Division of C.R. Bard, Billerica, Mass.) has a malecot design in the proximal end to prevent migration (Fig 68–9). The high friction coefficient of Silastic makes introduction of this stent difficult. Dilation of the tract two French sizes larger than the stent diam-

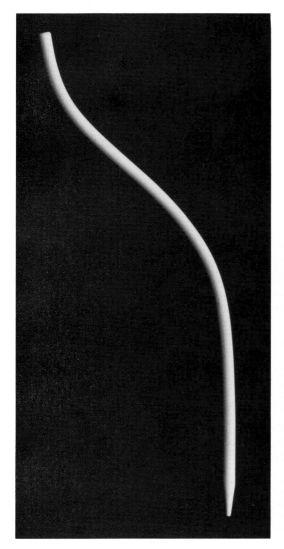

FIG 68–8.
Amplatz stent.

eter and maturation of the tract by 2 or 3 weeks facilitates introduction of the stent. The main advantage of silicone endoprostheses is their longer patency rate, as in this patient with metastatic colon carcinoma (Fig 68–10). Thirteen months after placement the endoprosthesis was patent, as shown by normal bilirubin levels.

Indications and Contraindications

Common indications for percutaneous biliary drainage include palliation in primary or metastatic malignant disease, benign strictures, sepsis associated with biliary obstruction, and preoperative decompression. Contraindications to percutaneous biliary drainage include bleeding diathesis. This can, however, be corrected by administration of fresh frozen plasma, vitamin K, platelets, or a specific blood coagulation compound. Sepsis is not a contraindication, because biliary drainage is the procedure of choice in the presence of cholangitis. However, to decrease the incidence of systemic sepsis intravenous antibiotics should be administered before and during the biliary drainage procedure and for a few hours after.

The presence of ascites makes biliary drainage procedures difficult but not impossible.

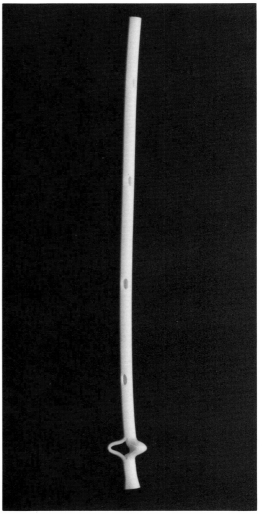

FIG 68–9.
Silicone stent.

CHAPTER 69

Percutaneous Management of Benign Bile Duct Strictures

Jeffrey C. Brandon, M.D.
Steven K. Teplick, M.D.

Case Presentation

A 77-year-old woman underwent a cholecystectomy and a T tube was inserted in the common bile duct 2 years prior to admission (Fig 69–1,A). She had obstructive jaundice and a stricture at the previous T tube site (Fig 69–1,B). The stricture was dilated with a 5 mm (15 French) balloon (Fig 69–1,C). Is this appropriate? What considerations should be entertained, and what might be done? What is the long-term success rate of percutaneous balloon dilation of benign strictures of the bile ducts?

DISCUSSION

Within the past decade the development of high-resolution imaging methods combined with improvements in a variety of interventional radiologic techniques and equipment have enabled the radiologist to offer nonoperative alternatives for the management of benign biliary tract strictures. For certain types of strictures these procedures hold promise for surpassing the efficacy and safety of traditional surgical repair and in some institutions are often the procedure of choice.

Most benign bile duct strictures are due to previous surgery.[1] The majority occur from inadvertent injury to the ducts during cholecystectomy, but strictures also may form at the anastomotic site after any biliary-enteric bypass procedure. Other benign causes include chronic pancreatitis, sclerosing chol-

angitis, infectious cholangitis, and common bile duct stone disease. The interval between ductal injury and the formation of a stricture is variable. Postsurgical strictures may develop in several days to several years.

Postsurgical strictures are solitary and involve the extrahepatic ducts either at the site of injury or at an anastomosis. Sclerosing cholangitis is a progressive inflammation of the bile ducts, usually resulting in multiple intrahepatic and extrahepatic strictures. Strictures from chronic pancreatitis occur at or near the distal common bile duct and are solitary; the degree of obstruction may be exacerbated with each episode of acute pancreatitis.

Can the cholangiogram distinguish a solitary benign stricture from a solitary malignant stricture? In our experience the radiographic appearance of the stricture can be misleading. Smooth tapered stric-

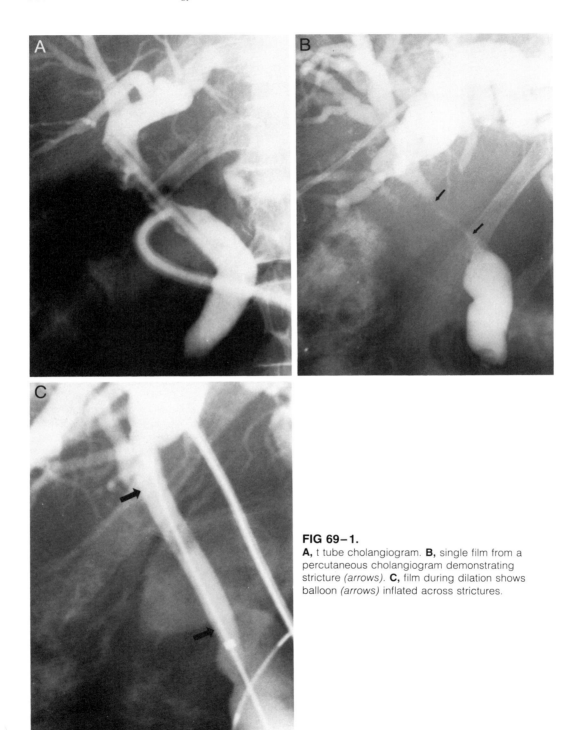

FIG 69–1.
A, t tube cholangiogram. **B,** single film from a
percutaneous cholangiogram demonstrating
stricture *(arrows).* **C,** film during dilation shows
balloon *(arrows)* inflated across strictures.

tures that look benign have on occasion proved to be malignant. Consequently needle aspiration biopsy of the stricture should be performed in most patients. The case presented illustrates this important point. The patient underwent a cholecystectomy and a T tube was inserted in the common bile duct 2 years before obstructive jaundice developed. A smooth stricture was demonstrated at the previous T tube site (Fig 69–1,B). The stricture was biopsied percutaneously, and the cytologic diagnosis was malignant disease. This changed the initial plan to dilate what appeared to be a benign stricture. Subsequently an internal stent was inserted.

Benign biliary strictures generally present as painless jaundice with or without episodes of cholangitis. If these strictures are untreated, progressive liver failure gradually develops. Occasionally emergent therapy is necessary when the patient has sepsis or possible liver abscesses.

In the past surgery was the only therapy. In addition to different types of surgical bypass procedures the stricture itself may be repaired. Choledochojejunostomy and jejunal Roux-en-Y hepatic jejunostomy have better success rates than other procedures, such as choledochoduodenostomy or primary ductal repair.[2–5] However, repeated operations frequently are needed, and the morbidity, mortality, and failure rates are significant. Stricture recurrence after reparative surgery ranges from 20% to 30%.[2–9] Among the factors that increase the likelihood of stricture recurrence are the presence of biliary cirrhosis, cholangitis, pericholangitis, and ductal scarring.[2]

In the mid-1970s the possibility of correcting biliary strictures nonsurgically became apparent with the introduction of the Gruntzig balloon angioplasty catheter. In addition, nonsurgical means of gaining access to the biliary system, such as percutaneous transhepatic biliary drainage and endoscopic retrograde cholangiopancreatography (ERCP), were gaining widespread acceptance. Initial reports introduced the plausibility and technical aspects of percutaneously dilating biliary strictures.[10–13] Subsequently larger series helped clarify appropriate patient selection, the risks and long-term benefits of the procedure, the appropriate techniques, and to a limited extent the success rate compared with that of surgery.[13, 14] The results for the nonsurgical approach seem favorable. However, insufficient data are available and many unanswered questions remain.

DIAGNOSIS

When a patient has jaundice, which noninvasive imaging studies are most helpful to differentiate hepatocellular disease from biliary obstruction? Current ultrasonography (US) equipment and computed tomographic (CT) scanners can readily detect dilated intrahepatic and extrahepatic bile ducts. However, these methods are less reliable for identifying the site and cause of the obstruction. Bile duct obstruction with no or minimal ductal dilation can occur. This is seen most often in patients with a ball valve type of obstruction due to common bile duct stones, but also can result from other causes, including benign strictures. Cholescintigraphy using technetium 99m–labeled iminodiacetic acid derivatives is useful when the ducts are not obviously dilated. The rate of small bowel opacification helps determine whether there is an obstruction.

When obstruction is diagnosed the patient frequently undergoes an invasive procedure. Percutaneous transhepatic cholangiography or ERCP demonstrates the cause and location of the obstruction. The interest and experience of the personnel at each institution determine the appropriate procedure. ERCP requires an experienced endoscopist and is technically more difficult than percutaneous transhepatic cholangiography. ERCP opacifies the nondilated biliary tree more often than does cholangiography; however, when the ducts are dilated the latter procedure is successful in nearly 100% of patients. Both percutaneous transhepatic cholangiography and ERCP can be followed by therapeutic procedures such as external biliary drainage, stone dissolution, and stricture dilation.

PERCUTANEOUS TRANSHEPATIC CHOLANGIOGRAPHY AND PERCUTANEOUS TRANSHEPATIC BILIARY DRAINAGE

All patients are pretreated with antibiotics to reduce the incidence of bacteremia. Sedation usually consists of local anesthesia and narcotics. However, in anxious patients or patients sensitive to pain, epidural anesthesia administered by the department of anesthesia usually provides complete pain relief. The needle generally is inserted at the tenth intercostal space in the mid-axillary line, with adjustments made under fluoroscopy to avoid traversing the pleura. The initial puncture is made with a 21- or 22-gauge "skinny needle" 6 to 8 inches long. The needle is inserted under fluoroscopic control and directed parallel to the table top toward the left axilla. Contrast material is injected as the needle is slowly withdrawn. If a bile duct is cannulated the entire biliary system usually can be opacified. The brisk washout of contrast material from the hepatic and portal veins readily distinguishes them from bile ducts. Opacified lymphatics empty slowly but have a reticulated, beaded appearance. In our experience the incidence of complications does not seem to increase with multiple needle insertions, so as many passes as necessary are made until the biliary tree is visualized. After opacification a catheter can be inserted. For strictures arising in the extrahepatic ductal system, either the right or left approach can be used; generally the left ductal system is more easily cannulated, because the needle is aimed directly down on and almost perpendicular to the left main duct. However, the angle the needle forms with the left duct occasionally makes subsequent catheter manipulations relatively difficult. For this reason entry into the right ductal system is often preferred, although it is technically more difficult. Biplane fluoroscopy simplifies cannulation of the right duct. A drainage catheter can be inserted in the opacified ducts through a second puncture site with an 18/19 Teflon sheath–needle combination and an 0.38 inch guidewire, or with an 0.18 inch guidewire through the 21- or 22-gauge needle used for the original transhepatic cholangiogram. Despite what seems to be complete biliary obstruction, a guidewire and catheter usually can be manipulated past the stricture site. If not, the stricture usually can be negotiated after several days of external drainage. If the patient has cholangitis or sepsis it is prudent to decompress the biliary system until the symptoms are controlled before attempting stricture dilation. This is best accomplished by keeping the catheter open to external drainage. Occasionally during the first few days after bile duct decompression bile output is excessive and may result in fluid and electrolyte imbalance. Accordingly, bile output should be monitored and appropriate fluid and electrolyte replacement therapy instituted when necessary.

The incidence of significant acute complications from percutaneous transhepatic cholangiography is slightly over 3%, with sepsis the most frequent complication, followed by bile leakage and intraperitoneal hemorrhage.[15, 16] If the procedure is combined with placement of a drainage catheter the incidence of complications increases.

There appear to be no absolute contraindications to percutaneous transhepatic cholangiography.

Patients with cholangitis or abnormal clotting are at greater risk, but the risk can be minimized by administration of antibiotics, fresh frozen plasma, or platelets. If during surgery there is suspicion of bile duct injury, a T tube inserted proximal to the suspected injured site reduces the risk and discomfort associated with a subsequent percutaneous transhepatic bile drainage should a stricture form. Negotiating guidewires and catheters through a tortuous T tube tract that forms an acute angle with the biliary system can be difficult, but usually no problems are encountered. Most T tube tracts are of sufficient caliber to accommodate the catheters and guidewires necessary for dilation, but the T tube tract should be allowed to mature for at least 4 weeks before any percutaneous manipulation.

Another percutaneous method to access the bile ducts is retrograde through the jejunal limb in patients with Roux-en-Y biliary-jejunal anastomoses.[17–19] The limb is entered through the anterior abdominal wall, and the guidewires and catheters are manipulated into the biliary system through the puncture site. The specific loop is localized with CT or by using percutaneous transhepatic cholangiography to fill its lumen with contrast material. The jejunal loop is fixed in place by postsurgical adhesions and clips, making cannulation easy and safe. Placing the end of the loop extraperitoneally during surgery just underneath the abdominal wall and marking its boundaries with clips for future fluoroscopic localization facilitates entry[18] and should further reduce the risks of hemorrhage and peritonitis. In 11 patients reported by Maroney and Ring,[19] there were no complications associated with manipulations through the jejunal loop route.

QUANTITATIVE EVALUATION OF BILIARY OBSTRUCTION

Before and after stricture dilation, biliary pressures and provocative perfusion tests determine the degree of obstruction and success of the procedure. Bile duct pressures are determined by placing a catheter above the stricture and connecting it to a saline solution–filled manometer via a three-way stopcock. The normal bile duct pressure is up to 20 cm saline solution. Perfusion rates are obtained by infusing specific quantities of saline solution into the bile duct. Normally the ducts accommodate at least 5 ml saline solution per minute. Generally bile duct pressures, flow rates, and serum bilirubin levels return to normal after successful dilation.

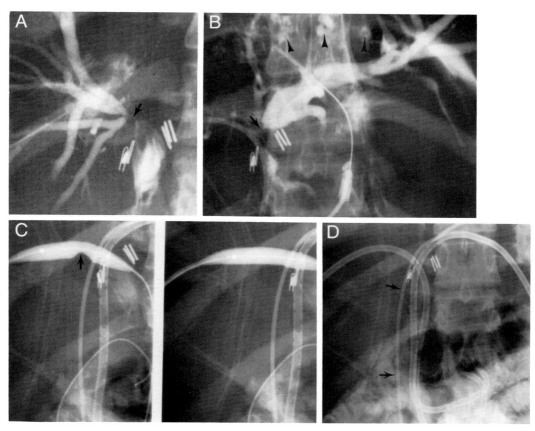

FIG 69–2.
A 17-year-old girl underwent a cholecystectomy 6 months before admission. During surgery the common hepatic duct was injured. The injury was realized, and the right and left hepatic ducts were individually anastomosed to the duodenum. She now has jaundice, cholangitis, and *Klebsiella* bacteremia. **A** and **B,** separate right and left transhepatic cholangiograms show strictures at both anastomoses *(arrows).* There are multiple intrahepatic abscesses on the left *(arrowheads).* **C,** balloon dilation of the right anastomotic stricture was accomplished using an 8 mm (24 French) balloon. There is a waist at the stricture site *(arrow).* The waist is broken with additional inflation. The left anastomotic stricture was also dilated. **D,** two internal-external catheters were inserted through the dilated strictures to act as long-term stents. A second catheter *(arrows)* was inserted into the left hepatic duct for better drainage of the abscess cavities.

STRICTURE DILATION (FIGS 69–2 THROUGH 69–4)

There are no criteria for dilating a benign bile duct stricture, and several questions concerning methods remain unanswered: (1) To what diameter should the stricture be dilated? (2) How often should it be dilated (once or multiple times)? (3) After dilation should the stricture be stented? If so, what size stent should be used, and for how long? (4) Should a catheter be inserted above the dilated stricture and clamped to see if it is functional? If so, for how long? The following discussion is a composite of our experience and the experience of others.

In general, prior to any manipulative procedure two guidewires should be inserted into the biliary tract to avoid losing access to the ducts should one of the guidewires come out.

Usually benign strictures are dilated with balloon catheters, but progressive dilation with sequentially larger dilators can be used. Almost any angioplasty catheter can be used, but we prefer the Blue Max catheter (Medi-Tech Inc., Watertown, Mass.). Balloon diameter and length are selected by determining the caliber of the nearest normal duct and

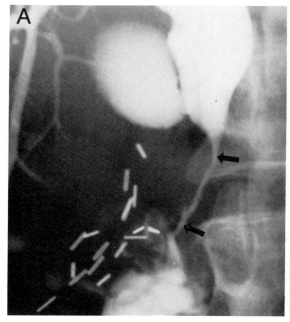

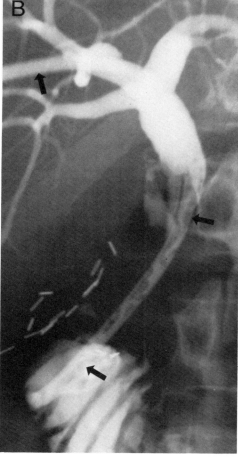

FIG 69-3.
A 40-year-old man had recurrent pancreatitis and abnormal liver function. Ultrasonography showed dilated bile ducts, gallbladder stones, and a possible common bile duct stone. **A,** a transhepatic cholangiogram demonstrated a benign appearing stricture of the distal common bile duct *(arrows),* consistent with chronic and recurrent pancreatitis. There were no ductal calculi. The stricture persisted when the current episode of pancreatitis subsided. The decision was made to try balloon dilation rather than a surgical bypass procedure. The stricture was dilated with a 5 mm (15 French) balloon. **B,** a 14 French catheter *(arrows)* was inserted through the dilated area to act as a stent and for internal drainage. The catheter will be left in place for at least several months.

the length of the stricture. Commonly used balloons have a maximal diameter between 5 and 10 mm (15 to 30 French) and should be longer than the stricture. The balloon catheter is placed over one of the guidewires, with the balloon centered in the stricture. The balloon is inflated and the pressure increased until the waistlike deformity caused by the stricture is effaced (usually 6 to 12 atm pressure). Inflation time is between 30 seconds and 3 minutes; repeated inflations may be necessary for the stricture to remain dilated. After dilation the catheter is removed, the system flushed free of any blood clots, and pressure and flow rates determined. A large-bore (12 to 16 French) drainage catheter with multiple side holes is then inserted through the dilated stricture to act as a stent. The external end of the stent is affixed to the skin and left open to external

drainage for 24 to 48 hours. At this point several alternate methods can be used. The stent can be replaced with a catheter situated proximal to the dilated area, and the stricture reevaluated as to patency, pressures, and flow rates. If the stricture appears to be functioning adequately the catheter can be removed or left above the stricture and clamped. The latter permits access to the bile ducts in case the stricture recurs in subsequent weeks. The stent through the dilated stricture can be left in place for several months, allowing the duct to heal around it. This method is advocated by most surgeons and is our preferred approach. However, catheter-related complications and patient intolerance may limit the time the stent remains in place.

The method chosen remains a matter of individual preference. At present there are no large se-

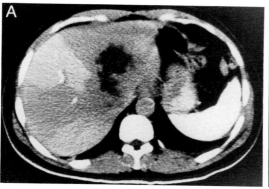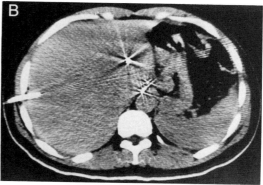

FIG 70–3.
A, computed tomographic scan of an irregular hypodense abscess. **B,** abscess has been totally drained. The catheter is placed in a slightly dependent posi-

tion to facilitate drainage. This patient's clinical condition improved significantly and drainage ceased. The catheter was removed in less than 48 hours.

GUIDANCE METHOD

US can be used for guidance if the lesions are large (5 cm or more), within 5 cm of the skin line, or in noncritical anatomic areas; CT is used for lesions that are smaller than 5 cm, more than 5 cm from the skin line, or in instances that require traversing. CT provides a better view of the entire abdomen and allows detection of other abscess sites. At our institution more than 90% of abscesses are drained with CT guidance.

If US is used for guidance the initial diagnostic aspiration is performed with a biopsy transducer device that corrects for the angle and determines the

skin entry site and distance the aspiration needle must traverse. The needle tip should be visible within the lesion before aspiration is begun.

If CT is used for guidance a marking catheter is placed over the patient's skin.[7] The correct CT slice for the precise route to the abscess is determined, and a repeat CT section is obtained at the appropriate table position. From the selected CT slice, the distance from the reference catheter to the skin entry site is calculated (Fig 70–4), as is the distance from the skin entry site to the abscess. Thus the computer provides both distance and angulation. This techniques can be performed relatively quickly.

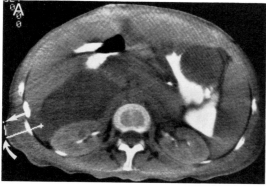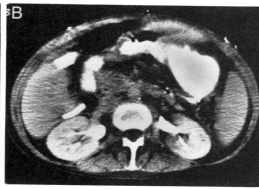

FIG 70–4.
A, computed tomographic scan demonstrates the marking catheter placed on the patient's skin *(arrow)*. From this catheter the skin entry site *(curved arrow)* is determined. Also, the distance from the skin entry site to the subhepatic biloma is determined. **B,** drain-

age of a biloma was accomplished with a single catheter. This catheter may remain in place for a significant time, because biliary defects usually take longer to heal.

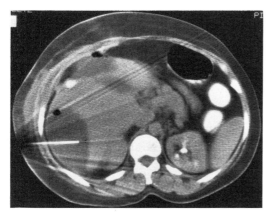

FIG 70−5.
Computed tomographic scan demonstrates diagnostic aspiration being performed with an 18-gauge sheathed needle. This is the first step in placement of a larger catheter using the Seldinger technique. The fluid obtained from this diagnostic aspiration is sent for culture and sensitivity testing. It also determines the viscosity of the fluid collection and therefore the size of catheter needed for proper drainage.

TECHNIQUE

Before percutaneous drainage is performed, broad-spectrum antibiotics are administered, through an intravenous line to lessen the chance of a severe anaphylactic reaction. A surgeon is alerted in case of a severe complication.

Seldinger Technique

The Seldinger technique is a two-step procedure. Diagnostic aspiration is performed with an 18-gauge sheathed needle and the fluid sent to the laboratory for culture and sensitivity analysis[8] (Fig 70−5). The sheath is left within the abscess and an 0.38 J guidewire placed into the lesion; the sheath is then removed and a drainage catheter placed over the guidewire into the abscess. The size of the drainage catheter used depends on the viscosity of the abscess material. Small catheters may be used with less viscous material; larger catheters are needed for viscous debris. Multiple dilators may be used to obtain the proper French size for the final catheter placement.

Trocar Technique

The trocar technique is a single-step procedure. The drainage catheter consists of a cannula and inner stylet.[8] This catheter configuration is then forced through the skin and liver into the abscess in one step. Once within the abscess, both the stylet and inner cannula are removed. This procedure is best reserved for large and superficial lesions, which are less likely to be missed by a single thrust. These abscesses are ideal candidates for the technique because they decrease the need for repetitive placement and possible complications.

CATHETER MANAGEMENT

Immediate catheter management is simple debridement of the abscess cavity with suction.[9, 10] After suction has decreased the cavity size, 5 to 10 ml aliquots of saline solution are introduced into the catheter for further debridement of the cavity (Fig 70−6). When the flush return clears, debridement

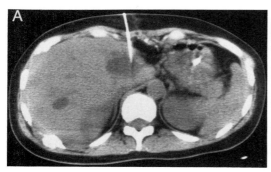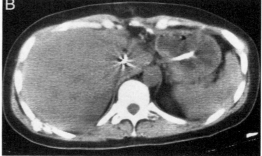

FIG 70−6.
A, computed tomographic scan demonstrates two low-density abscesses within the liver. A drainage catheter has just been placed in the larger abscess in the left hepatic lobe. **B,** after suction removal of the fluid collection the remaining cavity is debrided further with 5 to 10 ml aliquots of saline solution. Repeat scan demonstrates no cavity, and the proper debridement technique increases the chances for cure.

with saline solution is terminated. The catheter is then left to dependent drainage. Whereas some have advocated acetylcysteine (Mucomyst) as a material for debridement,[11] we believe it is unnecessary and offers little advantage over normal saline solution.

Further catheter management is important, requiring that the radiologist take a more active role in patient management. Monitoring the catheter return and the patient's clinical condition determines whether the catheter has become occluded from debris and that it remains in proper position.[12] The radiologist should advise the primary clinician on re-evaluation techniques, such as sinography or repeat imaging, and when to perform such studies.

If the catheter continues to drain significant amounts of fluid the possibility of a fistula should be considered.[13] Although a fistula may not be present on the initial examination, it may be visualized 2 to 4 days after the first drainage. If a fistula is present the drainage catheter can be placed near its orifice or a second catheter placed into the abscess for primary fistula drainage. The catheter should not be removed until the patient's condition has improved significantly, drainage has ceased, and the cavity has been obliterated. Removal of the catheter from a hepatic abscess may be possible within 36 hours or may not be feasible for 2 months or more, depending on the organism involved, whether fistulas are present, and on the general condition of the patient.[14] Also, more time usually is required in patients who have postoperative bilomas (biliary fistula; see Fig 70–3). Usually an imaging study precedes removal of the catheter.

THERAPEUTIC RESULTS

Cure

Cure rates of 50% to 100% have been reported for percutaneous hepatic abscess drainage.[1–3, 12, 13, 15, 16] However, it is important to analyze these data further. The lowest rate was reported in pediatric patients, whereas two patients not cured were improved significantly prior to more definitive therapy.[15] The higher rate was achieved in a selected patient population with amebic abscesses.[3] The initial cure rate was 85%. The final cure rate of 100% was achieved after second catheter placement in three patients.

Thus when all the data are examined, the cure rate for percutaneous hepatic abscess drainage at least equals the surgical cure rate, with less morbidity and mortality.

Temporizing (Partial Cure)

In some instances percutaneous drainage may be not definitive therapy. However, it may allow the patient's condition to improve metabolically so that a definitive surgical procedure can be initiated later. The percentage of such cases varies with the patient population. These patients are usually critically ill, and close cooperation between radiologist and surgeon is essential.

COMPLICATIONS

In a large series of abdominal abscess drainages the complication rate was 10.4%, but only 2.8% were major.[13] Hepatic abscess complication rates are similar or lower. The most common complications are bleeding and sepsis. Because this complication rate is better than that of repetitive surgery, we recommend percutaneous drainage as the primary technique for hepatic abscess drainage.

REFERENCES

1. Johnson RD, Mueller PR, Ferrucci JT Jr, et al: Percutaneous drainage of pyogenic liver abscesses. *Am J Roentgenol* 1985; 144:463–467.
2. Bernardino ME, Berkman WA, Plemons M, et al: Percutaneous drainage of multiseptated hepatic abscesses. *J Comput Assist Tomogr* 1984; 8:38–41.
3. vanSonnenberg E, Mueller PR, Schiffman RR, et al: Intrahepatic amebic abscesses: Indications for and results of percutaneous catheter drainage. *Radiology* 1985; 156:631–635.
4. Mueller PR, Dawson SL, Ferrucci JT Jr, et al: Hepatic echinococcal cyst: Successful percutaneous drainage. *Radiology* 1985; 155:627–628.
5. Francis IR, Glazer GM, Amendola MA, et al: Hepatic abscesses in the immunocompromised patient: Role of CT in detection, diagnosis, management, and follow-up. *Gastrointest Radiol* 1986; 11:257–262.
6. Miller JH, Greenfield LD, Wald BR: Candidiasis of the liver and spleen in childhood. *Radiology* 1982; 142:375–380.
7. Bernardino ME: Percutaneous biopsy. *Am J Roentgenol* 1984; 142:41–45.
8. vanSonnenberg E, Mueller PR, Ferrucci JT, et al: Sump catheter for percutaneous abscess and fluid drainage by trocar or Seldinger technique. *Am J Roentgenol* 1982; 139:613–614.
9. Mueller PR, vanSonnenberg E, Ferrucci JT Jr, et al: Percutaneous drainage of abdominal ab-

scesses and fluid collections in 250 diseases. II: Current procedural concepts. *Radiology* 1984; 151:343–347.

10. Martin EC, Karlson KB, Fankuchen E, et al: Percutaneous drainage in the management of hepatic abscesses. *Surg Clin North Am* 1981; 61:157–167.

11. vanWaes PFGM, Feldberg MAM, Mali WPTM, et al: Management of loculated abscesses that are difficult to drain: A new approach. *Radiology* 1983; 147:57–63.

12. Lang EK, Springer RM, Glorioso LW III, et al: Abdominal abscess drainage under radiologic guidance: Causes of failure. *Radiology* 1986; 159:329–336.

13. vanSonnenberg E, Mueller PR, Ferrucci JT Jr, et al: Percutaneous drainage of abdominal abscesses and fluid collections in 250 cases. I: Results, failures and complications. *Radiology* 1984; 151:337–341.

14. Rifkin MD, Heffelfinger D, Kurtz AB, et al: Outpatient therapy of intra-abdominal abscesses following early discharge from the hospital. *Radiology* 1985; 155:333–334.

15. Stanley P, Atkinson JB, Reid BS, et al: Percutaneous drainage of abdominal fluid collections in children. *Am J Roentgenol* 1984; 142:813–816.

16. Martin EC, Karlson KB, Fankuchen EI, et al: Percutaneous drainage of postoperative intraabdominal abscesses. *Am J Roentgenol* 1982; 138:13–15.

CHAPTER 71

Radiologic Imaging and Intervention for Pancreatic Inflammatory Disease

Nigel Anderson, M.B.ChB, F.R.A.C.R.
Eric vanSonnenberg, M.D.
Giovanna Casola, M.D.
Robert R. Varney, M.D.

Case Presentation

A middle-aged man with a known history of alcoholism had worsening abdominal pain. Computed tomography (CT) was performed (Fig 71–1). What is the diagnosis? What is the differential diagnosis of pancreatic fluid collections? What is the best method to image and follow them? How should pancreatic fluid collections be managed? Are there any differences between large and small pancreatic fluid collections? Is there a critical size? What is pancreatic necrosis? Should it be managed differentially by the radiologist than a pancreatic pseudocyst or abscess?

DISCUSSION

Pancreatic fluid collections occur within, around, or remote from the pancreas, and are manifestations and complications of severe acute pancreatitis. The emphasis of this chapter is on the appearances and management of complicated acute pancreatitis. In the appropriate clinical setting, the diagnosis usually is straightforward. If the fluid collection is detected without a history of acute pancreatitis, there may be both a diagnostic and therapeutic dilemma.

The management of pancreatic fluid collections, rather than their diagnosis, continues to be a clinical challenge. The timing and approach of treatment of pseudocysts, in particular, remain controversial.[1-3] A flow chart for the management of pancreatic fluid collections is presented, based on literature review, integrated with our experience.

CT is the most useful imaging technique for diagnosis and follow-up of complications of acute pancreatitis.[4-7] The timing of imaging, as well as the relative merits of CT, ultrasound (US), and magnetic resonance imaging (MRI), are addressed. The integrated roles of interventional radiology and surgery are discussed with reference to percutaneous

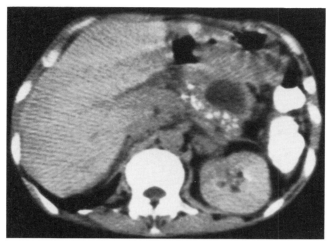

FIG 71–1.
Computed tomogram at level of body and tail of the pancreas.
What are the findings? What is your diagnosis?

versus open drainage of pseudocysts, phlegmons, and abscesses. Fluid collections associated with pancreatic transplants are common, and their diagnosis and treatment are highlighted. Finally, cystic pancreatic neoplasms, pseudoaneurysms, and other differential diagnoses for pancreatic pseudocysts are addressed.[8]

ACUTE AND CHRONIC PANCREATITIS

Pancreatitis has been categorized as acute, acute relapsing, and chronic. However, in terms of managing and treating the disease it is more useful to subdivide pancreatitis into acute, obstructive, and chronic.

Acute pancreatitis implies that the pancreas will return to normal. Obstructive pancreatitis implies an obstructive cause, such as papillary stenosis or pancreas divisum. Chronic pancreatitis implies chronic progressive fibrosis within the pancreas, whether associated with acute exacerbations or not.

Acute Pancreatitis

Causes of acute pancreatitis include alcohol, gallstones, trauma, surgery, hyperlipidemia, drugs, familial causes, post-parturition, systemic lupus erythematosus, and postcardiac pump. Most epi-

sodes of acute pancreatitis are self-limited; however, complications occur in 18% of cases,[5] with considerable morbidity and mortality. A severe form of complicated pancreatitis is hemorrhagic or necrotizing pancreatitis; this entity may be predicted in many instances from clinical and laboratory signs early in the course of the disease.[9] In the early stages of severe pancreatitis profound shock and hypovolemia require vigorous supportive measures. The next phase of pancreatitis is marked by persistent symptoms from necrosis or from unresolved fluid collections that form pseudocysts. Abscesses usually occur later in the course of the disease. The third phase is persistent pseudocyst or abscess, usually after 2 to 3 weeks of clinical symptoms.[10, 17] The distinction between pseudocyst and abscess is prognostically important.

The precise mechanism of the initial insult in acute pancreatitis is unknown; however, following pancreatic injury autodigestion of pancreatic and peripancreatic tissues occurs. The peripheral effects of pancreatic autodigestion are parenchymal necrosis, due to phospholipase A; fat necrosis, due to lipase and phospholipase A; vessel injury, due to elastase.[12]

These effects may result in small vessel hemorrhage, and hemorrhagic pancreatitis may ensue. Pancreatic duct rupture leads to pancreatic fluid collections,[13, 14] and sequestration of calcium in fat necrosis due to calcium soap formation accounts for hypocalcemia.[12]

If the sinus tract from the ruptured pancreatic duct remains open, ongoing pancreatic enzyme accumulation occurs. This leads to more extensive fat and tissue necrosis. If the fluid collection is adjacent to a visceral artery, pseudoaneurysms may form.[15] A collection adjacent to bowel wall may produce stenosis, necrosis, or fistula.[16]

Chronic Pancreatitis

Chronic pancreatitis may present insidiously or as an acute attack clinically identical to that described for acute pancreatitis. Pathologically, the gland fails to return to normal and becomes hard, fibrotic, and often contains multiple calcifications. Acute pancreatitis can be superimposed on chronic pancreatitis, as shown in Figure 71–1, which shows stippled calcifications through the body and tail, indicating chronic pancreatitis, and a 4 × 3 cm pseudocyst, indicating a resolving acute process. Alcohol is the usual precipitating factor. Inasmuch as the entire gland is abnormal, extensive pancreatic resections may lead to pancreatic insufficiency.

Pancreatic fluid collections seen in chronic pancreatitis are pseudocysts and chronic effusions resulting from pancreatic fistulas to peritoneum, pleura, or pericardium. These fistulous communications are seen more in chronic than in acute pancreatitis and may occur in the absence of any acute inflammatory episode. Elevated protein (> 3 gm/dl) amylase, and lipase levels in these fluid collections differentiate them from other effusions.[17, 18]

COMPLICATIONS OF PANCREATITIS

Ambiguity in terminology and overlap in pathologic features contribute to imprecision in defining complications of pancreatitis. The following are definitions of commonly encountered complications:

Phlegmon.—An inflammatory mass in peripancreatic tissues or in the pancreas itself. It may resolve completely or lead to necrosis, liquefaction, or abscess.

Loculated Fluid Collection.—A localized collection of pancreatic fluid seen early in the course of acute pancreatitis may be found within the pancreas, lesser sac, or retroperitoneum or may spread remotely into the groin, mediastinum, pleura, or pericardium. These resolve completely (53%) or persist as pseudocysts.

Pseudocyst (Fig 71–2).—Localized collection of pancreatic fluid confined by a capsule of fibrous and granulation tissue. Pseudocysts lack a true epithelial lining. The features distinguish it from a true cyst or cystic neoplasm. Pseudocysts frequently resolve completely if smaller than 4 cm. Persistent pseudocysts may rupture, become infected, bleed, or result in pseudoaneurysm formation.

Abscess.—Bacterial infection of a pancreatic phlegmon or of necrosis is pancreatic abscess. The

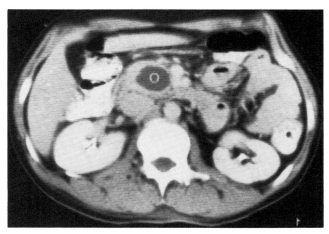

FIG 71–2.
Acute pancreatitis with low-density pseudocyst in the head of the pancreas.

mortality is 100% unless the abscess is drained. An abscess should not be confused with a secondarily infected pseudocyst; the natural history and sequelae of the two conditions differ.

Pancreatic Necrosis.—Nonviable pancreatic tissue may regenerate if small, but large areas often become infected as pseudocysts unless surgically healed.

Pancreatic Hemorrhage.—Massive hemorrhage may accompany a ruptured pseudocyst or pseudoaneurysm. Bleeding also may occur with pancreatic ascites or from a pseudocyst wall following drainage. Mortality with pancreatic hemorrhage is high.

Less life-threatening hemorrhage occurs at the onset of hemorrhagic pancreatitis. Minor bleeding may occur from the wall of a nondrained pseudocyst or after percutaneous drainage.

Gastrointestinal hemorrhage may occur from rupture of a pseudoaneurysm into the pancreatic duct either directly or via a pseudocyst[14]; a pseudocyst also may rupture or erode into the gastrointestinal tract.

Pseudoaneurysm.—Localized dilation of a visceral artery related to inflammatory weakening of the arterial wall by transudation of pancreatic enzymes liberated in acute pancreatitis. A pseudoaneurysm usually is associated with a pseudocyst. The splenic and gastroduodenal arteries are involved most frequently; however, any artery in contact with a pancreatic fluid collection may be affected. Hemorrhage either into a pseudocyst or into the pancreatic duct, presenting as a gastrointestinal hemorrhage, may be intermittent and repetitious or sometimes massive.[19]

Pancreatic Ascites.—Ongoing outpouring of pancreatic fluid from a disrupted pancreatic duct via a fistula into the peritoneal cavity. The fistula may occur with an episode of acute pancreatitis; more commonly it forms at a time remote from the acute event and as a complication of chronic pancreatitis. Endoscopic retrograde cholangiopancreatography (ERCP) may document the site of leakage prior to definitive surgery. Diagnosis is made by the triad findings of elevated amylase (and lipase) levels in the ascites and in the serum (due to passive absorption from the ascites), and elevated protein levels in the ascitic fluid (> 3 gm/dl).[17]

Pancreatic Pleural Effusion.—Pleural effusions commonly accompany pancreatitis and are usually sympathetic. Rarely a painless pleural effusion with high amylase and protein content is due to a pancreaticopleural fistula tracking via the aortic or esophageal hiatus into the mediastinum. A fistula is best demonstrated by CT performed immediately after ERCP.[20] Treatment usually requires excision of the involved part of pancreas.[18, 20]

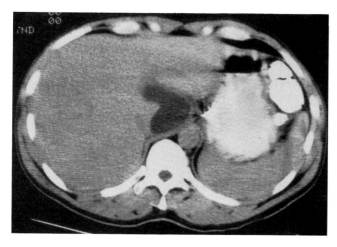

FIG 71–3.
Remote location of a pancreatic pseudocyst. Pancreatic fluid has dissected up into the liver in the superior recess of the lesser sac, where it is defined as a pseudocyst.

PANCREATIC FLUID COLLECTIONS

The pancreas lacks a well-defined capsule, and fluid collections tend to escape from it, and may dissect along tissue planes adjacent to the pancreas or continue to remote sites. These fluid collections are confined to the pancreas in only one third of patients. Potential sites for pancreatic fluid collections logically follow from anatomic pathways. More than one abdominal compartment usually is involved in any given patient. Specifics of each compartment follow.

Lesser Sac

The lesser sac is the commonest site of a pancreatic fluid collection, because of its anatomic proximity to the pancreas.[11] Fluid in the superior recess may be seen adjacent to the gastroesophageal junction. Apparent extension into the liver via the ligamentum venosum may also be seen (Fig 71-3). More commonly the fluid is seen behind the stomach (Fig 71-4).

Anterior and Posterior Pararenal Space

The anterior pararenal space, lying around and posterior to the pancreas,[11] is the second most common site of fluid collection. The ascending or descending colon may be involved. The anterior pararenal space communicates with the posterior pararenal space below Gerota's fascia. Fluid collections may occur anywhere in the retroperitoneum and may extend down to the groin or scrotum. Gerota's fascia tends to protect the kidneys and adrenal glands from involvement.[21]

Mesenteric Attachments and Gastrointestinal Tract

The transverse mesocolon with its broad pancreatic origin and the small bowel mesentery with its smaller attachment commonly are sites of pancreatic inflammation. Dissection along these mesenteries accounts for involvement of the transverse colon and small bowel loops (Fig 71-5). This inflammation results in the well-known "colon cutoff sign" and "sentinel loop," plain film signs of acute pancreatitis.

More serious bowel complications occur in about 1% of patients and include fistula, stenosis, or necrosis. In order of occurrence, fistulas are seen to the stomach, duodenum, colon, and esophagus. Stenosis and necrosis tend to be confined to the colon, presumed to be on the basis of small vessel thrombosis.[16] Small bowel infarction is rare,[22] perhaps surprising in view of the proximity of the superior mesenteric artery and vein to an inflammatory process.

Mediastinum and Pleura

Extension into the mediastinum can occur via the esophageal hiatus from the lesser sac or via the aortic hiatus from the retroperitoneum. These pancreatic collections may extend cephalad into the neck. Rarely they may rupture into one or both

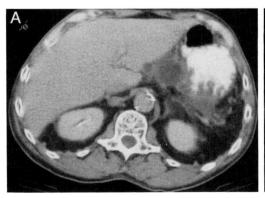 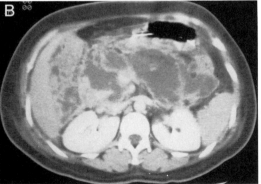

FIG 71-4.
Acute pancreatitis developing into a pseudocyst in the lesser sac. **A,** ill-defined intrapancreatic and extrapancreatic fluid collections posterior to the stomach. Note thickened rugal folds. **B,** three weeks later a defined pseudocyst is seen in the lesser sac on this more caudal scan.

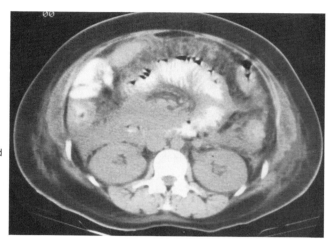

FIG 71-5.
Severe acute pancreatitis: Note marked thickening of areas in the mesentery extending into the small bowel wall. Dilation of the small bowel due to ileus is present. Inflammation extends into the abdominal musculature and soft tissue fascia.

pleural spaces. Usually a collection in the chest either remains localized to the mediastinum or ruptures into the pleural space.[17, 18, 20]

Peritoneum

A pancreaticoperitoneal fistula resulting in pancreatic ascites is uncommon. Peritoneal fluid usually is a sympathetic effusion if caused by acute pancreatitis; alternatively, it may represent a transient pancreatic fluid collection entering from the lesser sac via the epiploic foramen. Caudal extension of pancreatic fluid from the peritoneum into the scrotum may occur.[11, 20]

IMAGING OF PANCREATIC FLUID COLLECTIONS

The main uses of imaging for pancreatic fluid collections are to identify fluid collections, assess extent and character (i.e., necrosis, infection), diagnose complications (e.g., biliary obstruction), and guide needle aspiration or percutaneous catheter drainage. US and CT are the imaging methods of choice, with CT offering better precision. MRI and radionuclide scintigraphy have no current utility in the diagnosis and management of pancreatic inflammation.[7, 23–25]

Imaging is necessary because clinical criteria alone are insufficient to adequately predict serious complications of pancreatitis.[4] Clinical grading by Ranson's criteria[9, 26] or modifications of the severity of acute pancreatitis serves as a useful marker in predicting outcome of pancreatitis. An abscess will develop in 12.5% of patients hospitalized with mild

pancreatitis.[27] All cases of pancreatic necrosis[28] or abscess[27] are preceded by an acute extrapancreatic fluid collection or phlegmon, visible on CT early in the disease. However, 53% of such fluid collections or phlegmons resolve spontaneously and without sequelae[11] (Fig 71-6). Dynamic contrast-enhanced CT has been advocated to improve specificity in predicting pancreatic necrosis or abscess.[29] Thus CT early in the clinical course, combined with clinical grading, is helpful in predicting those patients at risk for serious complications (i.e., pseudocyst, necrosis, abscess).[1, 4, 27, 28]

Ultrasound

The main uses of ultrasound in pancreatic fluid collections and pancreatitis are to assess the bile ducts and to follow progression of a potential pseudocyst.[29] In practice, sonography frequently is the initial screening test in acute pancreatitis because of its ready availability compared with CT. Gallstones, biliary dilation, and fluid collections can be reliably detected, except when bowel gas obscures the fluid collections; this occurs in 36% of examinations.[5] In those examinations providing good to excellent visualization of the pancreas and retroperitoneum, the pancreatic tail as a rule is obscured,[5] so that even large masses or fluid collections may be missed. Recent hemorrhage (i.e., hemorrhagic pancreatitis) appears hyperechoic[30]; if this echogenic hematoma can be differentiated from surrounding normal structures, a complicated course may be predicted.[31] After seven days, pancreatic hemorrhage becomes hypoechoic and is indistinguishable from other fluid collections.[30]

Late in the disease course, as the small bowel

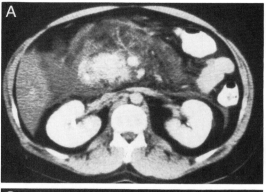

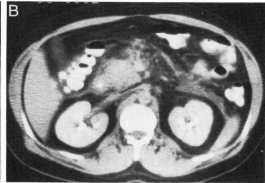

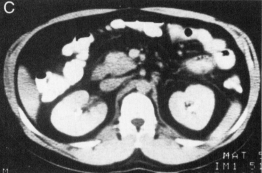

FIG 71–6.
Resolution of pancreatic inflammatory changes. **A,** on this enhanced computed tomographic scan note extensive peripancreatic, poorly-defined edematous and phlegmonous changes. **B,** two weeks later the inflammation has improved markedly. Ill-defined inflammatory changes are seen around the pancreatic head and the mesenteric artery and vein. **C,** four weeks later there is complete resolution.

ileus resolves, pancreatic visualization on US tends to improve, so that US is ideal for following development of a pseudocyst (Fig 71–7). Sonography can assess the size and internal consistency of pseudocysts, aiding treatment planning[32] (Fig 71–8).

Pseudocyst aspiration for diagnosis of infection can be done under US guidance.[3, 14, 33, 34] Because transgression of bowel should be avoided, CT-guided aspiration usually is preferred, especially inasmuch as catheter drainage may be required.[3, 14, 35, 36] Intraoperative US has a significant role in surgery for inflammatory pancreatic disease, allowing nonpalpable fluid collections and abscesses to be located.[37]

Computed Tomography

CT best displays the retroperitoneum and therefore is the method of choice for assessing complications of pancreatitis.[6, 7, 11] It is also the preferred guidance method for directing interventional procedures, because bowel, ureters, and viscera are best displayed and avoided.[7, 14, 33, 36, 38, 39]

CT rarely results in a nondiagnostic scan (2%), compared with US (36%).[5, 32] Technical problems usually are related to lack of patient cooperation resulting in scan artifacts.

CT resources do not allow for all patients with acute pancreatitis to be scanned, nor should they be. Patients who should undergo CT include all those with clinically severe pancreatitis, and they should be scanned early; any patient with pancreatitis not resolving within the first week; any patient with pancreatitis and a persisting or enlarging pleural effusion (to look for either abscess or pancreaticopleural fistula)[18]; any patient whose clinical condition deteriorates after improving initially.[4, 27, 40]

If CT is performed in the first 7 days of the acute episode, scans before and after intravenous injection of contrast material are ideal. Hemorrhage appears hyperdense during the first week, but becomes indistinguishable from other fluid collections after that (a pattern similar to that seen on US).[30] Comparison scans allow assessment of contrast enhancement of the pancreas and the phlegmon. The likelihood of complications correlates well with the presence of pancreatic fluid collections[5, 31, 39, 41] but even better with contrast enhancement of a phlegmon.[4, 27, 28, 41]

Problems with CT include differentiating abscess from phlegmon and necrosis, and assessing

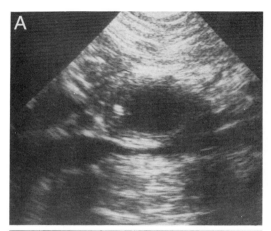

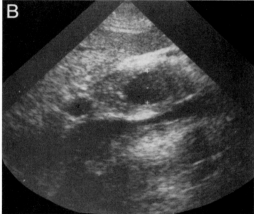

FIG 71–7.
Sonography for pancreatic pseudocyst. **A,** a 4 cm pseudocyst with a thick wall and an echogenic focus, likely representing calcification. **B,** two weeks later the pseudocyst is smaller.

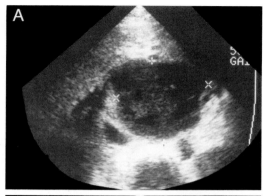

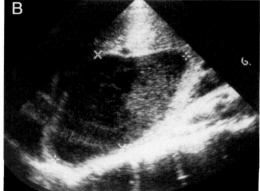

FIG 71–8.
Large debris-filled pancreatic pseudocyst seen in transverse **(A)** and longitudinal **(B)** sections. The pseudocyst extended into and through the diaphragm and into the mediastinum.

"drainability" of a collection.[38] CT reliability detects gas within the pancreatic tissues, but not all abscesses contain gas[27, 38, 40]; conversely, not all gas implies abscess.[42, 43] Gas may occur within a collection that has spontaneously fistulized into the gastrointestinal tract.[42]

Drainable fluid collections are hypodense on CT. Not all hypodense collections are abscess or pseudocyst; some are due to necrosis with liquefaction.[28]

Possible abscesses and potentially drainable fluid collections should undergo diagnostic needle aspiration. CT alone is not sufficiently specific to assess them.[14, 33, 44, 45]

Magnetic Resonance Imaging

MRI is not as useful as CT in imaging pancreatic inflammatory disease because of its poorer spatial resolution, problems with respiratory motion, difficulty with tissue characterization,[24, 46, 47] and less accessibility.

All pancreatic fluid collections have long T_2 relaxation times. It was initially thought that T_1 would be discriminatory for types of fluid collections,[25, 48] but with further experience a wide overlapping range of T_1 relaxation times has been seen in all inflammatory pancreatic processes.[24] Pancreatic phlegmon is difficult to distinguish from normal pancreas[24, 47] by relaxation time criteria. The extent and margins of extrapancreatic fluid collections are seen better on CT. Another problem with MRI is relative insensitivity to pancreatic calcifications.[24, 46, 47] Surface coil imaging improves spatial resolution and reduces respiratory motion artifact; these advantages are not enough to alter the overall inferiority of MRI compared with CT with inflammatory pancreatic disease.[24, 46]

In summary, MRI has no role at present in imaging complications of acute pancreatitis. CT performs the same function, but with added sensitivity and specificity.

Endoscopic Retrograde Cholangiopancreatography

The purposes of ERCP in pancreatic fluid collections are to (1) outline abnormalities in the biliary and pancreatic ducts after acute biliary pancreatitis,[49] (2) define pancreatic ductal anatomy prior to surgery for chronic pancreatitis,[50] (3) demonstrate the site of a pancreatic fistula to the pleura, pericardium, or peritoneum, (4) diagnose pancreas divisum,[51] and (5) demonstrate whether a pseudocyst communicates with or obstructs the pancreatic duct.[52] This last function is less important now that percutaneous drainage of pseudocysts allows this information to be ascertained by catheter sinography.[14] An emerging role for ERCP is early diagnosis of bile duct stones with urgent sphincterotomy in cases of acute biliary pancreatitis.[29] The procedure should be done within the first 24 hours. An early report suggests reduced morbidity and mortality from acute biliary pancreatitis.[53] Although this role still is considered controversial, it is likely to become more widely accepted.

The complication rate with ERCP is 2% to 3% in experienced hands, comprising pancreatitis and sepsis most commonly, and the risks of endoscopy.[53, 54] Sphincterotomy has a 0.5% to 1.5% mortality.[43] Pseudocysts filling via ERCP are prone to sepsis and should be drained within 24 hours of the procedure to limit this complication.[52]

If a pancreaticopleural fistula is suspected, ERCP followed by CT is the most effective diagnostic approach. ERCP demonstrates the site of leakage, allowing preoperative planning for surgical resection; CT demonstrates the size and exact course of the fistula.[14, 20]

In summary, ERCP has its greatest role in the workup of biliary pancreatitis and in preoperative planning for pancreatic resection in patients with chronic pancreatitis or pancreatic fistulas to the chest or peritoneum. An emerging role is urgent decompression of the biliary tree in acute biliary pancreatitis due to common duct stones.

Indium 111 Scintigraphy

Indium 111–labeled white cell imaging is sensitive in detecting pancreatic necrosis but cannot distinguish necrosis from abscess,[23] so CT still is required. Its major disadvantages are that other pancreatic fluid collections are not imaged and it does not display anatomy. Indium 111 leukocyte imaging, then, can reliably distinguish complicated acute pancreatitis from the uncomplicated disease, but is unable to differentiate between abscess, necrosis, and pseudocyst. Pancreatic scintigraphy is unlikely to have a major role in diagnosis of pancreatic fluid collections.

DIAGNOSTIC NEEDLE ASPIRATION

Establish Diagnosis of Cystic Pancreatic Mass.—Most cystic pancreatic masses are pseudocysts.[8, 55, 56] Amylase levels in the cyst fluid almost always distinguish pseudocyst from cystic neoplasm. Conversely, cytologic findings may be positive for cystadenocarcinoma. If there is a solid portion of the cystic mass, it should be biopsied as well.[8, 14, 55, 57]

Diagnosis of Infection.—The clinical diagnosis of infection in a pancreatic collection is difficult, because fever and leukocytosis are common to almost all complications of acute pancreatitis. Infected pancreatic fluid collections rarely are pathognomonic by imaging studies. Gas, present in 30% of abscesses, is a helpful but unreliable sign; gas may be seen when a fistula to bowel is present[2, 42, 58] or with sterile necrosis.[43] Timely diagnostic needle aspiration can answer the clinical question of whether infection is present.[7, 44] Aspiration is 90% to 95% accurate.[14, 45] Gram stain of infected fluid aspirate reveals abundant white cells and may identify an organism. Aerobic and anaerobic cultures are mandatory. Although the color, texture, and odor of an infected collection often are unmistakable, uninfected necrosis can be misleading. Early diagnosis expedites early treatment, which improves the prognosis.[4, 40]

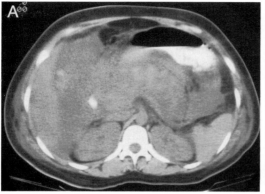

FIG 71–9.
Use of intravenous contrast to assess fluid content and predict drainability. **A,** changes of acute pancreatitis with isodense material in the pancreatic and lesser sac regions. **B,** after administration of intravenous contrast material, low-density mass is seen in the lesser sac region. This indicates that at least part of this complex can be drained percutaneously.

Assess Drainability.— By imaging criteria, low-density material after contrast administration usually can be evacuated by percutaneous catheter (Fig 71–9). Collections that have low density on CT or are echo poor on US may be necrotic or very viscous, and occasionally cannot be aspirated. Conversely, some collections that are moderately dense on CT or echogenic on US may have at least a portion that is drainable.[38, 39] High-density material almost assuredly cannot be drained percutaneously.

In most instances a 22-gauge needle will suffice to aspirate material; this indicates drainability and whether infection is present (Fig 71–10). Occasionally a larger needle (20 or 18 gauge) may be required if the material is viscous. If a thick fibrous wall surrounds the collection a firm puncture may be required to penetrate the wall.[14, 38, 39] If fluid cannot be aspirated with an 18-gauge needle the collection is deemed unsuitable for percutaneous drainage.[38]

Technique, Guidelines, and Problems.— For diagnostic aspiration of a possibly noninfected collection, bacteria-containing bowel should not be violated.[14, 34, 36, 38] In most cases the access route for aspiration should be planned with potential drainage in mind. CT usually is used to plan access routes, because of its superior display of anatomy.

Complications are unusual; transient episodes of bacteremia may occur when infected collections

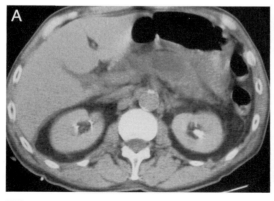
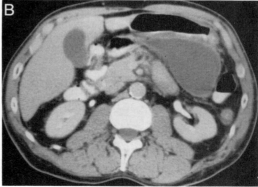

FIG 71–10.
Intrapancreatic fluid collection with surrounding inflammatory changes. **A,** small poorly-defined infected pseudocyst is present. **B,** more caudally is a large well-defined pseudocyst.

CHAPTER 73

Gastrointestinal Bleeding

David F. Hunter, M.D.
Robert J. Boudreau, M.D., Ph.D.

Case Presentation

A previously healthy middle-aged man had bright red rectal bleeding. His hematocrit was stable when he was admitted. Colonoscopy could not be completed because the scope could not reach the right colon. Blood was seen coming from the bowel proximal to the scope. What would you recommend? Why? How accurate are nuclear medicine studies? When would you recommend arteriography and interventional techniques? What are the success rates of the various interventional techniques? What are their complications?

NUCLEAR MEDICINE STUDIES

The first investigation in a patient suspected of having active upper gastrointestinal bleeding is endoscopy. Usually it has already been performed before the radiologist is consulted. Colonoscopy is usually not recommended with active lower gastrointestinal bleeding because the blood in the bowel can obscure the source. If acute hemorrhage is suspected, the next investigation of choice is a technetium 99m–labeled red blood cell (RBC) study. It is important not to introduce barium into the gastrointestinal tract, because this will seriously interfere with subsequent investigations. Originally there was considerable controversy as to whether gastrointestinal bleeding studies should be performed with Tc 99m–sulfur colloid or Tc 99m–labeled RBCs.[1, 2] Tc 99m–sulfur colloid had the advantage of being a quicker study to perform. Also, because the colloid is rapidly cleared from the circulation, the study is sensitive to small hemorrhages and the results easier to interpret. However, the patient must be actively bleeding at the time of the injection. In clinical practice this is usually not the case, and the

sensitivity of this study in routine clinical use is poor. Tc 99m–labeled RBC imaging can be conducted for up to 24 hours after injection, which greatly improves its sensitivity for the detection of gastrointestinal hemorrhage. In a recent study the sensitivity of the Tc 99m–sulfur colloid test was only 12%, compared with 93% for Tc 99m–labeled RBCs.[3] A common question arises as to when to terminate the Tc 99m–labeled RBC study. In the previously cited study 83% of the studies that ever yielded positive results did so within 90 minutes after injection. Another investigator[4] found the positivity rate of the RBC study to be 55% at 4 hours after injection. Of the remaining 45% of the studies that eventually yielded positive results, the vast majority did not appear until 12 to 24 hours after injection. Our current policy is to image until 2 hours after injection. If the patient appears stable and the study results are negative, a delayed image is obtained at 4 hours or the following morning. Imaging can be continued for up to 24 hours. Imaging also can be done any time if there is evidence of acute hemorrhage.

It was only recently that the bleeding rate necessary for detecting acute gastrointestinal bleeding with Tc 99m–labeled RBCs was determined. Animal experiments with Tc 99m–sulfur colloid had shown that bleeding rates as low as 0.05 to 0.01 ml/min could be detected. Angiography is supposedly only able to detect hemorrhage rates greater than 0.5 ml/min, although the limitations inherent in the study from which this figure is derived probably underestimate the capabilities of modern selective angiographic methods. A recent animal experiment performed by Thorn et al.[4] using Tc 99m–labeled RBCs showed that bleeding rates as low as 0.2 ml/min were detected within 10 minutes and those as low as 0.04 ml/min were seen by 55 minutes. Slower rates of bleeding were not detected. They also calculated that a minimum volume of 2 or 3 ml labeled blood was necessary to detect bleeding in the dog. Based on these results it would appear that Tc 99m–labeled RBCs are sensitive for low bleeding rates in the dog model. If results of this study are negative it is probably wise to defer angiography. Winzelberg et al.[2] found that of 17 angiograms performed in a face of negative results of a Tc 99m–labeled RBC study only one showed extravasation. However, five of these 17 studies showed abnormalities such as angiodysplasia or aneurysms but not hemorrhage. Thus the likelihood of demonstrating disease is significantly diminished in the face of negative Tc 99m–labeled RBC study results.

The Tc 99m–labeled RBC study in the case presented is shown in Figure 73–1. These images show an intense accumulation of radioactivity in the right lower quadrant that later migrates up through the ascending colon. Note that it is the pattern of migration of the activity that allows identification of the location of the bleeding site. In this patient it was not clearly seen on the first angiogram, but was seen on the second angiogram when the patient rebled (Fig 73–2,A and B). In contradistinction to the colonic bleeding site, a small bowel bleed will show migration from the left upper quadrant to the right lower quadrant, following the normal distribution of the small bowel. However, caution is advised in interpreting the exact anatomic location of the site of the hemorrhage. The RBC study is only 83% accurate in identifying the location of the hemorrhage.[1]

Not all RBC studies reveal a localized gastrointestinal hemorrhage. In Figure 73–3 a study is shown in which diffuse activity appeared throughout the bowel. This patient had immunoproliferative small intestinal disease, and the study was being performed to determine if the hemorrhage was diffuse or localized. The next example is a case in which the angiogram did not show extravasation but nonetheless revealed the abnormality. A definite right upper quadrant accumulation of RBCs is seen (Fig 73–4). The large cold spot in the center of the image is an infusion pump. An angiogram showed a collection of abnormal vessels in this location in the liver in addition to a possible ascending colon angiodysplasia. Although no extravasation was seen, a vasopressin (Pitressin) infusion was commenced, with subsequent control of the hemorrhage. Occasionally the hemorrhage is not into the bowel but intraperitoneal. Figure 73–5 shows a patient with

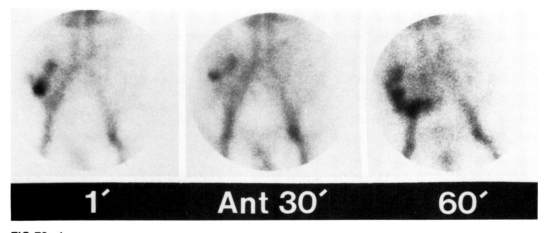

FIG 73–1.
Technetium 99m–labeled red blood cell study shows intense accumulation of radioactivity in the right lower quadrant that later migrates up the ascending colon.

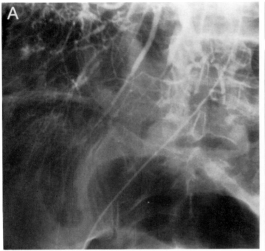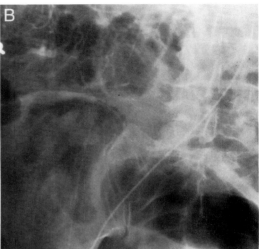

FIG 73–2.
A, arterial phase of a superior mesenteric artery injection shows early extravasation from a branch of the right colic artery into the ascending colon. **B,** venous phase shows the classic appearance of an expanding, irregular contrast collection.

Fanconi's anemia, declining hemoglobin level, and increasing abdominal girth. The RBC study initially shows a paucity of bowel activity within a distended abdomen, consistent with abdominal fluid. Subsequent images show a collection of red cells medial to the spleen, which then progresses inferomedially, diffusing into the peritoneal cavity. Subsequent exploratory surgery showed intraperitoneal hemorrhage originating from the inferior portion of the spleen.

There are numerous pitfalls in interpreting results of RBC studies. Because the entire vascular

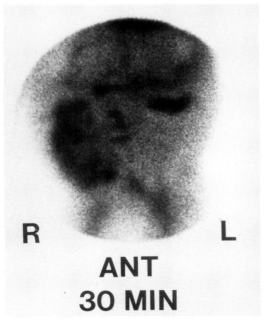

FIG 73–3.
Diffuse extravasation of labeled red cells is seen in this patient with immunoproliferative small intestinal disease.

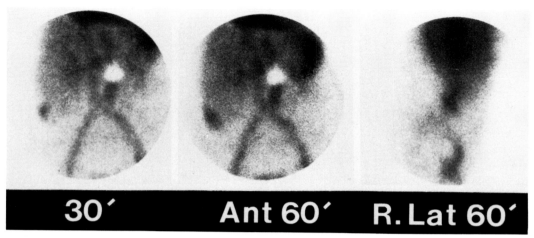

FIG 73–4.
Accumulation of tracer in the right upper quadrant is seen. Angiography revealed a vascular lesion of the liver and possible angiodysplasia of the colon. The central cold spot represents an infusion pump.

pool of the body is being imaged, a keen awareness of normal variations is required. Two articles have recently addressed the pitfalls of gastrointestinal bleeding studies.[5, 6] That by Dorfman et al.[6] contains numerous examples of both normal and abnormal studies and can serve as a reference for those with little experience in interpreting these studies. Technical problems can also compromise the study. Figure 73–6 shows an example of incomplete labeling of the red cells. Note the accumulation of tracer in the stomach and salivary glands related to free pertechnetate. If activity in the stomach is allowed to pass into the bowel the study results are invalidated. Consideration should be given to passing a nasogastric tube when large amounts of such activity are visualized.

In the pediatric population one specific cause of gastrointestinal hemorrhage that must be considered is Meckel's diverticulum. Tc 99m pertechnetate accumulates in gastric mucosa. Inasmuch as

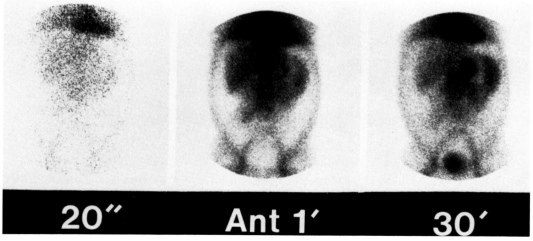

FIG 73–5.
Study shows an abdominal fluid collection as evidenced by a paucity of bowel activity. A focus of activity medial to the spleen migrates inferiorly into the peritoneal cavity. This patient had a peritoneal hemorrhage from the inferior portion of the spleen.

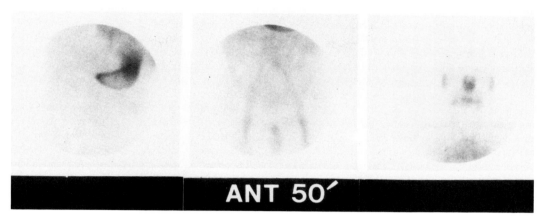

FIG 73–6.
Study shows patterns of a poor red blood cell tag.

most Meckel's diverticula that cause symptoms and hemorrhage do contain gastric mucosa, they are visualized on the study. These are usually located in the right lower quadrant in the distal ileum. Occasionally duplication cysts may also contain ectopic gastric mucosa and may also be identified. It is important that the diverticulum be visualized at the same time as the stomach, because this activity will gradually leave the stomach and progress through the small bowel. Various authors have used pharmacologic stimulation with cimetidine, secretin, and glucagon to increase the sensitivity of the study.[7–10] These pharmacologic manipulations should be considered in a patient who initially has negative study results but in whom there is strong clinical suspicion of disease.

ANGIOGRAPHIC DIAGNOSIS

In the last decade angiography has lost its role as the principal diagnostic tool in the evaluation of gastrointestinal bleeding. Angiography rose to preeminent position in the early 1960s after a series of superb articles by Baum, Nusbaum, Waltman, Athanasoulis, Margulis, and others that clearly showed the ability of angiography to localize and occasionally characterize lesions and therefore to significantly reduce surgical morbidity and mortality as well as postoperative rebleeding rates. With the advent of modern endoscopy and improved nuclear medicine techniques, however, angiography has become a third-order test used in selected patients and for specific reasons. In one study that included patients examined between 1972 and 1982, specific

mention was made of the fact that during that time angiography had lost its role as a tool in the localization of bleeding sites.[11] There are, however, two definite categories of patients for whom angiography is particularly useful: hemodynamically stable patients, in whom angiography is used after negative endoscopic studies in an attempt to more accurately establish the location and nature of the bleeding lesion prior to definitive transcatheter or surgical therapy,[12] and unstable or massively hemorrhaging patients, in whom angiography is required to rapidly locate the bleeding site prior to emergency surgery or in whom it is hoped that transcatheter control of the bleeding will either obviate surgery or allow a safer, more elective, and more selective surgery at a future date.

For patients in the first group we always request an RBC-tagged nuclear study prior to angiography unless a defined bleeding site has been seen endoscopically. Knowing the general area of the hemorrhage significantly reduces the amount of contrast agent and the number of x-ray exposures required to establish a diagnosis. As suggested by others,[6] we do not do angiography if the red cell study results are negative at 24 hours unless there is a strong clinical suspicion that the patient has a lesion, such as a tumor or angiodysplasia, that may be angiographically evident even without frank bleeding. A more selective guided approach to angiography increases the percentage of positive angiograms, which in one study increased from 30% prior to 1980 to 60% after 1980.[13] Although localization of the bleeding site is usually helpful to the angiographer, red cell scans can have problems with accuracy, particularly in cases where different sections of bowel overlap; when a hemorrhage occurs between two delayed scans and therefore may have occurred at a time and place remote from its location on the scan in which it is found; where bowel overlaps organs that may themselves be bleeding, such as the liver or pancreas; or where bowel overlies areas where there may be vascular abnormalities, such as an aneurysm or varices.[6] There is no argument that red cell studies are more sensitive than angiography in the detection of gastrointestinal bleeding, but the exact reason is less clear. The purported reason is the ability of the RBC study to detect bleeding at rates of 0.1 ml/min or less, significantly lower than the historically quoted 0.5 ml/min for angiography. Recent experimental evidence would suggest that this difference may be less than was thought,[14] and although angiographic detectability clearly parallels the rapidity with which the nuclear study becomes positive,[15] much of the increased sensitivity of the nuclear study is probably related to the tracer's persistence in the bloodstream, which allows it to detect intermittent bleeding.

The unstable or massively bleeding patient must be managed rapidly and smoothly using the history and physical findings as the guide to the most likely bleeding source. The shortcomings of the history and physical examination as indicators of the exact diagnosis have been fairly well substantiated. Even with the existence of a sophisticated computer model,[16] a careful prospective evaluation of 95 patients with upper gastrointestinal tract bleeding showed that an accurate diagnosis can be made only 60% of the time. Lower tract hemorrhage can be equally elusive, because rapid small bowel bleeding as occurs with jejunal diverticula[17] is almost always misdiagnosed as colon bleeding. Nonetheless, historical clues combined with examination of the nasogastric aspirate and the stool, and anoscopy and sigmoidoscopy[18] will usually give the angiographer an excellent idea about which of the three vessels to study first. Anesthesiology support is obtained in most cases, both to monitor the patient and to prepare the patient for a quick transfer to the operating room if necessary.

Several signs have been described as indicative of bleeding. The only truly definitive sign is contrast extravasation that persists, or in many cases increases, in intensity into the venous phase of the study (Fig 73–7,A through D). Filming must be continued for 15 to 20 seconds in order to distinguish between subtle extravasation and prominent mucosal staining or angiodysplasia. The shape of the extravasation can sometimes make interpretation difficult, particularly if the contrast material flows rapidly away from the source, producing the "pseudovein" appearance (Fig 73–7,C) or simply diluting to invisibility. Signs other than extravasation, such as intense staining and abnormal vessels, only indicate a site of pathologic change that may be responsible for bleeding. This is particularly true for Meckel's diverticula, which are usually noted only by their increased vascularity and staining.[19] Such ancillary findings have also been suggested to be important in the diagnosis of bleeding due to gastritis, where in one series an intense stain was the only positive finding in 95 of 216 positive examinations.[11] Such signs must be interpreted with caution, because the actual cause of bleeding may be quite different.[15]

Angiodysplasia, although a well-documented cause of bleeding, is particularly troublesome for angiographers. Criteria for the angiographic diagnosis have been fairly clearly established[19–23] as an abnormal cluster of vessels with an intense stain, an early draining vein, and prolonged intense vein opacification. Of these signs, the one we have seen most commonly is a prolonged, intense draining vein (Fig 73–8). Whether accurate diagnoses have been made in the reported series is, however, questionable. Much of the problem results because there is no clearly accepted histopathologically distinct definition of angiodysplasia that differentiates it from an arteriovenous malformation and the terms are clearly used interchangeably by many authors. Pathologic specimens show lesions with vessel sizes as small as capillaries, less than 1 mm, and colonoscopy indicates that vessels can range from 2 to 10 mm in diameter.[23] This range of vessel size is rarely seen at angiography (Fig 73–9). In addition, recent reports indicate that these acquired lesions are frequently multiple,[22, 23] and in one study of lower gastrointestinal bleeding sites the most common finding in patients with angiodysplasia was bilateral lesions,[23] which differs from the traditional angiographic claim that angiodysplasia is most often an isolated right-sided lesion. In most reported series where the angiographic diagnosis of angiodysplasia could be definitely made and no other bleeding site was found the angiodysplasia has been identified on the basis of surgical results as the bleeding site.[20, 23, 24] Nonetheless, the actual diagnosis of the abnormal tangle of vessels can be difficult and frequently requires magnification views as well as some imagination (Fig 73–10). Even with a firm angiographic diagnosis, the fact that there is a prev-

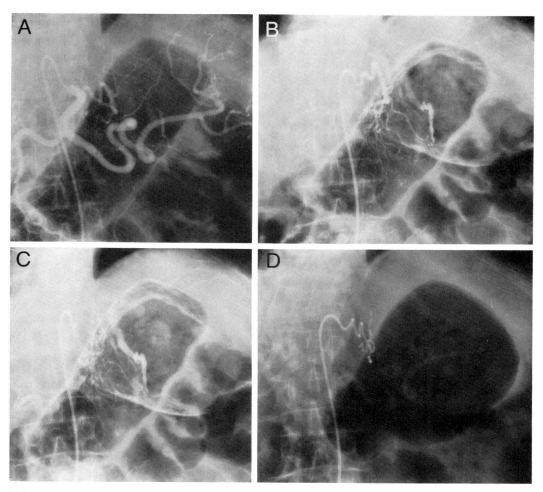

FIG 73–7.

A, celiac artery injection shows early rapid extravasation from a small artery into the body of the stomach. From this nonselective injection it is difficult to tell which of the main branches of the celiac artery leads to the bleeding vessel. The catheter used for the injection is a sidewinder type. Note that the tip of the catheter has been positioned just slightly inside the origin of the vessel, thereby filling nicely the left gastric artery, which originates close to the origin. Slight reflux is seen into the descending aorta. **B,** selective injection into the left gastric artery nicely demonstrates extravasation from the bleeding vessel, clearly seen to be a branch of the left gastric artery. Note the classic appearance of the "pseudovein."

The sidewinder catheter has been exchanged for a left gastric artery catheter. This catheter is shaped like a sidewinder and passes easily into the celiac artery. As it is slowly withdrawn the tip points upward, as in this case, engaging the orifice of the left gastric artery. **C,** later phase in the same injection shows an even more "veinlike" appearance to the extravasation, with a prominent mucosal blush noted in other portions of the stomach. **D,** twenty minutes after initiation of vasopressin at 0.2 U/min there is marked reduction in antegrade flow through the left gastric artery and complete cessation of bleeding from the small terminal branch. Faint opacification of small gastric mucosal arteries can nonetheless be seen.

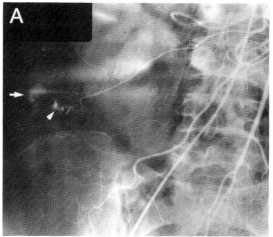
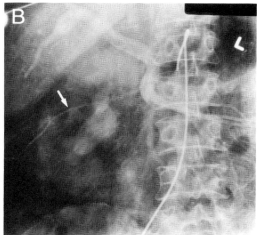

FIG 73–8.
A, early arterial phase of a nonselective superior mesenteric artery injection shows rapid extravasation in the ascending colon from a branch of the right colic artery *(arrow)*. The prominent tangle of vessels *(arrowhead)* at the site of the extravasation represents the classic appearance of an angiodysplasia. **B,** venous phase of the superior mesenteric artery injection shows intense prolonged opacification of the vein *(arrow)* draining the angiodysplasia. This finding has been the most common and most reliable indicator of angiodysplasia in our patients.

alence of approximately 1.4% of angiodysplasia in asymptomatic older individuals[22] and that these lesions occur in an older age group in which potential causes for bleeding such as diverticular disease and malignancy are also more common means that finding an angiodysplasia angiographically does not automatically imply that it is the source of bleeding. There are now ways to corroborate the diagnosis intraoperatively using the light of the colonoscope to transilluminate the bowel wall.[25] This obviates the cumbersome and technically demanding attempts to correlate specimen radiographs or latex-injected samples with the preoperative angiogram.

The technical approach to the angiographic study, which used to be fairly standardized, now varies with each patient in an attempt to tailor the examination to the specific problem as defined by the preliminary clinical findings and endoscopic and red cell studies. Abdominal aortography without magnification is only occasionally used to get an overview of the visceral arterial anatomy. It is performed with a pigtail or end-occluded catheter with the side holes in the lower thoracic aorta (T11 to T12 level). Only very rapid bleeding is seen on aortography, and vascular overlap often makes localization difficult. Others have found aortography equally profitless,[26, 27] and because it adds a significant contrast load to what is usually a high contrast

procedure, should be restricted to cases where bleeding may be arising from the aorta, such as with an aortoduodenal fistula, or cases in which vascular disease or technical problems have raised questions about visceral arterial patency or location. This is particularly true in cases in which it is desirable to do selective studies of a hard-to-find inferior mesenteric artery (IMA). The possibility of a vasculoenteric fistula must always be entertained in patients with a history of vascular grafting, especially in cases that involve the abdominal aorta. The diagnosis of an aortoduodenal fistula may be assisted by doing lateral aortography with the patient in the prone position.[28] Although arterial digital angiographic techniques would seem to be well suited to a study in which the primary finding is extravasation or hyperintense mucosal staining, digital angiography has not proved useful in those few cases in which we have tried it. The problems have arisen from gastrointestinal motion, which is difficult to totally suppress even with intravenous glucagon; respiratory motion that invariably occurs over the extended time necessary for an entire film series; and the small size of the more common abnormalities, such as angiodysplasia. Plain film subtraction is, however, often useful, particularly for subtle areas of extravasation that are superimposed on bone.

In the usual situation, the first study is a selec-

The statistics in the small bowel and colon are even more difficult to evaluate. Overall accuracy for angiography is probably in the range of 50% to 60%,[13, 27] although the number will clearly be higher for active or massive bleeding, 72% in one series,[24] and will clearly be lower for subtle lesions such as inflammatory disorders in children, tumors, and superior mesenteric vein thrombosis.[47, 57] As angiography is applied more selectively to patients with positive nuclear studies accuracy should improve, as was noted in one study, which found that angiographic positivity increased from 30% prior to 1980 to 60% after 1980.[13] One problem with deriving overall angiographic diagnostic accuracy data from the more modern studies, however, is that they frequently limit their analysis to lesions that have been treated with transcatheter techniques, which implies that an angiographic diagnosis has been made. In one such paper the authors stated that 12 of 13 angiograms showed extravasation at the bleeding site.[49] However, there was no mention of any patients with bleeding who had a negative angiogram during the same period.

Further difficulty with assessing overall angiographic accuracy in the lower tract has arisen from the uncritical acceptance of angiography as the gold standard in the diagnosis of angiodysplasia. In one study[22] the authors claimed that 100% of angiodysplasias had been detected angiographically. It is true that colonoscopy has historically had difficulty diagnosing angiodysplasia, with positive findings even in good studies being seen in only 21%[23] and 35%,[20] but in others careful endoscopy when carried fully to the cecum is reported to be 81%[22] and 73%[25] accurate. As colonoscopy has developed and the technique of intraoperative endoscopy has become more widely used, the true nature of this elusive problem has become clearer. Earlier reports stressed isolated right-sided lesions as the rule for angiodysplasia. Although there still appears to be a right colon preponderance, possibly as high as 75% to 89%,[20, 22] other articles stress the widely varied presentations that are possible, including the following: (1) There is often a multiplicity of lesions, as many as 2.1 per patient, with lesions appearing in the left and right colons in one series in nine patients, compared with seven patients with isolated lesions in the cecum or ascending colon.[23] (2) The frequency of small bowel lesions is probably higher than has been reported. In one series they were seen in six of 16 patients,[46] and in another series in nine of 21 patients.[19] (3) The lesions can be seen frequently in the upper portions of the small bowel in

children.[55] (4) Angiodysplasia may often be a more extensive lesion than it appears on either angiography or colonoscopy, particularly when it occurs in the left colon.[20, 25]

In one very careful study that appears to establish intraoperative endoscopy with transillumination for external inspection as a reasonable gold standard in the diagnosis of angiodysplasia,[25] six of eight patients with a definitely positive angiogram had right-sided lesions. Of all probably positive angiograms in 13 patients, 21 lesions were detected, of which 15 (71%) were in the right colon. Intraoperative findings indicated 32 lesions, of which 18 (56%) were right sided. More important, four patients with negative angiograms had angiodysplasias found at surgery. Five angiograms were completely wrong about the lesion location, and the operation was changed on the basis of intraoperative findings. Five angiograms were partially correct in that only minimal changes had to be made at the time of operation. Only four angiograms, or 50% of the eight definitely positive angiograms, were entirely correct. Angiography had similar diagnostic problems in one study of upper tract angiodysplasia in which only four of eight (50%) of the lesions were detected.[21]

ANGIOGRAPHIC THERAPY

The first and possibly most important step for the interventional radiologist to take to treat gastrointestinal bleeding effectively is to understand the clinical problem and integrate himself or herself into a closely cooperating team of radiologist, surgeon, and endoscopist. Without this "team approach," as espoused by Dorfmann,[18] appropriate treatment is often delayed or denied. One important group of patients for whom the angiographer can play a critical role as a team member is those with rapid bleeding from an unknown site. If emergency angiography localizes the bleed, the site can be marked with a small (2 ml) subselective (but not wedged) injection of methylene blue (Fig 73–15), a technique which has been shown to be easy, safe, and effective in a clinical and experimental study.[58] This technique should be more accurate and cause fewer complications than leaving a catheter in place for intraoperative injections of dyes or fluorescein or simply sending the angiograms and a verbal description of the probable site.

The basics of the clinical problem are easily grasped and will not only guide the radiologist in

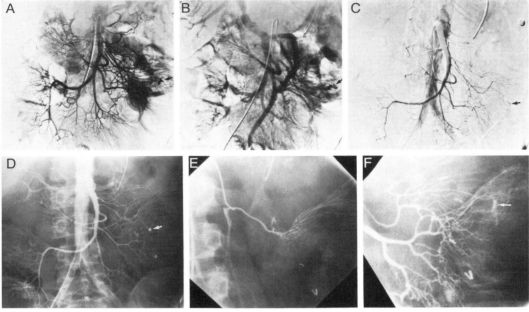

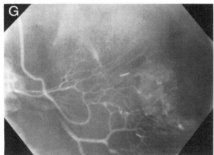

FIG 73–15.

A, patient had recently received a liver transplant, at which time a choledochojejunostomy was created with a Roux-en-Y anastomosis. Approximately 3 days after surgery severe gastrointestinàl bleeding developed, which required massive replacement to maintain adequate blood pressures. An endoscope was unable to traverse the bowel for sufficient length to discover the source of the bleeding. Gastric bleeding was ruled out by both nasogastric return and endoscopy. A selective superior mesenteric artery angiogram was obtained using a sidewinder catheter. Note that the tip of the catheter is possibly slightly too far into the superior mesenteric artery. However, the injection rate is adequate to reflux into the aorta so that the proximal branches to the pancreas, duodenum, transverse colon, and upper small bowel are well filled. An irregular collection of extravasated contrast *(arrow)* is clearly seen in the mid-left abdomen, which on films was noted to be at the staple site where the jejunojejunal anastomosis had been created. **B,** venous phase of the superior mesenteric artery angiogram shows that the contrast collection in the left mid-abdomen is enlarging *(arrow)*. The superior mesenteric vein is patent. The slight stenosis at the portal vein anastomosis for the liver transplant is nicely identified. **C,** in view of the patient's recent surgery, it was believed that embolization might be slightly risky. Therefore vasopressin infusion was attempted. Twenty minutes after vasopressin infusion at 0.2 U/min the superior mesenteric artery angiogram demonstrates nicely a diffuse decrease in vascular caliber. There was a faint suggestion of extravasation in the same location in the left mid-abdomen *(arrow)*. **D,** twenty-four hours after attempted surgical oversewing of the bleeding site at the anastomosis severe gastrointestinal bleeding again developed. A repeat superior mesenteric artery angiogram shows that the vessel had reopened; extravasation was identified in the exact same location in the left mid-abdomen *(arrow)*. In view of the fact that vasopressin therapy had failed on an earlier attempt, it was elected to accept the slightly increased risk of embolization in the postoperative patient if a subselective position could be obtained. Note the multiple vessels that arise from the superior mesenteric artery and pass in the direction of the bleeding site. On the basis of the angiogram it was not clear which of these vessels most directly supplied the bleeding point. The tangle of vessels is due primarily to the operative anatomy, which positions two loops of jejunum on top of each other. **E,** the sidewinder catheter was exchanged for a Berenstein catheter, which was easy to selectively maneuver into each of the branches feeding the left mid-abdomen. A selective injection into the uppermost branch demonstrated that it does not supply the bleeding site. If this branch had indeed supplied the site, it would have been an ideal candidate for embolization, be-

the performance of the angiogram but also assist him or her to manage the patient intelligently while the patient is on the angiographic table. Eighty percent to 90% of all gastrointestinal hemorrhages stop spontaneously with conservative treatment. The subgroup of variceal bleeds does less well; only 30% to 50% stop spontaneously.[18]

As blood loss continues the patient loses both volume and red cell mass. Red cell loss leads to decreased oxygenation of the tissues, and all patients with potential or known cardiac or respiratory problems should be kept on oxygen. Volume loss leads to hypotension, with secondary adrenergic stimulation. A loss of 10% to 20% of intravascular volume will result in orthostatic changes of approximately 10 mm Hg in the peak systolic pressure.[59] This assumes that the loss of volume occurs over a somewhat extended period; rapid loss of 10% of intravascular volume can result in shock. The vital signs, especially heart rate, respiratory rate, and blood pressure, are the best clues to the patient's status.[59] Laboratory tests such as hemoglobin and hematocrit take at least 6 hours to stabilize and are relatively useless in the acute blood loss situation. Blood gases, although useful, can be misleading. Tachypnea following red cell loss may cause an early respiratory alkalosis. Eventually, however, decreased tissue oxygenation secondary to hypotension, peripheral vasoconstriction, and loss of red cell mass will elevate the blood lactate concentration and cause metabolic acidosis. Although replacement of volume is clearly more important to saving the patient's life, red cell mass needs to be replaced if the blood loss is ongoing, and in cases of massive losses the only adequate replacement is whole blood or its equivalent.

A positive nasogastric aspirate almost always indicates an upper tract hemorrhage. A negative return is, however, less specific, having been found in 16 of 214 patients with an endoscopically proved upper tract hemorrhage.[60] It is unclear from this study, however, how many of these patients had duodenal hemorrhages. Nasogastric aspirate positive for bile but negative for blood would seem to effectively rule out an upper tract hemorrhage. If necessary the nasogastric tube could be passed into the duodenum under fluoroscopic control to improve the accuracy of this test. In the same study, 30% of patients with coffee ground emesis, which should imply a prior but inactive hemorrhage, had active bleeding at the time of endoscopy. Melena, or stool which is both black and tarry, should indicate at least 200 ml of upper tract or small bowel bleeding.[59] Black stool can arise from right colon bleeding, and bright red or maroon stool from any level, depending on the rate of bleeding.

Angiographic therapy starts very simply with a good diagnostic study. As soon as selective angiography began to be used to accurately localize bleeding sites, patient survival began to improve. As early as the late 1960s undirected surgery for emergency bleeding had decreased in one center from 26.6% to 3.1%.[61] The importance of this change can be seen in the historical statistics that show that mortality for surgery for bleeding of uncertain cause ranged from 28% to 50%[13, 24, 48, 62] and dropped to 10% to 15% when surgery followed angiography with or without a trial of vasopressin.[13, 24, 48] Of interest, however, the overall mortality for gastrointestinal hemorrhage has remained unchanged at approximately 10%. There have been suggestions that this may be related to a change in the patient population or to a change in the timing and type of surgery.[63, 64] A more plausible explanation is that it may also be related to a statistical problem of inadequate numbers of patients in any one study. In an

---

cause there is not an extensive intercommunication between this branch and adjacent branches. Embolization of this branch could be easily achieved with injection of a single piece of gelfoam into the main trunk. **F,** injection into a lower branch (the largest of the three branches opacified in this injection) shows the bleeding site arising from the long artery in the middle of this extensive arcade *(arrow)*. The multiple intercommunications between the three arteries passing into this area are beautifully demonstrated. **G,** catheter was repositioned into the middle branch, and selective injection into that branch demonstrates marked extravasation into the jejunum from the long branch, which is fed both from this artery and from the smaller artery in the arcade just above it. On the basis of the angiographic findings, it was determined that selective embolization could not be successfully done. An infusion guidewire was passed coaxially through the Berenstein catheter into the distal portion of the middle vessel in the arcade. It was elected to infuse methylene blue through the guidewire for operative localization of the bleeding site. Two milliliters of undiluted methylene blue was infused over 5 minutes. At the time of surgery the anastomotic region was widely opened. The blue stain at the site of the surgical anastomotic line was clearly identified. The entire anastomosis was resected and a new anastomosis was created. No further gastrointestinal bleeding occurred.

analysis of why modern upper gastrointestinal endoscopy has failed to show any effect on upper tract bleeding mortality,[33] the fact that the majority of deaths are in patients with bleeding varices, who often have end-stage liver disease and in whom therapy is only palliative, means that series of 3,000 to 6,000 patients would be required to find a statistically significant change.

Angiographic intervention utilizes primarily the infusion of vasopressin or embolization. The choice of therapy depends on the location of the lesion, the nature of the lesion, and the condition of the patient.

Surgery remains the definitive treatment for many upper tract hemorrhages, especially those associated with duodenal ulcer. Many upper tract bleeds are also now treated very successfully by endoscopy, especially those arising from one or a few medium to small vessels. Success rates of 80% to 95% for injection techniques and 87% to 94% for electrocautery or laser cautery have been reported, with rebleeding rates of only 17% to 24%.[65] Upper tract bleeds for which angiography still plays an important role include Mallory-Weiss tears, diffuse

gastritis, multiple gastric ulcers, and large vessel bleeds, especially those in the duodenum in patients who are not good surgical risks. Mortality rates for patients in whom upper tract bleeding can be controlled by angiographic techniques are significantly lower (27%) than for those in whom hemorrhage cannot be stopped (48%).[11]

One special category of patients who can have either upper or lower tract bleeding for whom angiographic intervention is clearly the procedure of first choice, if not the only choice, is those with the source of bleeding in or around the liver or pancreas. Hematobilia is usually iatrogenic and is most commonly associated with a pseudoaneurysm in 58% to 65% of cases.[66] For this and other pseudoaneurysms vasopressin is ineffective and embolization is the preferred treatment (Fig 73–16). Superselective coils or gelfoam plugs are preferred. Detachable balloons can be used if superselective positioning is not possible. Getting the balloon to "flow" to the pseudoaneurysm, however, may be difficult, because unlike hepatic artery to portal vein fistulas, which can also be a source of gastrointestinal bleeding (often because of varices), the flow to a

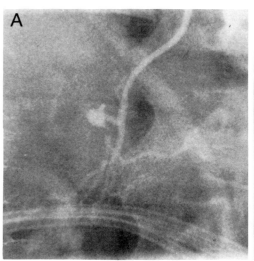 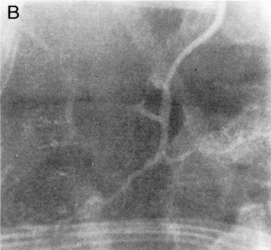

FIG 73–16.
A, patient with severe pancreatitis and multiple operative procedures for drainage of abscesses and lysis of adhesions began having severe crampy upper abdominal pain and gastrointestinal bleeding. Upper gastrointestinal endoscopy was unsuccessful because of operative deformity of the stomach and duodenum. Using a left axillary artery approach, a Cobra catheter was advanced selectively into the superior mesenteric artery, where an injection suggested the possibility of a small pseudoaneurysm in the region of the head of the pancreas. The catheter was selectively placed into a pancreaticoduodenal artery, and a selective injection clearly shows the pseudoaneurysm arising from the first large branch. **B,** after injection of two pledgets of gelfoam, each approximately 3 × 3 × 3 mm, a repeat injection of contrast shows elimination of the pseudoaneurysm. No further gastrointestinal bleeding occurred.

pseudoaneurysm is not markedly increased. In patients who are unstable or bleeding rapidly, central hepatic artery or large branch occlusions can be successful. Peripheral embolization with small particles should be avoided, as should any embolization of the hepatic artery branch giving rise to the gallbladder, because collateral vessels to the gallbladder are scant.[66] In one series of 19 visceral artery aneurysms, the most common cause in 13 (68%) was pancreatitis (see Fig 73–16).[67] Patients with gastrointestinal bleeding in association with pancreatitis often have bleeding into the pancreatic duct, which like bleeding into the biliary duct can cause colicky right upper quadrant pain and jaundice. Not treating these visceral artery aneurysms results in 100% mortality, and surgery, especially in the vicinity of the head of the pancreas, is associated with up to 50% mortality.[67] Vasopressin is ineffective.[68] Embolization, on the other hand, in one series was successful in 79%, with only three major complications.[67]

Selective embolization in the celiac and mesenteric arteries can be difficult. Getting the catheter to the desired location is the primary problem. We have found several techniques particularly useful. From the femoral approach, the catheter that we always try first is one with a Cobra shape. Used with a floppy-tipped guidewire, this high-torque catheter can often be maneuvered selectively into branches of any of the three visceral arteries. It is particularly well suited to the splenic artery, the gastroduodenal artery (see Fig 73–14), small bowel branches of the SMA, and the inferior branch of the IMA. If entry into the primary artery (such as the hepatic artery) is a problem, the 6 French Cobra is particularly well suited to the large loop technique, which is not only helpful in the hepatic artery but also for branches of the SMA, including the pancreaticoduodenal artery, the middle and transverse colic arteries, and the superior branch of the IMA. If the large loop technique is unsuccessful, more specifically shaped catheters, such as a selective hepatic, sidewinder, or inferior mesenteric catheter, can be used to place an exchange wire into the desired vessel over which the Cobra or other torque control preshaped or steam-shaped catheter can be inserted. Such exchanges, which are usually around sharp bends into downward directed mesenteric vessels, are made markedly easier by the use of a stiff exchange wire. Of the various high-torque catheters available, it seems that those with the simplest shapes are often the most successful. In addition to the Cobra, the other catheter we have found most useful is the Be-

renstein, with its simple 45-degree angle tip at the end of the flexible 5 French segment (see Fig 73–15). The tip of the Berenstein catheter can also be easily steam shaped to fit special circumstances, such as vessels that arise from a main trunk at 90-degree or steeper angles, like the right gastric from the left hepatic artery and the colonic or pancreaticoduodenal branches from the SMA. Once a catheter has passed around one or more tight curves or even several gentle curves, much of the torque control is lost. Selective catheterization then often requires the use of a torque control guidewire. Such guidewires come in a variety of sizes, and although the larger ones with greater stiffness are preferred for easier catheter advancement, smaller vessels and tighter curves often necessitate a smaller, 0.016 inch or 0.018 inch floppy-tipped guidewire. Once such a small wire is in position, however, the stainless steel shaft is often inadequate for catheter advancement. To further stiffen the wire, a 3 French Teflon catheter, which is unfortunately difficult to see, can be passed coaxially over the wire inside the angiographic catheter. Alternatively a tapered torque wire (0.035 or 0.038 inch shaft with a 0.018 inch floppy tip) can be used. If all of these maneuvers fail the usual cause is a very steep visceral artery origin from the aorta. In such cases an axillary artery approach will usually prove much easier.

Another major problem with visceral artery embolization is avoiding complications. As with any arterial embolization, the procedure should always be done through an introducer sheath. In the event that the catheter becomes obstructed by the embolic agent or the catheter tip is dislodged into a "nontarget" vessel, the entire catheter can be simply removed and arterial access is preserved.

Avoiding "spillover" or embolization of nontarget vessels can be important. One method of ensuring this is to avoid nonselective embolization. It is tempting occasionally to use nonselective techniques for hepatic and splenic artery hemorrhage, because achieving a selective position can be difficult. Complications, however, can result, especially infarction of the gallbladder, which has limited collateral supply,[66] hepatic abscess,[69] pancreatitis, and infarction and abscess of the spleen.[11] There have been suggestions that increased flow would allow mesenteric hemorrhages to be embolized from nonselective catheter positions.[70] The potentially disastrous results of long segment bowel infarction argue strongly against this practice. Indeed, we have not infrequently noticed spasm in vessels leading to bleeding sites, which might tend to divert embolic particles to adjacent arcades.

The most feared complication of visceral artery embolization is infarction of the embolized tissue, whether it is a segment of bowel or an abdominal organ. This is of very little concern in the esophagus, stomach, duodenum, and liver, all of which have more than one source of vascular supply. In cases, however, where alternative supply routes are compromised, such as previous surgery, severe atherosclerosis, or multivessel embolization, infarction has resulted.[27, 50, 71] Even in these well-perfused organs supplied by the celiac artery, traditional wisdom suggests that small particle embolization is inadvisable, because occlusion of the small terminal branches would prohibit collateral development. However, several investigators have performed experimental and clinical upper tract embolizations with gelfoam powder,[71] Ivalon,[72, 73] and bucrylate[25, 69, 74] without a marked increase in ischemic complications. In one series of 14 patients using bucrylate, 10 patients died; in six of these histologic material was obtained at autopsy.[25] Two of these six patients had evidence of bucrylate in small vessels at the site of the embolized lesion. One patient had a gastric ulcer but no evidence of ischemic changes in the adjacent portions of the stomach. The other patient had bucrylate in the spleen and tail of the pancreas and had developed areas of splenic infarction. Of 14 patients treated with gelfoam powder,[71] two had ischemic injuries. Both of these patients had had prior surgery and were undergoing embolization for the second time. Of 23 patients treated with Ivalon,[73] none had ischemic complications. This may be due to the size of the Ivalon particles, which were greater than 420 μm. Previous experimental work[72] had indicated that particle sizes greater than 300 μm would probably be safe in the upper tract because the small vessels forming the submucosal and muscularis collateral plexus would remain patent. Even with these relatively benign results, the threat of a potentially catastrophic ischemic injury and the fact that results with smaller particles are not significantly better than with larger particles would indicate that larger particles should be used except possibly in certain extreme instances, such as diffuse gastric bleeding in association with a coagulopathy.

Ischemia is more clearly a problem in the small bowel and colon, and early anecdotal reports recommended that embolization of mesenteric vessels be avoided entirely. Now that series with larger numbers of patients have been reported, more realistic statistics concerning ischemic injury have emerged, with rates for clinically evident ischemic injury varying from 11% to 33%.[46, 49–51, 62, 75, 76] The exact magnitude of the postembolization ischemic problem is probably understated in most of these series. Several series report temporary clinical problems such as ileus[75] or pain and fever[49] following mesenteric embolization, which may eventually result in long-term problems such as stricture formation. Another series noted that one patient who was totally asymptomatic was found to have an area of ischemic stricture at the time of surgery.[46] In one experimental series of ileal embolizations in five dogs,[77] only one dog had symptoms (diarrhea), and yet when they were killed at 3 to 4 weeks, four of the five dogs had attached omentum with no evidence of perforation, three of the five had a stricture with loss of the muscularis propria, and one of the five had a scar without stricture. Only one was histologically normal. The clinical implications of this are unclear, however, because dogs have fewer collaterals between arcades and adjacent vasa recta than humans do.

In another sense, however, the magnitude of the postembolization ischemic problem may be significantly overstated, because few of the reported ischemic injuries led to immediate necrosis, perforation, and emergency surgery, but to delayed infarction without perforation. At the time that the delayed infarction became apparent, surgery in the now hemodynamically stable patient with a well-localized area of injury was much safer.

Avoiding mesenteric infarction demands a thorough knowledge of the anatomy of the mesenteric arteries, an understanding of the mechanism of embolization, and careful technique. The literature reflects one difficulty with terminology concerning anatomy in the development of collaterals. Although the IMA with both SMA and pelvic collaterals may have a more secure collateral supply,[46] the interarcade and intramural collaterals that sustain the bowel wall in cases of subselective embolization are more numerous in the small bowel (see Fig 73–15,F and G), particularly toward the ileum.[27, 48, 49, 51, 78, 79] Nonetheless, rates of ischemic complication appear currently to be roughly equal in the small bowel and colon.[46] The mechanism of ischemic injury appears to be embolization of too many or too small vessels rather than progressive postembolization thrombosis, since angiographic evidence of collaterals immediately after

TABLE 73–1.

Reported Effectiveness of Treatment for Gastrointestinal Bleeding

Site/Disease	Vasopressin					Embolization			
	Reference	No of Patients	% Success	% Rebleed	% Recontrol	Reference	No of Patients	% Success	% Rebleed
Upper tract in general	27	33	58			27	16	75	
						50	15	93	
						82	9	78	14
Mallory-Weiss tear	87	4	100			71	3	100	
Stomach	11	156	75	18	62	11	14	71	
						53	9	100	33
						69	15	93	21
	75	9	89	25		73	5	100	40
	87	26	77			75	5	60	0
						87	6	83	
Duodenum	51	1	0			69	18	72	46
	75	5	40	100		75	6	67	25
	87	13	62			87	7	57	
	89	46	33	33		89	7	43	
Lower tract in general	46	24	75	28		46	28	93	15
						49	13	85	8
						50	4	50	
	51	9	78	29		51	4	100	25
	75	9	67	0		75	3	100	0
						78	3	100	33
Small bowel	87	7	71			49	2	100	0
						50	1	100	0
						56	2	100	0
						78	3	100	33
Colon	24		91	50		49	11	82	9
	87	12	83						
	92	57	75	15	50	50	3	100	67
						56	1	100	0
						75	3	100	0
Angiodysplasia	25	6	67			46	5	80	75
	46	1	100						
Colon diverticula	46	16	63			13	2	100	100
	93	23	96			46	13	100	8
						48	2	100	0
Pancreatitis or aneurysm	74		0			69	9	100	22
						74	12	75	
						94	14	93	8

culature or bowel wall. For the same reasons, embolization appears to be more effective in children in the only series dealing with that subgroup.[55]

A sampling of reported effectiveness and rebleeding rates for vasopressin and embolization in various areas or for different diseases is reported in Table 73–1. The data are clearly scattered, and a best policy is not obvious for each location or disease. Our current thinking parallels that of Gomes et al.,[75] who advocated embolization as the treatment of choice for upper tract bleeding that comes to angiographic attention, and vasopressin therapy for lower tract bleeding, followed by embolization if necessary.

REFERENCES

1. Alavi A: Detection of gastrointestinal bleeding with[99mTc]–sulfur colloid. *Semin Nucl Med* 1982; 12:126–138.
2. Winzelberg GG, McKusick KA, Froelich JW, et al: Detection of gastrointestinal bleeding with [99mTc]-labeled red blood cells. *Semin Nucl Med* 1982; 12:139–146.
3. Bunker ST, Lull RJ, Tanasescu DE, et al: Scintigraphy of gastrointestinal hemorrhage: Superiority of [99mTc] red blood cells over [99mTc] sulfur colloid. *AJR* 1984; 143:543–548.
4. Thorne DA, Datz FL, Remley K, et al: Bleeding rates necessary for detecting acute gastrointestinal bleeding with technetium-99m-labeled red blood cells in an experimental model. *J Nucl Med* 1987; 28:514–520.
5. Lecklitner ML, Hughes JJ: Pitfalls of gastrointestinal bleeding studies with [99mTc]-labeled RBCs. *Semin Nucl Med* 1986; 15:151–154.
6. Dorfman GS, Cronan JJ, Staudinger KM: Scintigraphic signs and pitfalls in lower gastrointestinal hemorrhage: The continued necessity of angiography. *Radiographics* 1987; 7:543–562.
7. Yeker D, Buyukunal C, Benli M, et al: Radionuclide imaging of Meckel's diverticulum: Cimetidine versus pentagastrin plus glucagon. *Eur J Nucl Med* 1984; 9:316–319.
8. Baum S: Pertechnetate imaging following cimetidine administration in Meckel's diverticulum of the ileum. *Am J Gastroenterol* 1981; 76:464–465.
9. Sagar VV, Piccone JM: The effect of cimetidine on blood clearance, gastric uptake, and secretion of 99mTc-pertechnetate in dogs. *Radiology* 1981; 139:729–731.
10. Petrokubi RJ, Baum S, Rohrer GV: Cimetidine administration resulting in improved pertechne-

tate imaging of Meckel's diverticulum. *Clin Nucl Med* 1978; 3:385–388.
11. Eckstein MR, Kelemouridis V, Athanasoulis CA, et al: Gastric bleeding: Therapy with intraarterial vasopressin and transcatheter embolization. *Radiology* 1984; 152:643–646.
12. Kerlan RK Jr, Pogany AC, Burke DR, et al: UCSF interventional radiology rounds. *AJR* 1986; 147:1185–1188.
13. Uden P, Jiborn H, Jonsson K: Influence of selective mesenteric arteriography on the outcome of emergency surgery for massive, lower gastrointestinal hemorrhage. A 15-year experience. *Dis Colon Rectum* 1986; 29:561–566.
14. Denham JS, Becker GJ, Siddiqui AR, et al: Detection of acute gastrointestinal bleeding by intra-arterial Tc-99m sulfur colloid scintigraphy in a canine model. Preliminary study. *Invest Radiol* 1987; 22:37–40.
15. Smith R, Copely DJ, Bolen FH: [99mTc] RBC scintigraphy: Correlation of gastrointestinal bleeding rates with scintigraphic findings. *AJR* 1987; 148:869–874.
16. Ohmann C, Thon K, Stoltzing H, et al: Upper gastrointestinal tract bleeding: Assessing the diagnostic contributions of the history and clinical findings. *Med Decis Making* 1986; 6:208–215.
17. Spiegel RM, Schultz RW, Casarella WJ, et al: Massive hemorrhage from jejunal diverticula. *Radiology* 1982; 143:367–371.
18. Dorfman GS: Integrated approach vital in managing GI hemorrhage. *Diagn Imaging* 1988; 1:102–109.
19. Sheedy PF II, Fulton RE, Atwell DT: Angiographic evaluation of patients with chronic gastrointestinal bleeding. *AJR* 1975; 123:338–347.
20. Miller KD Jr, Tutton RH, Bell KA, et al: Angiodysplasia of the colon. *Radiology* 1979; 132:309–313.
21. Quintero E, Pique JM, Bombi JA, et al: Upper gastrointestinal bleeding caused by gastroduodenal vascular malformations. *Dig Dis Sci* 1986; 31:897–905.
22. Richter JM, Hedberg SE, Athanasoulis CA, et al: Angiodysplasia. *Dig Dis Sci* 1984; 29:481–485.
23. Smith GF, Ellyson JH, Parks SN, et al: Angiodysplasia of the colon. *Arch Surg* 1984; 119:532–536.
24. Browder W, Cerise EJ, Litwin MS: Impact of emergency angiography in massive lower gastrointestinal bleeding. *Ann Surg* 1986; 204:530–536.
25. Bowden TA Jr, Hooks VH III, Mansberger AR Jr: Intestinal vascular ectasias: A new look at an old disease. *South Med J* 1982; 75:1310–1317.

26. Lesak F, Andresen J: The value of angiography in gastrointestinal and urological bleeding. *Diagn Imaging Clin Med* 1986; 55:126–131.

27. Rahn NH III, Tishler JM, Han SY, et al: Diagnostic and interventional angiography in acute gastrointestinal hemorrhage. *Radiology* 1982; 143:361–366.

28. Pingoud EG, Pais SO: Usefulness of the prone position for aortography of aortic graft-intestinal fistulae. *AJR* 1979; 132:836–837.

29. Meschan I: Small intestine, colon, and biliary tract, in Meschan I (ed): *An Atlas of Anatomy Basic to Radiology*. Philadelphia, WB Saunders Co, 1975, p 878.

30. Ruzicka FF, Rossi P: Normal vascular anatomy of the abdominal viscera. *Radiol Clin North Am* 1970; 8:3–29.

31. Michels NA (ed): *Blood Supply and Anatomy of Upper Abdominal Organs with Descriptive Atlas*. Philadelphia, JB Lippincott Co, 1955, pp 242–243.

32. Alpert M, Brody S: The detection of massive colonic haemorrhage by selective coeliac arteriography. *Br J Radiol* 1987; 60:190–192.

33. Erickson RA, Glick ME: Why have controlled trials failed to demonstrate a benefit of esophagogastroduodenoscopy in acute upper gastrointestinal bleeding? A probability model analysis. *Dig Dis Sci* 1986; 31:760–768.

34. Kelemouridis V, Athanasoulis CA, Waltman AC: Gastric bleeding sites: An angiographic study. *Radiology* 1983; 149:643–648.

35. Athanasoulis CA: Upper gastrointestinal bleeding of arteriocapillary origin, in Athanasoulis CA, Pfister RC, Greene RE, et al (eds): *International Radiology*. Philadelphia, WB Saunders Co, 1982, pp 55–89.

36. Waltman AC, Courey WR, Athanasoulis CA, et al: Technique for left gastric artery catheterization. *Radiology* 1973; 109:732–734.

37. Meschan I: The upper alimentary tract, in Meschan I (ed): *An Atlas of Anatomy Basic to Radiology*. Philadelphia, WB Saunders Co, 1975, pp 834–836.

38. Briley CA Jr, Jackson DC, Johnsrude IS, et al: Acute gastrointestinal hemorrhage of small-bowel origin. *Radiology* 1980; 136:317–318.

39. Casarella WJ, Galloway SJ, Taxin RN, et al: "Lower" gastrointestinal tract hemorrhage: New concepts based on arteriography. *AJR* 1974; 121:357–368.

40. Athanasoulis CA: Lower gastrointestinal bleeding, in Athanasoulis CA, Pfister RC, Greene RE, et al (eds): *Interventional Radiology*. Philadelphia, WB Saunders Co, 1982, pp 115–148.

41. Baum S, Athanasoulis CA, Waltman AC, et al: Angiodysplasia of the right colon: A cause of gastrointestinal bleeding. *AJR* 1977; 129:789–794.

42. Baum S, Nusbaum M, Blakemore WS, et al: The preoperative radiographic demonstration of intraabdominal bleeding from undetermined sites by percutaneous selective celiac and superior mesenteric arteriography. *Surgery* 1965; 58:797–805.

43. Casarella WJ, Kanter IE, Seaman WB: Right sided colonic diverticula as a cause of acute rectal hemorrhage. *N Engl J Med* 1972; 286:450–453.

44. Koehler PR, Salmon RB: Angiographic localization of unknown acute gastrointestinal bleeding sites. *Radiology* 1967; 89:244–249.

45. Reuter SR, Bookstein JJ: Angiographic localization of gastrointestinal bleeding. *Gastroenterology* 1968; 54:876–883.

46. Sebrechts C, Bookstein JJ: Embolization in the management of lower-gastrointestinal hemorrhage. *Semin Intervent Radiol* 1988; 5:39–48.

47. Soper NJ, Rikkers LF, Miller FJ: Gastrointestinal hemorrhage associated with chronic mesenteric venous occlusion. *Gastroenterology* 1985; 88:1964–1967.

48. Goldberger LE, Bookstein JJ: Transcatheter embolization for treatment of diverticular hemorrhage. *Radiology* 1977; 122:613–617.

49. Uflacker R: Transcatheter embolization for treatment of acute lower gastrointestinal bleeding. *Acta Radiol* 1987; 28:425–430.

50. Jander HP, Russinovich AE: Transcatheter gelfoam embolization in abdominal, retroperitoneal, and pelvic hemorrhage. *Radiology* 1980; 136:337–344.

51. Walker WJ, Goldin AR, Shaff MI, et al: Per catheter control of haemorrhage from the superior and inferior mesenteric arteries. *Clin Radiol* 1980; 31:71–80.

52. Rosch J, Kozak BE, Keller FS: Unusual sources of gastrointestinal bleeding. *Semin Intervent Radiol* 1988; 5:64–72.

53. Morris DC, Nichols DM, Connell DG, et al: Embolization of the left gastric artery in the absence of angiographic extravasation. *Cardiovasc Intervent Radiol* 1986; 9:195–198.

54. Rosch J, Kozak BE, Keller FS: Interventional diagnostic angiography in acute lower-gastrointestinal bleeding. *Semin Intervent Radiol* 1988; 5:10–17.

55. Meyerovitz MF, Fellows KE: Angiography in gastrointestinal bleeding in children. *AJR* 1984; 143:837–840.

56. Waltman AC: Transcatheter embolization versus vasopressin infusion for the control of arteriocapillary gastrointestinal bleeding. *Cardiovasc Intervent Radiol* 1980; 3:289–297.

57. Meyerovitz MF, Fellow KE: Typhlitis: A

cause of gastrointestinal hemorrhage in children. *AJR* 1984; 143:833–835.

58. Jasinski RW, Smith DC, Chase DR, et al: Angiographic preoperative bowel segment localization using methylene blue, isosulfan blue, and fluorescein. *Invest Radiol* 1987; 22:462–466.

59. Schaffner J: Acute gastrointestinal bleeding. *Med Clin North Am* 1986; 70:1055–1066.

60. Silverstein FE, Gilbert DA, Tedesco FJ: The national ASGE survey on upper gastrointestinal bleeding. *Gastrointest Endosc* 1981; 27:73–102.

61. Mitty WF, Befeler D, Grossi CE: Combined approach to upper gastrointestinal bleeding. *Am J Gastroenterol* 1969; 51:377–386.

62. Rosenkrantz H, Bookstein JJ, Rosen RJ, et al: Postembolic colonic infarction. *Radiology* 1982; 142:47–51.

63. Gogel HK, Tandberg D: Emergency management of upper gastrointestinal hemorrhage. *Am J Emerg Med* 1986; 4:150–162.

64. Greenburg AG, Saik RP, Bell RH, et al: Changing patterns of gastrointestinal bleeding. *Arch Surg* 1985; 120:341–344.

65. Keeffe EB, Lieberman DA: Endoscopic management of gastrointestinal hemorrhage. *Semin Intervent Radiol* 1988; 5:85–92.

66. Rosch J, Putnam JS, Keller FS: Diagnosis and management of hemobilia. *Semin Intervent Radiol* 1988; 5:49–60.

67. Mandel SR, Jaques PF, Mauro MA, et al: Nonoperative management of peripancreatic arterial aneurysms. A 10-year experience. *Ann Surg* 1987; 205:126–128.

68. Steckman ML, Dooley MC, Jaques PF, et al: Major gastrointestinal hemorrhage from peripancreatic blood vessels in pancreatitis. Treatment by embolotherapy. *Dig Dis Sci* 1984; 29:486–497.

69. Feldman L, Greenfield AJ, Waltman AC, et al: Transcatheter vessel occlusion: Angiographic results versus clinical success. *Radiology* 1983; 147:1–5.

70. Lawler G, Bircher M, Spencer J, et al: Embolisation in colonic bleeding. *Br J Radiol* 1985; 58:83–84.

71. Rosch J, Keller FS, Kozak B, et al: Gelfoam powder embolization of the left gastric artery in treatment of massive small-vessel gastric bleeding. *Radiology* 1984; 151:365–370.

72. Castaneda-Zuniga WR, Jauregui H, Rysavy J, et al: Selective transcatheter embolization of the upper gastrointestinal tract: An experimental study. *Radiology* 1978; 127:81–83.

73. Kusano S, Murata K, Ohuchi H, et al: Low-dose particulate polyvinylalcohol embolization in massive small artery intestinal hemorrhage.

Experimental and clinical results. *Invest Radiol* 1987; 22:388–392.

74. Waltman AC, Luers PR, Athanasoulis A, et al: Massive arterial hemorrhage in patients with pancreatitis. Complementary roles of surgery and transcatheter occlusive techniques. *Arch Surg* 1986; 121:439–443.

75. Gomes AS, Lois JF, McCoy RD: Angiographic treatment of gastrointestinal hemorrhage: Comparison of vasopressin infusion and embolization. *AJR* 1986; 146:1031–1037.

76. Palmaz JC, Walter JF, Cho KJ: Therapeutic embolization of the small-bowel arteries. *Radiology* 1984; 152:377–382.

77. Cho KJ, Schmidt RW, Lenz J: Effects of experimental embolization of superior mesenteric artery branch on the intestine. *Invest Radiol* 1979; 14:207–214.

78. Chalmers AG, Robinson PJ, Chapman AH: Embolisation in small bowel haemorrhage. *Clin Radiol* 1986; 37:379–381.

79. Ross JA: Vascular patterns of small and large intestine compared. *Br J Surg* 1952; 39:330.

80. Morris DC, Nichols DM, Connell DG, et al: Embolization of the left gastric artery in the absence of angiographic extravasation. *Cardiovasc Intervent Radiol* 1986; 9:195–198.

81. Vinters HV, Galil KA, Lundie MJ, et al: The histotoxicity of cyanoacrylates: A select review. *Neuroradiology* 1985; 27:279–291.

82. Freeny PC, Mennemeyer R, Kidd R, et al: Long-term radiographic-pathologic follow-up of patients treated with visceral transcatheter occlusion using isobutyl 2-cyanoacrylate (bucrylate). *Radiology* 1979; 132:51–60.

83. Athanasoulis CA: Therapeutic applications of angiography (First of two parts). *N Engl J Med* 1980; 302:1117–1125.

84. Greenfield AJ, Waltman AC, Athanasoulis CA, et al: Vasopressin in control of gastrointestinal hemorrhage: Complications of selective intra-arterial vs. systemic infusions (abstract). *Gastroenterology* 1979; 76:1144.

85. Groszmann RJ, Kravetz D, Bosch J, et al: Nitroglycerin improves the hemodynamic response to vasopressin in portal hypertension. *Hepatology* 1982; 2:757–762.

86. Conn HO, Ramsby GR, Storer EH, et al: Intraarterial vasopressin in the treatment of upper gastrointestinal hemorrhage: A prospective, controlled clinical trial. *Gastroenterology* 1975; 68:211–221.

87. Clark RA, Colley DP, Eggers FM: Acute arterial gastrointestinal hemorrhage: Efficacy of transcatheter control. *AJR* 1981; 136:1185–1189.

88. Keller FS, Rosch J: Embolization for acute

gastric hemorrhage. *Semin Intervent Radiol* 1988; 5:25–31.

89. Waltman AC, Greenfield AJ, Novelline RA, et al: Pyloroduodenal bleeding and intraarterial vasopressin: Clinical results. *AJR* 1979; 133:643–646.

90. Baum S, Rosch J, Dotter CT, et al: Selective mesenteric arterial infusions in the management of massive diverticular hemorrhage. *N Engl J Med* 1973; 288:1269–1272.

91. Walter WJ, Goldin AR, Shaff MI, et al: Per catheter control of haemorrhage from superior and inferior mesenteric arteries. *Clin Radiol* 1980; 31:71–80.

92. Walker TG, Waltman AC: Vasoconstrictive infusion therapy for management of arterial gastrointestinal hemorrhage. *Semin Intervent Radiol* 1988; 5:18–24.

93. Baum S, Athanasoulis C, Waltman A: Angiographic diagnosis and control of large bowel bleeding. *Dis Colon Rectum* 1974; 17:447–453.

94. Avila-Varguez JE, Alvarado-Monterrubio B, Castaneda-Zuniga C: Angiographic management of severe gastrointestinal bleeding in the immediate postoperative period. *Semin Intervent Radiol* 1988; 5:93–97.

Index